The Lacrimal System

The Lacrimal System

Diagnosis, Management, and Surgery

Edited by

Adam J. Cohen, MD

Consulting Surgeon, Eyelid and Facial Aesthetic and Reconstructive Surgery, Craniofacial Surgery, Neuro-Ophthalmology, Evanston, Illinois

Michael Mercandetti, MD, MBA, FACS

Attending Staff, Department of Surgery, Doctor's Hospital, Sarasota, Florida

Brian G. Brazzo, MD

Clinical Assistant Professor, Department of Ophthalmology, Weill Medical College of Cornell University, New York, New York; Director, Oculoplastics Service, Department of Ophthalmology, Maimonides Medical Center, Brooklyn, New York; Director, Oculoplastics Service, Department of Ophthalmology, Lincoln Hospital, Bronx, New York; Attending Surgeon, Department of Ophthalmology, The New York Eye and Ear Infirmary, New York, New York

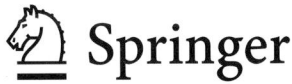 Springer

Adam J. Cohen, MD
Consulting Surgeon, Eyelid and Facial Aesthetic and Reconstructive Surgery, Craniofacial Surgery, Neuro-Ophthalmology, Evanston, IL 60201, USA

Michael Mercandetti, MD, MBA, FACS
Attending Staff, Department of Surgery, Doctor's Hospital, Sarasota, FL 34239, USA

Brian G. Brazzo, MD
Clinical Assistant Professor, Department of Ophthalmology, Weill Medical College of Cornell University, New York, NY 10021; Director, Oculoplastics Service, Department of Ophthalmology, Maimonides Medical Center, Brooklyn, NY 11219; Director, Oculoplastics Service, Department of Ophthalmology, Lincoln Hospital, Bronx, NY 10451; Attending Surgeon, Department of Ophthalmology, The New York Eye and Ear Infirmary, New York, NY 10003, USA

Library of Congress Control Number: 2005938668

ISBN-10: 0-387-25385-8   e-ISBN 0-387-35267-8
ISBN-13: 978-0387-25385-5

Printed on acid-free paper.

Printed in the United States of America.   (BS/MVY)

9 8 7 6 5 4 3 2 1

springer.com

To our families and mentors.

Foreword

Drs. Brazzo, Cohen, and Mercandetti have honored me by inviting me to write the Foreword to their new textbook on *Lacrimal Surgery* and I am honored to do so. Although there has been a recent proliferation of new publications in the field of ophthalmic and facial plastic surgery, the expansion of our specialty, the refinement of surgical procedures, and new technology warrant the production of these new works.

The authors, with whom I am well acquainted, are gifted and innovative surgeons in their own right. They have invited an illustrious group of surgeons to produce a work that is well organized and well written. The concepts and techniques presented represent the state of the art of lacrimal diagnosis and surgery.

There is mention of lacrimal infection dating back to the Code of Hammurabi in 2250 BC, but it was not until the late 1800s that real progress began to be made. Toti, an ENT surgeon in Florence, Italy, described external dacryocystorhinostomy (DCR) with turbinectomy and creation of an osteotomy in the early 1900s. Around 1911, Whitnall described the anatomy. Subsequently, endonasal procedures were described and more recently, the use of lasers was introduced.

Transcanalicular laser-assisted DCR, although in its infancy, represents an incredible breakthrough in the field. Our own group, while working at the University of Oviedo in Spain, has for five years been working with this procedure and the results, albeit not long-term, have been gratifying.

This work truly represents the "codification" of the developments in the field. The authors and editors are to be congratulated for producing a work of this quality. I am sure it will endure for years to come.

Frank A. Nesi, MD

Foreword

Preface

"What medicines do not heal, the lance will; what the lance does not heal, fire will."
—Hippocrates

Tearing disorders are among the most common dilemmas that ophthalmologists and oculofacial surgeons encounter. When patients present with tears streaming down their cheek or an acute infection of the lacrimal sac, diagnosis is usually straightforward. Frequently, this is not the case and evaluation of a "wet eye" can be complicated by structures that are not easily visualized and diagnostic tests that are often difficult to interpret. Restoration of lacrimal system patency and tear flow often involves surgical techniques that are challenging to master and frequently have unpredictable results.

Our attempt is to provide a comprehensive textbook on the diagnosis, management, and surgery of lacrimal system disorders with input by the world's experts. The anatomy of the lacrimal system and intranasal anatomy are presented in exquisite detail. Etiologies and evaluation of congenital and acquired tear duct obstructions are presented in a clear and comprehensive manner by leading authorities. The surgical technique section is the most comprehensive of any lacrimal textbook to date with all procedures described in marvelous detail and imagery by the world's experts. The contributions from all of these outstanding physicians allow for the creation of this unique tome, for without their efforts the book would not have come to fruition.

We hope this effort will afford surgeons at all echelons to gain from their valuable and timely insights.

Adam J. Cohen, MD
Michael Mercandetti, MD, MBA, FACS
Brian G. Brazzo, MD

Contents

Section One: Anatomy

Section Two: Diagnosis

Section Three: Management and Surgical Techniques

Contributors

Joshua Amato, MD
Resident, Department of Ophthalmology, Saint Louis University Health Sciences Center, St. Louis, MO 63104, USA

Bruce B. Becker, MD
Clinical Professor, Department of Ophthalmology, Jules Stein Eye Institute, University of California School of Medicine, Los Angeles, CA 90095, USA

Brian G. Brazzo, MD
Clinical Assistant Professor, Department of Ophthalmology, Weill Medical College of Cornell University, New York, NY 10021; Director, Oculoplastics Service, Department of Ophthalmology, Maimonides Medical Center, Brooklyn, NY 11219; Director, Oculoplastics Service, Department of Ophthalmology, Lincoln Hospital, Bronx, NY 10451; Attending Surgeon, Department of Ophthalmology, The New York Eye and Ear Infirmary, New York, NY 10003, USA

Cat N. Burkat, MD
Assistant Professor, Department of Ophthalmology, Oculoplastics Service, University of Wisconsin – Madison, Madison, WI 53792, USA

Jorge G. Camara, MD
Chairman, Department of Ophthalmology, St. Francis Medical Center, University of Hawaii School of Medicine, Honolulu, HI 96817, USA

Susan R. Carter, MD
Department of Ophthalmology and Visual Science, University of Medicine and Dentistry New Jersey, Newark, NJ 07103, USA

Marco Carvessacio, MD
The Ocular Suface, Ethis Communications Inc., New York, NY 10038, USA

Francois Codere, MD
Associate Professor, Department of Ophthalmology, McGill University, and Royal Victoria Hospital, Montreal, Quebec, Canada

Adam J. Cohen, MD
Consulting Surgeon, Eyelid and Facial Aesthetic and Reconstructive Surgery, Craniofacial Surgery, Neuro-Ophthalmology, Evanston, IL 60201, USA

Steven C. Dresner, MD
Associate Clinical Professor, Keck School of Medicine, University of Southern California; Fellowship Director, Ophthalmic Plastic and Reconstructive Surgery, Eyesthetica, Los Angeles, CA 90033, USA

Mark T. Duffy, MD, PhD
Orbital, Oculoplastic, Facial and Reconstructive Surgery, Green Bay Eye Clinic, Green Bay, WI 54307, USA

Jonathan J. Dutton, MD, PhD
Professor and Vice Chair, Department of Ophthalmology, University of North Carolina at Chapel Hill, Chapel Hill, NC 27599, USA

Karl-Heinz Emmerich, Priv.Doz.
Direktor der Augenklinik, Klinikum Darmstadt – Akad. Lehrhospital der Universitäten Frankfurt und Mannheim-Heidelberg – Heidelberger Landstr. 379, 64297 Darmstadt, Germany

Irene D. Enriquez, MD
Fellow in Ophthalmic Plastic and Reconstructive Surgery, University of Hawaii School of Medicine, Honolulu, HI 96817, USA

Robert G. Fante, MD
Clinical Assistant Professor, Fante Eye and Face Center, Department of Ophthalmology and Otolaryngology, University of Colorado Medical School, Denver, CO 80205, USA

Roberta E. Gausas, MD
Director of Oculoplastic and Orbital Surgery, Scheie Eye Institute, Department of Ophthalmology, University of Pennsylvania, Philadelphia, PA 19104, USA

Geoffrey J. Gladstone, MD, FACS
Clinical Professor, Department of Ophthalmology, Michigan State University School of Medicine, East Lansing, MI 48824; Assistant Clinical Professor, Department of Ophthalmology and Otolaryngology, Kresge

Eye Institute, Wayne State University School of Medicine, Detroit, MI 48201; Co-director, Oculoplastic Surgery, Department of Ophthalmology, William Beaumont Hospital, Royal Oak, MI 48073; and Consultants in Ophthalmic and Facial Plastic Surgery, Southfield, MI 48034, USA

John D. Griffiths, MD, FACS
Clinical Associate Professor, Department of Ophthalmology, University of Nebraska College of Medicine, Omaha, NE 68198, USA

Richard H. Hart, MD, MBChB, FRANZCO
Adnexal Fellow, Moorfields Eye Hospital, London, England

Morris E. Hartstein, MD
Associate Professor, Department of Ophthalmology and Surgery, St. Louis University Eye Institute, St. Louis, MO 63104, USA

Jan Lei Iwata, Pharm D, DO, MS
Attending Medical Staff, Advocate-Illinois Masonic, Medical Center, Oculoplastics Service, Chicago, IL 60657, USA

Reynaldo M. Javate, MD, FICS
Professor of Ophthalmology, Chief, Oculofacial, Orbit, and Lacrimal Section, Department of Ophthalmology, University of Santo Tomas, Manila, The Philippines

James A. Katowitz, MD
Professor, Department of Ophthalmology and Director of Oculoplastic and Orbital Surgery at The Children's Hospital of Philadelphia and the Edwin and Fannie Gray Hall Center for Human Appearance, University of Pennsylvania School of Medicine, Philadelphia, PA 19104, USA

William R. Katowitz, MD
Resident, Department of Ophthalmology. The Scheie Eye Institute and The Children's Hospital of Philadelphia, University of Pennsylvania, Philadelphia, PA 19104, USA

Jennifer S. Landy, MD
Brandon Eye Associates, 1463 Oakfield Drive, Brandon, FL 33511, USA

Susan Irene E. Lapid-Lim, MD, DPBO
Visiting Consultant, Department of Ophthalmology, University of Santo Tomas, Manila, Philippines

Michael A. Lemp, MD
Clinical Professor, Department of Ophthalmology, Georgetown University, Washington, DC 20016; Clinical Professor, Department of Ophthalmology, George Washington University, Washington, DC 20016, USA

Mark J. Lucarelli, MD
Director, Oculoplastics Service, and Associate Professor, University of Wisconsin – Madison, Madison, WI 53792, USA

Harry Marshak, MD
Clinical Instructor, Department of Ophthalmology, Doheny Eye Institute, Keck School of Medicine of the University of Southern California, Los Angeles, CA 90033, USA

Michael Mercandetti, MD, MBA, FACS
Attending Staff, Department of Surgery, Doctor's Hospital, Sarasota, FL 34239, USA

Hans-Werner Meyer-Rüsenberg, Prof. Dr. Med.
Direktor der Universitäts-Augenklinik, St. Josefs-Hospital Hagen Universität Witten/Herdecke, Deutschland

Joseph P. Mirante, MD, MBA, FACS
Clinical Assistant Professor, Department of Otolaryngology, University of South Florida, Tampa, FL 33620; Attending Otolaryngologist, Halifax Medical Center, Daytona Beach, FL 32114, USA

Showkat Mirza, BmedSci, FRCSEd
Senior Specialist Registrar, Queens Medical Center, Nottingham, United Kingdom

Frank A. Nesi, MD, FAACS
Assistant Clinical Professor, Department of Ophthalmology and Otolaryngology: Co-Director, Oculoplastic Surgery, Kresge Eye Institute, Wayne State University School of Medicine, Detroit, MI 48201; Clinical Professor, Department of Ophthalmology and Neurology, Michigan State University, Lansing, MI 48824; Director, Oculoplastic Surgery, Department of Ophthalmology, William Beaumont Hospital, Royal Oak, MI 48073; and Consultants in Ophthalmic and Facial Plastic Surgery, Southfield, MI 48034, USA

Niall P. O'Donnell, FRCS, FRCOphth
Oculoplastic and Orbital Surgeon, Leicester Royal Infirmary, University Hospitals Leicester, United Kingdom

Jay Justin Older, MD, FACS
Affiliate Professor, Department of Ophthalmology, University of South Florida College of Medicine, Tampa, FL, USA

John Pak, MD, PhD
Department of Ophthalmology and Visual Sciences, University of Illinois Eye and Ear Infirmary, Chicago, IL 60611, USA

Ferdinand G. Pamintuan, MD
Clinical Faculty, Department of Otorhinolaryngology, University of Santo Tomas, Manila, Philippines

Jerry K. Popham, MD, FACS
Park Avenue OculoPlastic Surgeons, St. Denver, CO 80218, USA

Suzanne Powrie, MRCS, LRCP, FRCA, FANZCA, DA
Consultant, Anaesthetist and Clinical Director, Department of Anesthesia, Moorfields Eye Hospital, London, United Kingdom

Andrew K. Robson, FRCS
Consultant, Cumberland Infirmary, Carlisle, United Kingdom

Geoffrey E. Rose, BSc, MBBS, MS, DSc, MRCP, FRCS, FRCOphth
Consultant, Orbital and Lacrimal Surgeon, Moorfields Eye Hospital, London, United Kingdom

David W. Rossman, MD
Fellow, Oculoplastic Surgery, Montreal, Canada

Daniel P. Schaefer, MD, FACS
Director, Department of Oculoplastic, Facial, Orbital, and Reconstructive Surgery, Clinical Professor, Department of Ophthalmology, and Clinical Assistant Professor, Department of Otolaryngology, School of Medicine and Biomedical Sciences, State University of New York at Buffalo, Buffalo, NY 14214, USA

David I. Silbert, MD, FAAP
Family Eye Group, Lancaster, PA 17604, USA

Hampson A. Sisler, MD
Manhattan Eye, Ear and Throat Hospital, New York, NY 10021, USA

Charles B. Slonim, MD, FACS
Affiliate Professor, Department of Ophthalmology, University of South Florida College of Medicine, Tampa, FL 33613, USA

Ajay Tripathi, MS, FRCS (Glasgow), FRCS (Edinburgh)
Oculoplastic and Orbital Surgeon, Southport and Ormskirk Hospitals, United Kingdom

Angelo Tsirbas, FRACO, AAFPS
Department of Ophthalmology, Flinders University, Adelaide, Australia; Department of Ophthalmology, Columbia University, New York, NY 10032, USA

F. Campbell Waldrop, MD
Oculoplastic Division, EYE-Q Vision Care, Fresno, CA 93720, USA

David A. Weinberg, MD, FACS
Associate Professor, Department of Surgery (Ophthalmology) and
Neurology, University of Vermont College of Medicine; Director,
Orbital and Ophthalmic Plastic Surgery and Neuro-Ophthalmology,
Fletcher Allen Health Care, Burlington, VT 05401, USA

Robert A. Weiss, MD, FACS
Director, Oculoplastic and Reconstructive Surgery Service, Advocate
Illinois Masonic Medical Center and Chicago Eye Institute, and Clini-
cal Associate Professor, Departments of Ophthalmology and Visual
Science, and Neurosurgery, University of Illinois at Chicago, Chicago,
IL 60612, USA

Jeffrey J. White, MD
Carolina Eye Associates, Southern Pines, NC 27378, USA

William L. White, MD
Associate Clinical Professor, Department of Pediatrics and Ophthal-
mology, Children's Mercy Hospital, University of Missouri, Kansas
City, Kansas City, MO 64108, USA

Peter John Wormald, MD, FRACS, FRCS, FCS (SA), MBChB
Chairman, Otolaryngology Head and Neck Surgery, Adelaide and
Flinders Universities, Adelaide, Australia

Mary Ann Yasay-Luis, MD
Fellow in Ophthalmic Plastic and Reconstructive Surgery, University
of Hawaii School of Medicine, Honolulu, HI 96817, USA

Section 1

Anatomy

Section 1

Anatomy of the Lacrimal System

Cat N. Burkat and Mark J. Lucarelli

Successful lacrimal surgery begins with a thorough history and preoperative clinical examination, both of which guide the surgeon to the correct diagnosis and appropriate management. A thorough understanding of the anatomy of the lacrimal system will further facilitate the chance of a successful surgical outcome.

The following components of the lacrimal drainage system anatomy will be discussed in detail:

1. Embryology
2. Osteology
3. Nasal and paranasal sinuses
4. Secretory system
5. Excretory system

Embryology

Familiarity with lacrimal system embryology is necessary to understand congenital abnormalities of the nasolacrimal drainage system. The orbital walls are embryologically derived from neural crest cells. Ossification of the orbital walls is completed by birth except at the orbital apex. The lesser wing of the sphenoid is initially cartilaginous, unlike the greater wing of the sphenoid and other orbital bones that develop via intramembranous ossification. The membranous bones surrounding the lacrimal excretory system are well developed at 4 months of embryologic age and ossify by birth.

The lacrimal gland begins development at the 22- to 25-mm embryologic stage as solid epithelial buds arise from the ectoderm of the superolateral conjunctival fornix.[1-5] Mesenchymal condensation around these buds forms the secretory lacrimal gland. The early epithelial buds form the orbital lobe in the first 2 months, whereas the secondary buds, which appear later in the 40- to 60-mm stage, develop into the palpebral lobe.[1-3] Canalization of the epithelial buds to form ducts occurs, on average, at the 60-mm stage, but may be seen in as early as the 28.5-mm stage.[1,3,5] The developing tendon of the levator palpebrae superioris muscle divides the gland into two lobes around the tenth week of development.[1,5] The lacrimal gland continues to develop until 3–4 years after birth.[3]

The excretory system begins its development at an earlier stage. In the 7-mm embryo, a depression termed the naso-optic fissure develops, bordered superiorly by the lateral nasal process and inferiorly by the maxillary process. The naso-optic fissure or groove gradually shallows as the structures bordering it grow and coalesce. Before it is completely obliterated, however, a solid strand of surface epithelium thickens along the floor of the rudimentary fissure extending from the orbit to the nose. The thickened cord of epithelium becomes buried to form a rod connected to the surface epithelium at only the orbital and nasal ends. This separation from the surface typically occurs at 43 days of embryologic age.[6] The superior end of the rod enlarges to form the lacrimal sac, and gives off two columns of cells that grow into the eyelid margins to become the canaliculi.[7,8]

Canalization of this nasolacrimal ectodermal rod begins at the fourth month or the 32- to 36-mm stage of development, proceeding first in the lacrimal sac, the canaliculi, and lastly in the naso-lacrimal duct.[7–9] The central cells of the rod degenerate by necrobio-sis, forming a lumen closed at the superior end by conjunctival and canalicular epithelium and closed at the inferior end by nasal and nasolacrimal epithelium. The superior membrane at the puncta is usually completely canalized when the eyelids separate at 7 months of gestation, and therefore is normally patent by birth. In contrast, the inferior membrane frequently persists in newborns, resulting in congenital nasolacrimal obstruction.[10–12] Abnormalities of development in this region, occurring typically after the fourth month of gestation, can result in congenital absence of any segment of the nasolacrimal system, supernumerary puncta, and lacrimal fistulae.[6–9,12–15]

Osteology

Whitnall[16] described the orbital rim as a spiral with its two ends over-lapping medially on either side of the lacrimal sac fossa. The medial orbital rim is formed anteriorly by the frontal process of the maxillary bone rising to meet the maxillary process of the frontal bone. The lac-rimal sac fossa is a depression in the inferomedial orbital rim, formed by the maxillary and lacrimal bones. It is bordered by the anterior lac-rimal crest of the maxillary bone and the posterior lacrimal crest of the lacrimal bone. The fossa is approximately 16-mm high, 4- to 9-mm wide, and 2-mm deep,[16,17] and is narrower in women.[18] The fossa is widest at its base, where it is confluent with the opening of the naso-lacrimal canal. On the frontal process of the maxilla just anterior to the lacrimal sac fossa, a fine groove termed the *sutura notha* or *sutura lon-gitudinalis imperfecta* of Weber, runs parallel to the anterior lacrimal crest (Figure 1.1).[16] It is a vascular groove through which small twigs of the infraorbital artery pass through to supply the bone and nasal

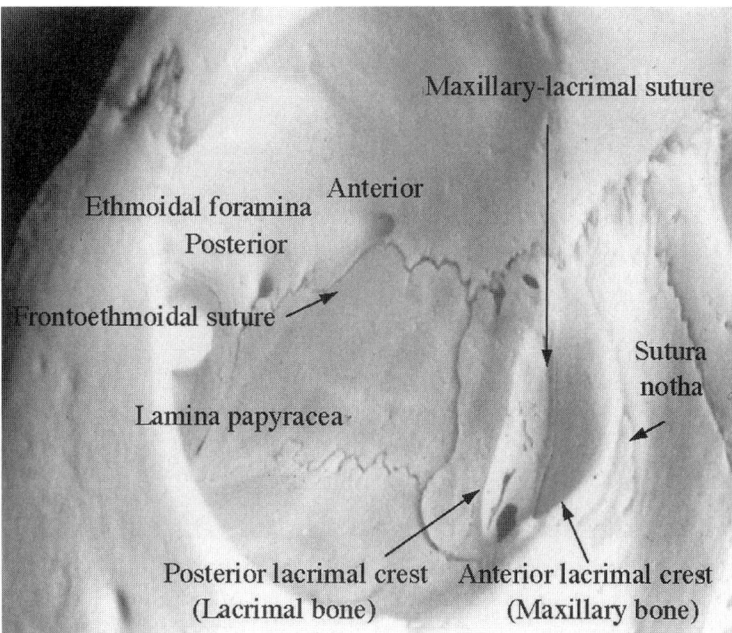

FIGURE 1.1. Bony anatomy of the lacrimal sac fossa and medial orbital wall. The anterior and posterior lacrimal crests are formed by the maxillary and lacrimal bones, respectively.

mucosa, and should be anticipated during lacrimal surgery to avoid bleeding.

The medial orbital wall is formed, from anterior to posterior, by the frontal process of the maxilla, the lacrimal bone, the ethmoid bone, and the lesser wing of the sphenoid bone. The thinnest portion of the medial wall is the lamina papyracea, which covers the ethmoid sinuses laterally. The many bullae of ethmoid pneumatization appear as a honeycomb pattern medial to the ethmoid bone (Figure 1.2). The medial wall becomes thicker posteriorly at the body of the sphenoid and again anteriorly at the posterior lacrimal crest of the lacrimal bone.

The frontoethmoidal suture is important in orbital bony decompression or lacrimal surgery as it marks the roof of the ethmoid sinus. Bony dissection superior to this suture may expose the dura of the cranial cavity. The anterior and posterior ethmoidal foramina conveying branches of the ophthalmic artery and the nasociliary nerve are located at the frontoethmoidal suture, 24- and 36-mm posterior to the anterior lacrimal crest, respectively (Figure 1.3).[19]

The anterior lacrimal crest is an important landmark during external dacryocystorhinostomy, as the anterior limb of the medial canthal tendon attaches to the anterior lacrimal crest superiorly. This attachment of the medial canthal tendon is often detached from the underlying bone along with the periosteum in order to gain better exposure during surgery.

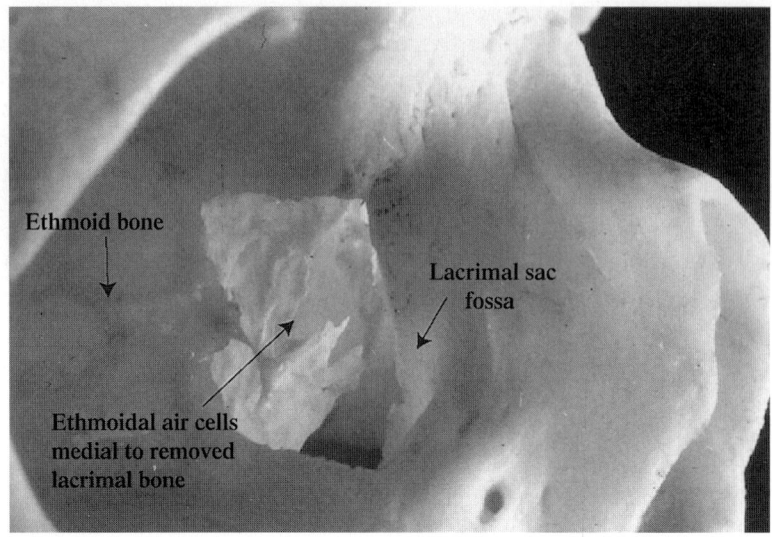

FIGURE 1.2. The ethmoidal air cells are medial to the removed lacrimal bone, and may extend anteriorly to pneumatize the maxillary bone of the lacrimal sac fossa.

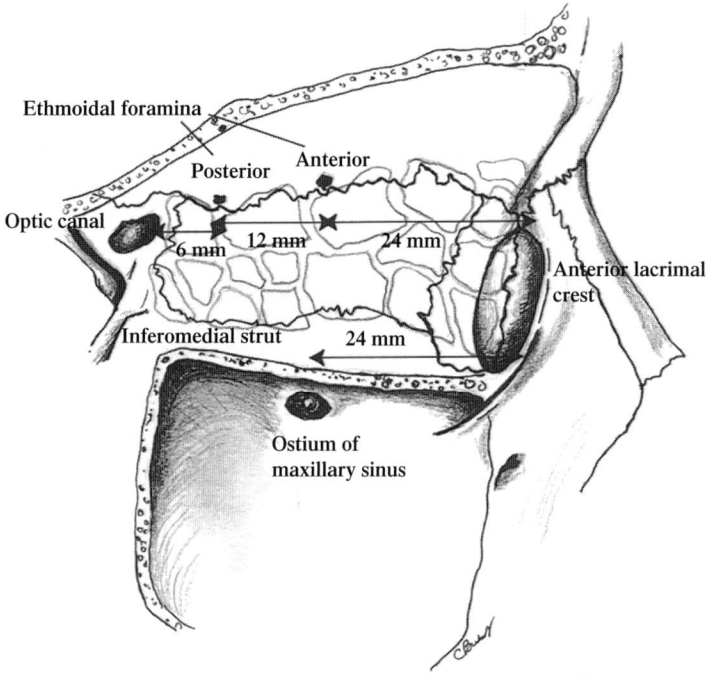

FIGURE 1.3. Anteroposterior distances of the foramina from the anterior lacrimal crest. The ostium of the maxillary sinus lies approximately in a vertical line to the anterior ethmoidal foramen.

A vertical suture runs centrally between the anterior and posterior lacrimal crests, representing the anastomosis of the maxillary bone to the lacrimal bone (see Figure 1.1). A suture located more posteriorly within the fossa would indicate predominance of the maxillary bone, whereas a more anteriorly placed suture would indicate predominance of the lacrimal bone. The lacrimal bone at the lacrimal sac fossa has a mean thickness of 106 microns, which allows it to be easily penetrated to enter the nasal cavity at surgery.[20] In a patient with a maxillary bone dominant fossa, the thicker bone makes it more difficult to create the osteotomy.

At the junction of the medial and inferior orbital rims, at the base of the anterior lacrimal crest, a small lacrimal tubercle may be palpated externally to guide the surgeon to the lacrimal sac located posterior and superior to it. In 28%–34% of orbits, the tubercle may project posteriorly as an anterior lacrimal spur.[16,21]

The nasolacrimal canal originates at the base of the lacrimal sac fossa, and is formed by the maxillary bone laterally and the lacrimal and inferior turbinate bones medially. The width of the superior opening of the canal measures, on average, 4–6 mm.[16] The duct courses posteriorly and laterally in the bone shared by the medial wall of the maxillary sinus and the lateral nasal wall for 12 mm to drain into the inferior meatus of the nasal cavity.[22]

Nasal and Paranasal Sinuses

Knowledge of nasal and paranasal sinus anatomy enhances the understanding of surgical relationships to the orbit, and is particularly important in endonasal approaches.

The bones forming the orbital floor, roof, and medial wall are pneumatized by air sinuses arising from the primitive nasal cavities. They retain communication with the nasal cavity and are thus lined by a continuation of the nasal mucous membrane. The sinuses appear in early childhood, increase actively during puberty, and may continue to grow until 30 years of age.[16]

The maxillary sinus is the largest of the paranasal sinuses, measuring 15 cc.[16] The roof of the maxillary sinus forms the orbital floor that declines from the medial wall to the lateral wall at an angle of approximately 30°. The maxillary sinus drains into the hiatus semilunaris within the middle meatus through an ostium located near the level of the orbital floor, immediately inferior to the midlength portion of the maxilloethmoidal orbital strut. The ostium measures, on average, 24 mm from the orbital rim, which is approximately in a vertical line to the anterior ethmoidal foramen in the medial orbital wall (see Figure 1.3).[23]

The ethmoid sinuses are the first to develop, reaching adult configuration at as early as 12 years of age.[24] Ethmoid bullae are particularly exuberant in their expansion, and may pneumatize the orbital plate of the frontal bone, and even develop as frontal sinuses. The growth of the ethmoid sinuses frequently extends past the suture of the ethmoid bone and even into the lacrimal and maxillary bones of the lacrimal sac fossa (see Figure 1.2).[25,26]

The ethmoid, sinuses are shaped like a rectangular box, slightly wider posteriorly where they articulate with the sphenoid sinus. The ethmoid sinuses comprise three main groups – the anterior, middle, and posterior ethmoidal air cells. The anterior and middle ethmoidal air cells drain into the middle meatus, whereas the posterior cells drain into the superior meatus.

The roof of the orbit slopes down as it travels medially, and this slope continues at the frontoethmoidal suture to become the roof of the ethmoid sinus, or *fovea ethmoidalis*. The ethmoid roof continues to slope inferiorly and medially to overlie the nasal cavity as the cribriform plate. The crista galli bisects the cribriform plate on its superior aspect, and continues inferiorly as the vertical nasal plate, or vomer. Because of this sloping, which is most prominent over the anterior ethmoid air cells, it is important to know the individual anatomy and variations before surgery to avoid inadvertent entry into the cranial cavity and cerebrospinal fluid leak, or more severe intracranial injury.[27]

The anatomic relationship of the anterior ethmoid air cells to the lacrimal sac fossa is important to understand before performing dacryocystorhinostomy, in order to avoid confusion between the ethmoid and nasal cavities during creation of the ostium. A close anatomic relationship between the anterior ethmoid air cells, termed the agger nasi cells, to the lacrimal sac fossa has been demonstrated in several past studies.[24–26,28–30] These agger nasi bullae may pneumatize the lacrimal bone, and rarely extend into the frontal process of the maxillary bone.

Whitnall[25] described in 1911 the relationship of the anterior ethmoid air cells directly medial to the lacrimal sac fossa in 86% of skulls. In 32% of skulls, the air cells extended anteriorly to the vertical maxillary-lacrimal suture, and in an additional 54%, the air cells extended even farther to the anterior lacrimal crest. The ethmoid cells were located consistently in the superior half of the fossa, with the inferior half of the fossa directly adjacent to the middle meatus of the nasal cavity. Similarly, Blaylock et al.[26] studied computed tomography (CT) scans of 190 orbits with normal ethmoid anatomy and found that in 93% of the orbits, the anterior ethmoid cells extended anterior to the posterior lacrimal crest, with 40% extending anterior to the maxillary-lacrimal bone suture and entering the frontal process of the maxilla. In only 7% of orbits was the nasal cavity directly adjacent to the entire lacrimal sac fossa. The anterior extension of the air cells is most prominent adjacent to the superior half of the lacrimal sac fossa.[24–26,28,30,31]

The ethmoid air cells and sinus mucosa should be removed to allow a proper osteotomy. Understanding the anatomic relationship of the lacrimal sac fossa to the ethmoid sinus also helps avoid complications such as inadvertent dacryocystorhinostomy fistulization into the ethmoid sinus, cerebrospinal fluid leakage, orbital hemorrhage, and trauma to and subsequent scarring of the nasal mucosa and nasal septum.[32]

The bony nose is formed by the frontonasal process during embryology. The nasal septum bisects the nasal cavity and comprises three portions: the bony perpendicular plate of the ethmoid (superoanterior) and the vomer (posterior and anteroinferior), a cartilaginous anterior triangle, and an inferior membranous columella that divides the nares anteriorly. Laterally, the nasal wall has three or more horizontal ridges termed turbinates, with a corresponding meatus below each (Figure 1.4). During the sixth week of embryologic development, before cartilage forms in the walls of the primitive nasal cavities, linear outgrowths of the lining epithelium occur on the sides and roof of each nasal side. Each outgrowing gutter becomes a meatus, whereas the ridges left behind form the turbinates.[8,16]

The inferior turbinate is the largest, arising from the medial wall of the maxillary sinus. The smaller and more posterior middle, superior, and supreme (if present) turbinates are outcroppings of the ethmoid bone. The supreme turbinate may be found in up to 65% of patients. The inferior turbinate is visualized by directing a nasal speculum parallel to the floor of the nasal cavity. The nasal vestibule is the large

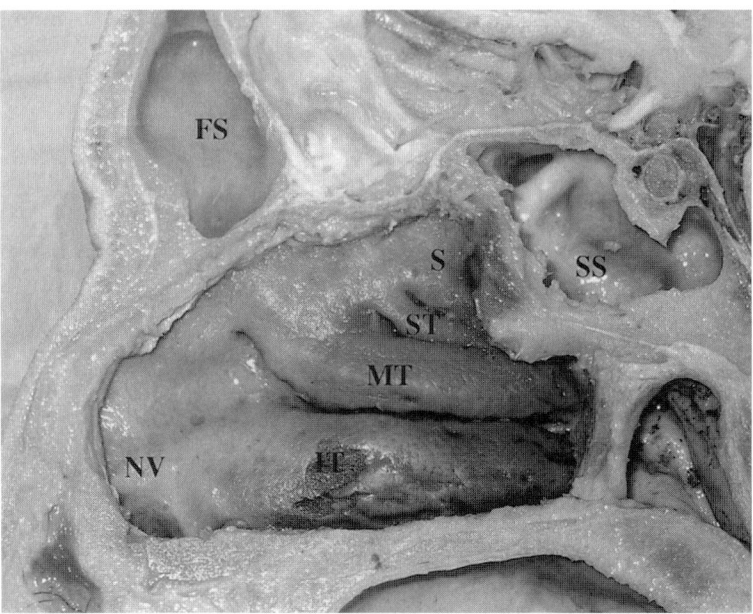

FIGURE 1.4. Endonasal sagittal view. Each nasal turbinate has a corresponding meatal space located immediately below. FS, frontal sinus; IT, inferior turbinate; MT, middle turbinate; NV, nasal vestibule; S, supreme turbinate; SS, sphenoid sinus; ST, superior turbinate.

cartilaginous anterior dilatation of the nose above the nares, covered by squamous epithelium with hair follicles, to which the silicone tubes may be secured during surgery.

The middle turbinate originates posteriorly from the roof of the nose at the cribriform plate, and arises anteriorly from the medial wall of the maxillary sinus. The lacrimal sac fossa lies anterior and lateral to the anterior tip of the middle turbinate, thus the entry in an external dacryocystorhinostomy is at the anterior tip of the middle turbinate (Figure 1.5). An ostium achieved by the endoscopic approach is usually more inferior to the routine external site.

Within the middle meatus lies a curvilinear gutter, the hiatus semilunaris, which houses the ostium of the maxillary sinus. It is bordered inferiorly by a bony ridge termed the uncinate process, and superiorly by the bulla ethmoidalis prominence which represents the most anterior ethmoid air cells (Figure 1.6).[33] The middle meatus receives the drainage of the ethmoid (anterior and middle), frontal, and maxillary sinuses. The frontonasal duct drains the frontal sinus into the anterosuperior portion of the hiatus semilunaris. The posterior ethmoid air cells drain into the superior meatus.

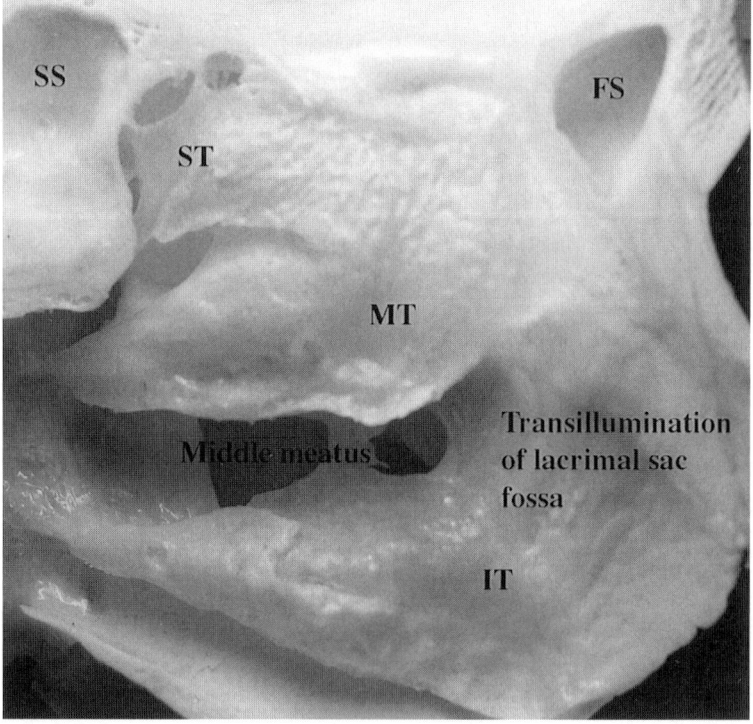

FIGURE 1.5. Endonasal site of a dacryocystorhinostomy ostium. Transillumination through the lacrimal sac fossa demonstrates its location at the anterior tip of the middle turbinate. FS, frontal sinus; IT, inferior turbinate; MT, middle turbinate; SS, sphenoid sinus; ST, superior turbinate.

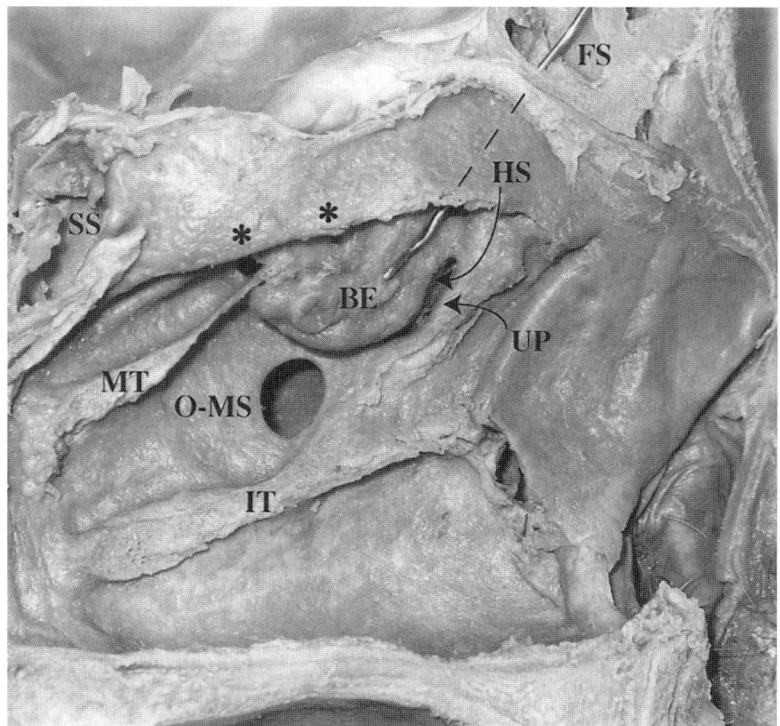

FIGURE 1.6. Endonasal view of lateral nasal wall with turbinates removed. BE, bulla ethmoidalis; FS, frontal sinus; HS, hiatus semilunaris; IT, inferior turbinate; MT, middle turbinate; O-MS, ostium of maxillary sinus; SS, sphenoid sinus; UP, uncinate process; *, ethmoid ostia.

Secretory System

Lacrimal Gland and Accessory Glands

The main lacrimal gland is located in the superotemporal orbit in a shallow lacrimal fossa of the frontal bone. The gland is composed of numerous acini that drain into progressively larger tubules and ducts. The acini are made up of a basal myoepithelial cell layer with inner columnar secretory cells. Contraction of the myoepithelial cells helps to force secretions into the tubules and drainage ducts.[34]

The gland measures $20 \times 12 \times 5$ mm and is divided by the lateral horn of the levator aponeurosis into a larger orbital lobe, and a lesser palpebral lobe below.[35,36] The orbital lobe is the larger of the two lobes and lies posterior to the orbital septum and preaponeurotic fat and anterior to the levator aponeurosis.[35] Two to six secretory ducts from the orbital lobe of the lacrimal gland pass through the palpebral lobe or along its fibrous capsule, joining with ducts from the palpebral lobe to form six to 12 tubules that empty into the superolateral conjunctival fornix 4–5 mm above the tarsus.[34,37]

Accessory lacrimal glands are located in the conjunctival fornices and along the superior tarsal border. There are approximately 20–40 accessory glands of Krause in the superior conjunctival fornix, and half that number present in the lower eyelid. Accessory glands of Wolfring are located along the superior tarsal border in the upper eyelid.[35,38]

The lacrimal gland receives innervation from cranial nerves V and VII, as well as from the sympathetics of the superior cervical ganglion.[39] The lacrimal branch of the ophthalmic division of the trigeminal nerve carries sensory stimuli from the lacrimal gland. The lacrimal gland receives arterial supply from the lacrimal artery, with contributions from the recurrent meningeal artery and a branch of the infraorbital artery. The venous drainage follows approximately the same intraorbital course of the artery and drains into the superior ophthalmic vein.

The course of the parasympathetic secretomotor innervation to the lacrimal gland is more complex. Parasympathetic secretomotor fibers originate in the lacrimal nucleus of the pons. These fibers travel a long course within the nervus intermedius, the greater superficial petrosal nerve, the deep petrosal nerve, and the vidian nerve to finally synapse in the pterygopalatine ganglion.[34] Postganglionic parasympathetic fibers leave the pterygopalatine ganglion via the pterygopalatine nerves to innervate the lacrimal gland.[40,41] In addition, some fibers may join the zygomatic nerve as it branches from the maxillary division of the trigeminal nerve and enters the orbit through the inferior orbital fissure. Branches of the zygomatic nerve may ascend and enter the posterior surface of the lacrimal gland either alone or in combination with the lacrimal nerve.[35] However, in a more recent anatomic study by Ruskell[42] in 2004, he found that parasympathetic fibers traveled along a branch of the middle meningeal artery through the superior orbital fissure before joining the ophthalmic or lacrimal artery to supply the lacrimal gland. This was in contrast to the traditional assumption that secretomotor nerves pass to the gland via the zygomatic and lacrimal nerves.

Sympathetic nerves arrive with the lacrimal artery and along with parasympathetics in the zygomatic nerve. The zygomatic branch of the maxillary trigeminal nerve gives off the lacrimal branch before dividing into zygomaticotemporal and zygomaticofacial branches. This lacrimal branch anastomoses with the lacrimal nerve of the ophthalmic trigeminal nerve or travels along the periorbita to independently enter the gland at its posterolateral aspect.

Excretory System

Lacrimal Drainage System

The lacrimal excretory pathway begins at a 0.3-mm opening on the medial portion of each eyelid termed the punctum.[16,37] Because of more rapid growth of the maxilla compared with the frontal bone during embryologic development, the lateral migration pulls the inferior canaliculus laterally, resulting in the lower eyelid punctum being located slightly lateral to the upper eyelid punctum.[8] The punctal opening widens into the ampulla, which is 2 mm in height and directed perpendicular to the eyelid margin, before making a sharp turn into the canaliculi. The canaliculi measure 8–10 mm in length and 0.5–1.0 mm in diameter, and course parallel to the eyelid margins (Figure 1.7). The canaliculi are lined with stratified squamous epithelium and surrounded by orbicularis muscle.

In more than 90% of individuals, the superior and inferior canaliculi merge to form a common canaliculus before entry into the nasolacrimal sac.[37,43] In a large study using digital subtraction dacryocystograms, the common canaliculus was present in 94% of lacrimal drainage systems. The upper and lower canaliculi joined at the wall of the lacrimal sac without a common canaliculus in an additional 4%, with only 2% of systems having completely separate drainage of the upper and lower canaliculi into the lacrimal sac.[44] The common internal punctum visualized within the lacrimal sac should be free of any mucosal membrane or stricture for success of the dacryocystorhinostomy surgery.

The functional valve between the common canaliculus and the lacrimal sac has traditionally been attributed to the valve of Rosenmüller, although some studies have been unable to document this structure.[6] Tucker demonstrated a consistent pattern of angulation within the canalicular system.[45] The canaliculi first angle posteriorly behind the medial canthal tendon. The canaliculi then bend at the canaliculus–common canaliculus junction at an angle of 118°, before passing anteriorly to enter the lacrimal sac at an acute angle of 58°. This consistent angulation may contribute to a valve-like effect that prevents retrograde flow from the lacrimal sac.

The nasolacrimal sac and duct are portions of the same continuous structure (Figures 1.7 and 1.8). The lacrimal drainage system is lined

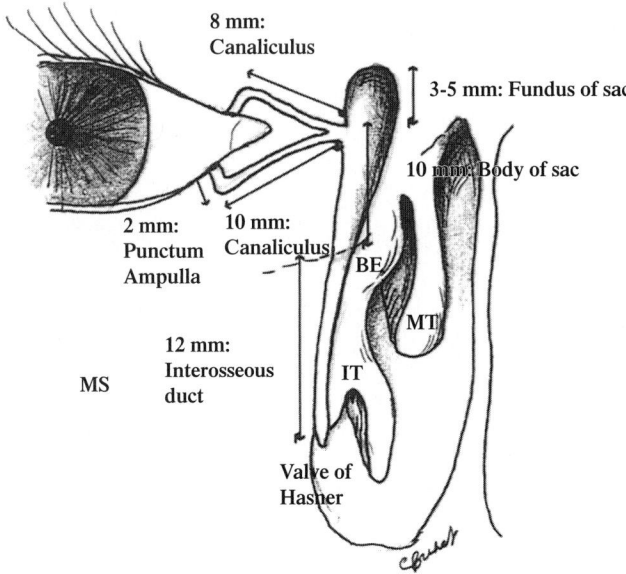

FIGURE 1.7. Approximate dimensions of the lacrimal excretory system. BE, bulla ethmoidalis; IT, inferior turbinate; MS, maxillary sinus; MT, middle turbinate.

by nonciliated columnar epithelium. The total sac measures a length of 12–15 mm vertically and 4–8 mm anteroposteriorly. The fundus of the sac extends 3–5 mm above the medial canthal tendon, and the body of the sac measures 10 mm in height.[37] The sac rests in the lacrimal sac fossa, with its medial aspect tightly adherent to the periosteal lining of the fossa. The lower nasolacrimal fossa and the nasolacrimal duct are narrower in females, which may account for the female predominance of nasolacrimal obstruction.[18] The nasolacrimal duct then travels inferolaterally and slightly posteriorly in its bony course to the inferior turbinate for an interosseous distance of 12 mm. The long axis of the duct and canal forms an angle of 15–25° posterior to the frontal plane, or in a line connecting the medial commissure to the first molar tooth (Figure 1.9).[16]

Wormald et al.[46] used CT dacryocystograms to evaluate the relationship of the lacrimal sac to the insertion of the middle turbinate on the lateral nasal wall in 76 patients. The mean height of the lacrimal sac

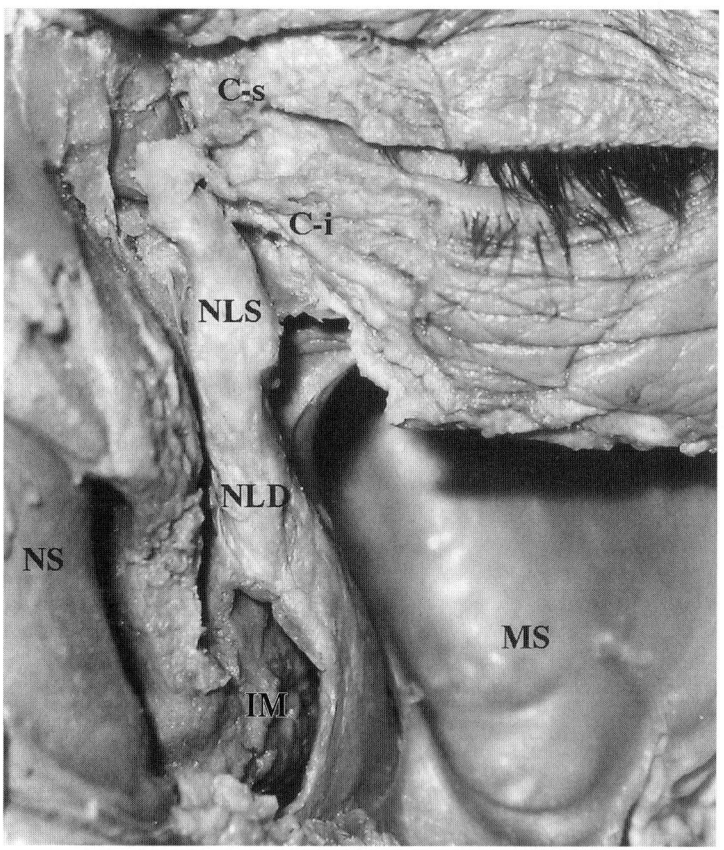

FIGURE 1.8. Anatomic dissection of the lacrimal drainage system within the bony wall between the nasal cavity and maxillary sinus. The nasolacrimal duct drains into the inferior meatus. C-i, inferior canaliculus; C-s, superior canaliculus; IM, inferior meatus; MS, maxillary sinus; NLD, nasolacrimal duct; NLS, nasolacrimal sac; NS, nasal septum.

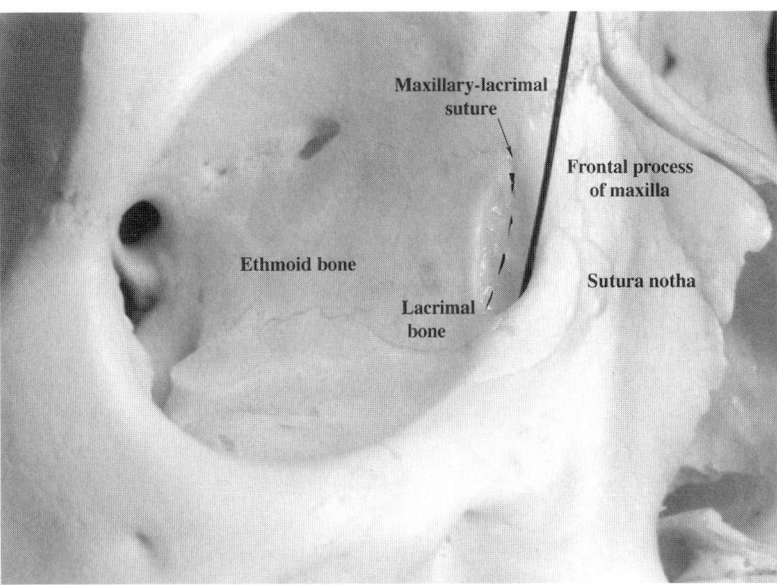

Maxillary-lacrimal suture

Frontal process of maxilla

Ethmoid bone

Sutura notha

Lacrimal bone

FIGURE 1.9. The nasolacrimal duct travels inferolaterally and slightly posteriorly in its bony course to the inferior turbinate, forming an angle of approximately 15–25° posterior to the frontal plane.

above the middle turbinate insertion was measured to be 8.8 mm and below it was 4.1 mm.

Multiple mucosal folds and sinuses have been reported within the lacrimal drainage system, although their role and presence are unclear. The previously mentioned valve of Rosenmüller is located at the junction of the common canaliculus and sac, and the valve of Krause between the sac and duct. A mucosal flap, Hasner's valve (or *plica lacrimalis*), may be present at the opening of the duct into the inferior meatus of the nose.[47] The nasolacrimal duct ostium within the inferior meatus is located 25–30 mm posterior to the lateral margin of the anterior nares.[16]

The inferior oblique muscle arises from a shallow depression in the orbital plate of the maxilla at the anteromedial corner of the orbital floor just lateral to the lacrimal excretory fossa.

The canaliculi are encased in superficial pretarsal orbicularis oculi muscle as they traverse the medial eyelids and medial canthal region. The lacrimal sac is ensheathed in the lacrimal fascia, which refers to the periorbital lining that splits at the posterior lacrimal crest into one layer that lines the fossa, and another layer that encases the lateral sac to reach the anterior lacrimal crest. Additionally, the lacrimal sac is wrapped by the thick anterior and thin posterior limbs of the medial canthal tendon. Almost immediately after the medial canthal tendon arises from the tarsal plates, it divides into a thicker anterior limb that wraps along the anterior upper half of the lacrimal sac before inserting onto the anterior lacrimal crest, and a very thin posterior limb that passes behind the sac to insert onto the posterior lacrimal crest (Figure 1.10). The deep portion of the pretarsal orbicularis muscle important

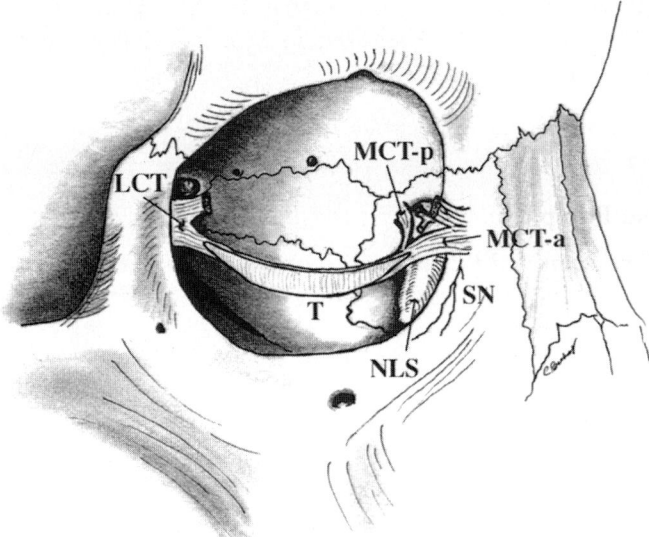

FIGURE 1.10. Relationship of the medial canthal tendon to the lacrimal sac. The thick anterior limb of the medial canthal tendon wraps along the anterior upper half of the lacrimal sac to insert onto the anterior lacrimal crest, whereas the thin posterior limb passes behind the sac to insert onto the posterior lacrimal crest. LCT, lateral canthal tendon; MCT-a, medial canthal tendon-anterior limb; MCT-p, medial canthal tendon-posterior limb; NLS, nasolacrimal sac; SN, sutura notha; T, tarsus.

in lacrimal outflow (Horner-Duverney muscle, *tensor tarsi*, or *pars lacrimalis*) passes posterior to the lacrimal sac and the posterior limb of the medial canthal tendon, and inserts onto the upper posterior lacrimal crest.[7,16,37,48] The orbital septum inserts along or just posterior to the inferior posterior lacrimal crest.

Creation of a large osteotomy helps to increase the chance of success of dacryocystorhinostomy surgery. As much as one-third of the lacrimal sac may lie above the medial canthal tendon; therefore, to create an adequate osteotomy for apposition of the entire lacrimal sac and nasal mucosa, the osteotomy should extend superior to the level of the medial canthal tendon. Bone may be removed with the rongeur until thickening of the frontal bone is noted. This point should generally lie 5mm or more above the common internal punctum.

Slightly above the level of the medial canthal tendon lies the anterior cranial fossa. Botek and Goldberg[49] found that the oblique distance between the common internal punctum and the most anterior aspect of the cribriform plate was 25 ± 3mm. Using a retrospective study of coronal maxillofacial CT scans from 40 adults, McCann and Lucarelli[50] found that the mean vertical dimension between the medial canthal ligament and the level of the cribriform plate was 17 ± 4mm.

The angular artery branch of the facial artery runs along the line of the nasojugal skinfold and passes superficial to the medial canthal tendon. The angular vein courses immediately lateral to the artery, with both vessels located approximately 5mm anteromedial to the anterior lacrimal crest, or 8mm medial to the medial commissure of the eyelids.[16]

Lacrimal Pump

Jones[7,37] popularized the lacrimal pump theory, in which he proposed that contraction of the pretarsal orbicularis muscle fibers during eyelid closure compresses and shortens the canaliculi, pumping tears toward the lacrimal sac. Furthermore, simultaneous lateral movement of the lateral lacrimal sac from contraction of the deep head of the preseptal orbicularis muscle was thought to generate a negative pressure within the lacrimal sac that draws tears into the sac from the canaliculi. In contrast, other anatomic and physiologic studies[48,51–55] have found that a positive-pressure mechanism, rather than a negative-pressure mechanism, is responsible for the lacrimal pump during eyelid closure. Thale used histological, immunohistochemical, and scanning electron microscopic techniques to demonstrate that the wall of the lacrimal sac is composed of collagen, elastic, and reticular fiber bundles arranged in a helical pattern. He proposed that the lacrimal sac distends and is pulled superolaterally because of its medial attachments when the lacrimal orbicularis muscle contracts with blinking. In addition, the helical collagen and elastic fibers encircling the sac may result in the sac being "wrung out" as another proposed mechanism for lacrimal drainage.[56,57]

References

1. Duke-Elder SS, Cook C. System of Ophthalmology. Normal and Abnormal Development. Part 1: Embryology. St. Louis: Mosby; 1963.
2. Jakobiec F, Iwamoto T. The ocular adnexa: introduction to lids, conjunctiva, and orbit. In: Jakobiec F, ed. Ocular Anatomy, Embryology, and Teratology. Philadelphia: Harper & Row; 1982:677–731.
3. Ozanics V, Jakobiec F. Prenatal development of the eye and its adnexa. In: Jakobiec F, ed. Ocular Anatomy, Embryology, and Teratology. Philadelphia: Harper & Row; 1982:11–96.
4. Wahl C, Noden DM. Defining the environment around the eye. In: Tasman W, Jaeger E, eds. Duane's Clinical Ophthalmology. Philadelphia: Lippincott-Raven; 2000.
5. de la Cuadra-Blanco C, Peces-Pena MD, Merida-Velasco JR. Morphogenesis of the human lacrimal gland. J Anat 2003;203:531–536.
6. Schaeffer JP. The genesis and development of the nasolacrimal passages in man. Am J Anat 1912;13:1–23.
7. Jones LT, Wobig JL. Congenital anomalies of the lacrimal system. In: Surgery of the Eyelids and Lacrimal System. Birmingham, AL: Aesculapius; 1976: 157–173.
8. Hurwitz JJ. Embryology of the lacrimal drainage system. In: Hurwitz JJ, ed. The Lacrimal System. Philadelphia: Lippincott-Raven; 1996:9–13.

9. Cassady JV. Developmental anatomy of the nasolacrimal duct. Arch Ophthalmol 1952;47:141–158.

10. Petersen RA, Robb RM. The natural course of congenital obstruction of the nasolacrimal duct. J Pediatr Ophthalmol Strabismus 1978;15:246–250.

11. Ffooks OO. Dacryocystitis in infancy. Br J Ophthalmol 1962;46:422.

12. Yuen SJ, Oley C, Sullivan TJ. Lacrimal outflow dysgenesis. Ophthalmology 2004;111:1782–1790.

13. Kirk RC. Developmental anomalies of the lacrimal passages: a review of the literature and presentation of three unusual cases. Am J Ophthalmol 1956;42:227–232.

14. Masi AV. Congenital fistula of the lacrimal sac. Arch Ophthalmol 1969;81: 701–704.

15. Sevel D. Development and congenital abnormalities of the nasolacrimal apparatus. J Pediatr Ophthalmol Strabismus 1981;18:13–19.

16. Whitnall SE. The Anatomy of the Human Orbit and Accessory Organs of Vision. New York: Oxford University Press; 1932:1–252.

17. Bailey JH. Surgical anatomy of the lacrimal sac. Am J Ophthalmol 1923;6: 665–671.

18. Groessl SA, Sires BS, Lemke BN. An anatomical basis for primary acquired nasolacrimal duct obstruction. Arch Ophthalmol 1997;115:71–74.

19. Lemke BN, Della Rocca R. Surgery of the Eyelids and Orbit: An Anatomical Approach. East Norwalk, CT: Appleton & Lange; 1990.

20. Hartikainen J, Aho HJ, Seppa H, Grenman R. Lacrimal bone thickness at the lacrimal sac fossa. Ophthalmic Surg Lasers 1996;27(8):679–684.

21. Whitnall SE. The naso-lacrimal canal: the extent to which it is formed by the maxilla, and the influence of this upon its caliber. Ophthalmoscope 1912;10:557–558.

22. Groell R, Schaffler G, Uggowitzer M, et al. CT: anatomy of the nasolacrimal sac and duct. Surg Radiol Anat 1997;19:189–191.

23. Kim JW, Goldberg RA, Shorr N. The inferomedial orbital strut. Ophthal Plast Reconstr Surg 2002;18:355–364.

24. Mattox DE, Delaney RG. Anatomy of the ethmoid sinus. Otolaryngol Clin North Am 1985;18:3–42.

25. Whitnall SE. The relations of the lacrimal fossa to the ethmoidal cells. Ophthal Rev 1911;30:321–325.

26. Blaylock WK, Moore CA, Linberg JV. Anterior ethmoid anatomy facilitates dacryocystorhinostomy. Arch Ophthalmol 1990;108:1774–1777.

27. McCormick CD, Bearden WH, Hunts JH, Anderson RL. Cerebral vasospasm and ischemia after orbital decompression for Graves ophthalmopathy. Ophthal Plast Reconstr Surg 2004;20(5):347–351.

28. Mosher HP. The surgical anatomy of the ethmoid labyrinth. Ann Otol Rhinol Laryngol 1929;38:869–901.

29. Bagatella R, Guiado CR. The ethmoid labyrinth: an anatomical and radiological study. Acta Otolaryngol (Stockh) 1983;403(suppl):1–19.

30. Terrier F, Weber W, Ruefennacht D, Porcellini B. Anatomy of the ethmoid: CT, endoscopic and macroscopic. Am J Radiol 1985;144:493–500.

31. Masala W, Perugini S, Salvolini U, et al. Multiplanar reconstructions in the study of ethmoid anatomy. Neuroradiology 1989;31:151–155.

32. Buus D, Tse D, Farris B. Ophthalmic complications of sinus surgery. Ophthalmology 1990;97:612–619.

33. Bridger MWM, Van Nostrand AWP. The nose and paranasal sinuses: applied surgical anatomy. J Otolaryngol 1978;suppl 6:1–33.

34. Lemke BN, Lucarelli MJ. Anatomy of the ocular adnexa, orbit, and related facial structures. In: Nesi FA, Lisman RD, Levine MR, Brazzo BG,

Gladstone GJ, eds. Smith's Ophthalmic Plastic and Reconstructive Surgery. 2nd ed. St. Louis: Mosby; 1998:3–78.

35. Dutton JJ. The lacrimal systems. In: Dutton J, ed. Atlas of Clinical and Surgical Orbital Anatomy. Philadelphia: WB Saunders; 1994:140–142.

36. Morton AD, Elner VM, Lemke BN, et al. Lateral extensions of the Müller muscle. Arch Ophthalmol 1996;114:1486–1488.

37. Jones LT. An anatomical approach to problems of the eyelids and lacrimal apparatus. Arch Ophthalmol 1961;66:111–124.

38. Seifert P, Spitznas M, Koch F, et al. Light and electron microscopic morphology of accessory lacrimal glands. Adv Exp Med Biol 1994;350: 19–23.

39. Walcott B. Anatomy and innervation of the human lacrimal gland. In: Albert DM, Jakobiec F, Robinson N, eds. Principles and Practice of Ophthalmology: Basic Sciences. Philadelphia: WB Saunders; 1994:454–458.

40. Ruskell GL. The distribution of autonomic post-ganglionic nerve fibers to the lacrimal gland in monkeys. J Anat 1971;109:229–242.

41. Ruskell GL. The orbital branches of the pterygopalatine ganglion and their relationship with internal carotid nerve branches in primates. J Anat 1970;106:323–339.

42. Ruskell GL. Distribution of pterygopalatine ganglion efferents to the lacrimal gland in man. Exp Eye Res 2004;78(3):329–335.

43. Lemke BN. Lacrimal anatomy. Adv Ophthal Plast Reconstr Surg 1984;3: 11–23.

44. Yazici B, Yazici Z. Frequency of the common canaliculus: a radiological study. Arch Ophthalmol 2000:118(10):1381–1385.

45. Tucker NA, Tucker SM, Linberg JV. The anatomy of the common canaliculus. Arch Ophthalmol 1996;114:1231–1234.

46. Wormald PJ, Kew J, Van Hasselt A. Intranasal anatomy of the nasolacrimal sac in endoscopic dacryocystorhinostomy. Otolaryngol Head Neck Surg 2000;123(3):307–310.

47. Aubaret E. The valves of the lacrymo-nasal passages (Les Replis valvulaires des canalicules et du conduit lacrymo-nasal, etc.). Arch d'Ophthal 1908;28: 211–236.

48. Ahl NC, Hill JD. Horner's muscle and the lacrimal system. Arch Ophthalmol 1982;100:488–493.

49. Botek AA, Goldberg RA. Margins of safety in dacryocystorhinostomy. Ophthalmic Surg 1993;24:320–322.

50. McCann DP, Lucarelli MJ. Radiologic analysis of the ethmoid bone-cribriform plate spatial relationship. Invest Ophthalmol Vis Sci 1998;39(4): S498. Abstract 2281.

51. Ploman K, Engel A, Knutsson F. Experimental studies of lacrimal passageways. Acta Ophthalmol 1928;6:55–90.

52. Rosengren B. On lacrimal drainage. Ophthalmologica 1972;164:409–421.

53. Maurice DM. The dynamics and drainage of tears. Int Ophthalmol Clin 1973;13:103–116.

54. Doane MG. Blinking and the mechanics of the lacrimal drainage system. Ophthalmology 1981;88:844–851.

55. Becker BB. Tricompartment model of the lacrimal pump mechanism. Ophthalmology 1992;99:1139–1145.

56. Thale A, Paulsen F, Rochels R, et al. Functional anatomy of the human efferent tear ducts: a new theory of tear outflow mechanism. Graefes Arch Clin Exp Ophthalmol 1998;236:674–678.

57. Paulsen F. The human nasolacrimal ducts. Adv Anat Embryol Cell Biol 2003;170:1–106.

2

Gender and Racial Variations of the Lacrimal System

Susan R. Carter and Roberta E. Gausas

Anatomic variations of the lacrimal system must be considered when surgery of this region is contemplated. Racial and gender differences seem to exist in the lacrimal region. Although not well described in the literature, because most anatomic descriptions of the lacrimal system in the Western literature refer to white populations, these differences are supported by surgical experience in this region. Gender and racial anatomic variations may exist in the lacrimal region with respect to both bone and soft tissue. The nasolacrimal canal may vary in width, length, bony thickness, and in proximity to ethmoidal air cells. External soft tissue may vary in skin thickness, presence or absence of epicanthal folds, and nasal projection. Differences between men and women and between the lacrimal systems in white, Asian, and black patients will be discussed as they pertain to external and endoscopic lacrimal surgery.

Lacrimal Region Variations: Bony Anatomy

Nasolacrimal Canal Width and Length

The primary difference between the lacrimal systems of men and women is thought to be the width and length of the nasolacrimal canal, which contains the membranous nasolacrimal duct. A narrower, longer nasolacrimal canal is thought to occur more frequently in women than in men. Groessl et al.[1] measured the nasolacrimal canal at three different levels in axial computed tomographic (CT) scans of 36 men and 35 women. The dimensions of the lower and middle canal were found to be smaller in women than in men. Janssen et al.[2] measured the minimum diameter of the nasolacrimal canal on axial CT scans in 50 male and 50 female controls and 19 individuals with primary acquired nasolacrimal duct obstruction (PANDO). The mean minimum diameter in women, 3.35 mm, was statistically smaller than that of men, 3.70 mm. Patients with PANDO had a mean minimum diameter of 3.0 mm.

These studies demonstrating a narrower nasolacrimal canal in women may explain the higher incidence of involutional stenosis and obstruction of the nasolacrimal duct seen in women as compared with men.

Racial differences in the nasolacrimal canal may also exist among white, Asian, and black patients. The nasolacrimal canal of Asians and blacks is thought to be shorter and wider than that of whites, which would lend credence to the observation that nasolacrimal obstruction occurs more often in whites than other races. Ni et al.,[3] in an article in the Chinese literature, examined the nasolacrimal canal in 80 half-skulls of Chinese adults and found the mean length to be 14.14 mm. However, Groell et al.,[4] examining CT scans from 147 patients at the Medical School in Austria with a presumably primarily white population, found the mean nasolacrimal duct length to be 11.2 mm with a range of 6–21 mm. Although the methods of measurement of the nasolacrimal canal differed, the Chinese nasolacrimal duct was not substantially shorter than that of the Austrian group. A well-controlled comparison study is needed to further address this issue, as well as that of the nasolacrimal canal diameter.

Lacrimal Bone Thickness

A second, possible, and frequently discussed difference in the lacrimal region of whites, Asians, and blacks pertains to lacrimal bone thickness. The lacrimal bone appears clinically thicker in Asians and blacks than in whites during dacryocystorhinostomy (DCR), although few studies exist to confirm this experience (Figure 2.1). In 69 lacrimal bones from 48 Finnish patients, Hartikainen et al.[5] found the mean lacrimal bone thickness to be 106 microns, leading him to conclude that the lacrimal bone at the lacrimal sac fossa is so thin that it is easily penetrated in most cases. However, Lui et al.[6] measured lacrimal bone thickness in 386 Taiwanese patients during DCR and found the average thickness to be 5.8 ± 0.9 mm in males, and 4.2 ± 0.8 mm in females.

Anticipation of lacrimal bone thickness by the lacrimal surgeon is important in selection of surgical approach. Adequate bony opening is critical in achieving surgical success. Paper-thin lacrimal bones easily lend themselves to large osteotomies with routine instruments, whereas achieving an adequate osteotomy in thick bone is more challenging and may require additional instrumentation, such as a drill. Selection of either an external or endoscopic approach to DCR should take into account anticipated lacrimal bone thickness.

Disease state itself may alter bone thickness. Hinton et al.[7] found evidence of active bone remodeling in 19% of bone pieces harvested from DCRs and conjunctivodacryocystorhinostomies. Additionally, lacrimal bone thickness and density have been found to correlate with systemic bone density, suggesting that low-density, thin lacrimal bone may be found during DCR in patients with osteoporosis.[8] Osteoporosis is more common in women than men, and this may contribute to the clinical experience of easier osteotomies in women than men.[9,10]

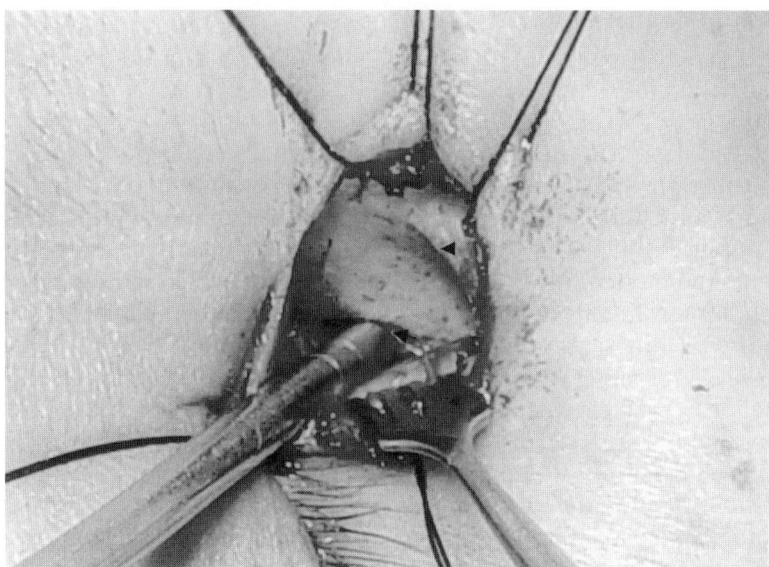

FIGURE 2.1. External DCR intraoperative view of lacrimal sac fossa in an Asian patient. Suction tip points to area of lacrimal bone suture line. The thick maxillary bony portion and anterior crest of the fossa lie above it. In this case, the maxillary bone is 2.5 to 3 times the width of the suction tip.

Lacrimal Sac Fossa Relationship to Ethmoidal Sinus

In 1964, Zhang and Lui undertook detailed measurements of 100 Chinese orbits and lacrimal fossas. In 56% of the specimens, they found ethmoidal air cell extension into the lacrimal sac fossa.[6,11] In 76% of the specimens, the anterior portion of the middle turbinate was also encountered in this area. An intervening ethmoid sinus between the lacrimal sac and the nose may cause confusion when performing a DCR leading to an inadequate or false passage. Ethmoid sinus mucosa can be differentiated from nasal mucosa by being much thinner. Entering the anterior portion of the middle turbinate surgically may cause excessive bleeding, and partial blockage of the ostium by the middle turbinate may lead to obstruction. Lui[6] suggests that such variations in nasal and lacrimal anatomy may account for the perceived difficulty of performing lacrimal surgery on Asian patients. However, initial entry into the ethmoid air cells rather than the nasal cavity was described in 23 of 50 DCRs (46%) by Talks of the United Kingdom in a presumably predominately white population.[12] Therefore, it behooves the lacrimal surgeon to understand the possible variations of nasal anatomy during all cases.

Lacrimal Sac Fossa Relationship to Cribriform Plate

Another surgically pertinent, possible difference between whites and Asians is the location of the cribriform plate with respect to the lacrimal apparatus. Botek and Goldberg,[13] in a dissection of five human cadaver heads, found the distance between the internal common punctum and the cribriform plate to be 25.1 ± 2.95 mm. Neuhaus and Baylis[14] performed DCRs and anatomic dissections on three fresh cadavers and found that the distance from a 15-mm vertical and 18-mm horizontal osteotomy to the floor of the anterior cranial fossa was 5.0 mm (range 1–7 mm). In a cadaver study of 28 Japanese skulls, Kurihashi and Yamashita[15] measured the distance from a point 10 mm posterior to the medial canthus superiorly to the anterior cranial fossa floor. Although the distance ranged from 1 to 30 mm, with an average of 8.3 mm, 21% had a distance of 3 mm or less. They recommended that surgeons not make a bony ostomy beneath the medial canthal tendon because of the possibility of violation of the cribriform plate.

Lacrimal Region Variations: Soft Tissue

External differences in the lacrimal region of whites, Asians, and blacks, particularly the absence or presence of epicanthal folds, the broad nasal bridge, and the thickness of the skin, clearly exist. Placement of skin incisions for an external DCR must take these factors into consideration. The broad nasal bridge of some Asians and blacks makes an incision more visible from a frontal view than in a white patient. Precise placement of the angle and length of the incision, particularly if a bilateral procedure is being performed, is essential for proper postoperative patient cosmesis. Because of the thicker skin of the nasal bridge, the incision should be placed closer to the medial canthus in the Asian and black patient than in the white patient. A less noticeable scar should occur in thinner skin. However, the epicanthal fold of some Asians must be avoided at all costs to prevent medial canthal webbing with scar contracture. An endoscopic DCR would avoid any potential problems arising from these external differences; however, one would need to take the thicker bone of the lacrimal region, often encountered in Asians and blacks, into consideration.

Conclusion

In summary, some differences between the lacrimal systems of males and females and those of different races have been well documented, such as the smaller nasolacrimal canal diameter of women as compared with men. However, further comparative studies are needed to fully address the anatomic differences, which would provide better surgical guidelines. Variations exist even within each gender and race. The key to being a successful lacrimal surgeon lies in the awareness of such nuances and the ability to adjust surgical technique when an anatomic variation is encountered in any patient.

References

1. Groessl SA, Sires BS, Lemke BN. An anatomical basis for primary acquired nasolacrimal duct obstruction. Arch Ophthalmol 1997;115(1):71–74.

2. Janssen AG, et al. Diameter of the bony lacrimal canal: normal values and values related to nasolacrimal duct obstruction – assessment with CT. AJNR Am J Neuroradiol 2001;22(5):845–850.
3. Ni C, et al. [The applied anatomy and measure of nasolacrimal duct]. Lin Chuang Er Bi Yan Hou Ke Za Zhi 1999;13(2):62–63.
4. Groell R, et al. CT-anatomy of the nasolacrimal sac and duct. Surg Radiol Anat 1997;19(3):189–191.
5. Hartikainen J, et al. Lacrimal bone thickness at the lacrimal sac fossa. Ophthalmic Surg Lasers 1996;27(8):679–684.
6. Lui D. Ethnic ophthalmic plastic surgery. In: Bosniak S, ed. Principles and Practice of Ophthalmic Plastic and Reconstructive Surgery. Vol II. Philadelphia: WB Saunders; 1996:691–701.
7. Hinton P, Hurwitz JJ, Cruickshank B. Nasolacrimal bone changes in diseases of the lacrimal drainage system. Ophthalmic Surg 1984;15(6): 516–521.
8. Oestreicher JH, Chung HT, Hurwitz JJ. The correlation of clinical lacrimal bone density and thickness, established at the time of DCR surgery, with systemic bone mineral densitometry testing. Orbit 2000;19(2):73–79.
9. Looker AC, et al. Prevalence of low femoral bone density in older U.S. adults from NHANES III. J Bone Miner Res 1997;12(11):1761–1768.
10. Looker AC, et al. Prevalence of low femoral bone density in older U.S. women from NHANES III. J Bone Miner Res 1995;10(5):796–802.
11. Zhang T, et al. [The clinical anatomy of lacrimal sac fossa]. Lin Chuang Er Bi Yan Hou Ke Za Zhi 2003;17(11):652–653.
12. Talks SJ, Hopkisson B. The frequency of entry into an ethmoidal sinus when performing a dacryocystorhinostomy. Eye 1996;10(pt 6):742–743.
13. Botek AA, Goldberg SH. Margins of safety in dacryocystorhinostomy. Ophthalmic Surg 1993;24(5):320–322.
14. Neuhaus RW, Baylis HI. Cerebrospinal fluid leakage after dacryocystorhinostomy. Ophthalmology 1983;90(9):1091–1095.
15. Kurihashi K, Yamashita A. Anatomical consideration for dacryocystorhinostomy. Ophthalmologica 1991;203(1):1–7.

3

Nasal Anatomy and Evaluation

Joseph P. Mirante

The nose is a significant organ of respiration and the primary organ of olfaction. The nasal septum is a cartilaginous and bony structure that divides the nose into two chambers. The anatomy of the lateral nasal wall is formed by a series of folds and spaces known respectively as the nasal conchae and meati. The effect of these structures on the inspired air-stream sets the parameters for nasal breathing and the treatment of air before it is directed down into the lungs. The turbulent airflow caused by the conchae adds to the perceived resistance of nasal airflow and the sensation of adequate breathing. Turbulent airflow allows for the wafting of molecules to the sensory cells of the olfactory system and thus aids the senses of taste and smell.

The paranasal sinuses, immediately adjacent to the nasal cavity, are air-filled spaces lined with respiratory epithelium in continuity with the epithelium of the nasal cavity. Within the confines of the nose and paranasal sinuses courses the collecting portion and the lower drainage portion of the lacrimal system and the lacrimal sac and duct, respectively. The complex relationship between nasal anatomy and the lacrimal system requires that the ophthalmologist has a good understanding to successfully approach the lacrimal system while avoiding complications in the nasal cavity.[1-4]

Anatomy

The External Nose

The external projection of the nose approximates a pyramid. The superior attachment at the forehead is known as the root. The inferior angular portion is known as the tip. The dorsum nasi is the intervening ridge. The nares are the paired openings to the nasal cavity each bounded medially by the septum and laterally by the alae. Each ala is formed by a rounded lower lateral cartilage.

The nasal skeleton is partially cartilage, part bone, and part membranous. Two paired nasal bones articulate with the frontal bones and rest firmly supported by the frontal process of the maxilla to support the bridge of the nose. The lower portion of the nasal pyramid is formed by several major and minor cartilages. The upper lateral cartilage is triangular in shape, extending from the paired nasal bones. The curved lower lateral cartilages overlie these and form the nasal opening. The medial portions of the lower cartilages sit anterior to the central septal cartilage.

The nasal cavity is divided into two nasal fossae. They are triangular in shape, opening anteriorly at the nares. The posterior openings into the pharynx are known as the choanae. The walls of the nasal cavity consist of the medial wall, formed by the septum; a lateral wall; and a floor. The most anterior portion of the nasal cavity is known as the vestibule. It is lined by squamous epithelium and has hairs, sweat glands, and sebaceous glands. The remainder of the nasal cavity is lined with respiratory epithelium, is highly vascular, and contains mucous and serous glands. The ciliated epithelium of the nasal cavity engages in active transport of mucous down into the nasopharynx.

The Nasal Septum

The nasal septum is formed by both bone and cartilage. The perpendicular plate of the ethmoid bone forms much of the posterior and superior portion of the nasal septum. The anterior portion is formed by the septal cartilage. Inferiorly lies the bony plate of the vomer, which rests on the nasal crests of the maxilla and the palatine bones. Variation in the anatomy, or deviation of the septum, can be attributed to the presence of bony protuberances, or septal spurs arising from the bony structures. The articulation of the septal cartilage can be angled from the nasal crest, causing a cartilaginous encroachment of the septum into the nasal cavity; clinically, this is known as a septal spur (Figure 3.1). The septal cartilage can also have a curved shape, causing narrowing of the nasal cavity, frequently referred to as septal deviation. These variations can be congenital in nature or acquired changes from nasal trauma.

The nerve supply of the nasal septum comes from the anterior ethmoidal and maxillary nerves with innervation coming via the sphenopalatine ganglion. Surgical treatment or trauma to the septum and resulting inflammation can lead to symptoms of numbness or pain of the upper incisors. The blood supply to the septum includes branches of the sphenopalatine artery, the ethmoidal artery, and the facial artery. The tissue is quite vascular and bleeding in surgery or from trauma can be quite brisk. Vasoconstrictive agents, topical and injected, are advisable when manipulation of the septum is necessary for surgical procedures.

The Lateral Nasal Wall

In contrast to the relatively simple medial wall, the lateral nasal wall in much more complex in both its anatomy and its involvement with the functions of respiration and drainage of the paranasal sinuses. It is the medial border of the paranasal sinuses and holds the projecting

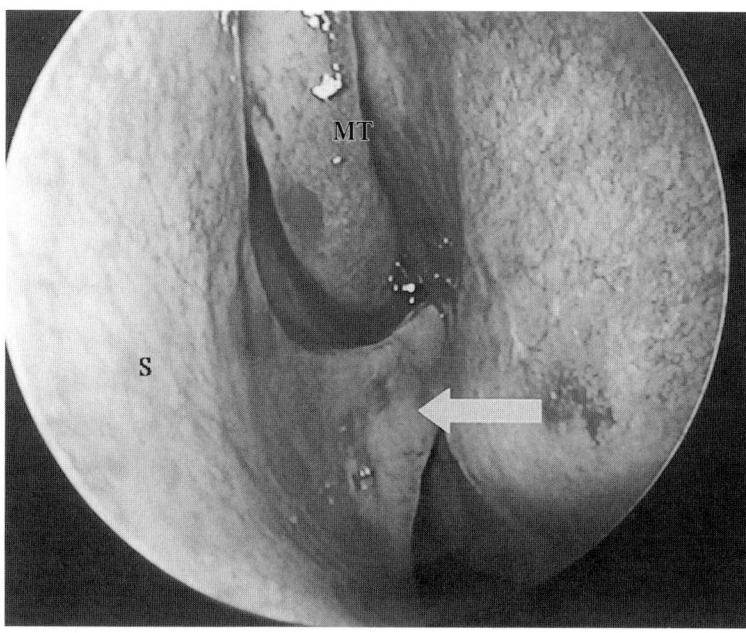

FIGURE 3.1. Septal spur. The arrow identifies a large septal spur. (S) identifies the nasal septum. (MT) identifies the middle turbinate.

ridges of bone known as the conchae or turbinates. These folds of respiratory mucosa over bone are named based on their relative position from below upward as the inferior, middle, and superior turbinate, respectively. In some cases, a fourth or supreme turbinate is present.

The inferior and middle turbinate are most important to discussions of the relationship between the lacrimal system and nasal anatomy. The spaces below the turbinates are known as meati and are named in accordance with the ridge to which they are related. The inferior meatus lies below the inferior turbinate, the middle meatus lies below the middle turbinate, and so on. The beginning of the space is at the anterior attachment or root of the turbinate.

The inferior turbinate consists of bone independent of the lateral wall (Figure 3.2). It is covered with a thick mucous membrane and contains a significant cavernous plexus which can be a source of brisk bleeding after surgical procedures. The inferior meatus, defined by the shape of the turbinate, is narrow anteriorly and posteriorly, and arched higher and wider in the center portion.

The structure of most importance in the inferior meatus is the opening of the nasolacrimal duct (Figure 3.3). Its shape is quite variable and has been described from rounded to more slit-like in appearance. The opening can be more raised from the surrounding tissue and papillae-like or can be more flattened and open into a deep groove or fossa. When the opening is more slit-like, it usually courses through a protective fold of mucous membrane known as the plica lacrimalis or

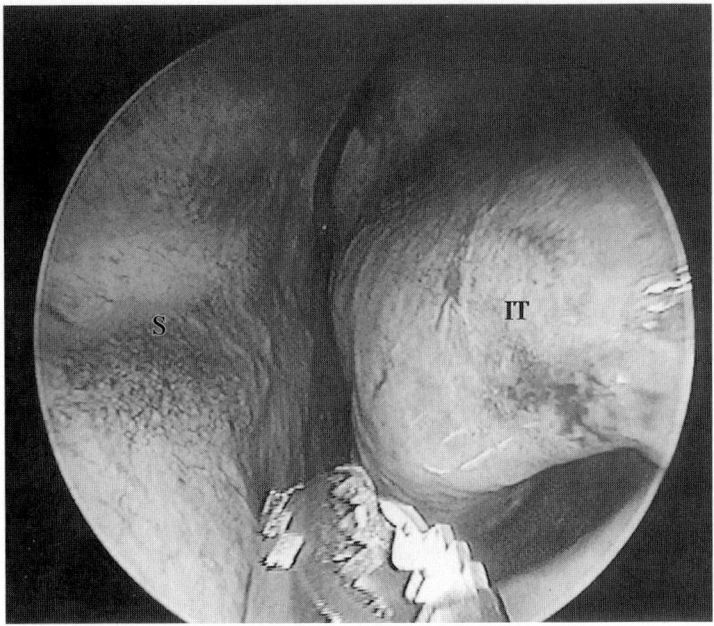

FIGURE 3.2. Inferior turbinate: (S) identifies the nasal septum. (IT) identifies the anterior portion of the inferior turbinate. A dissecting microdebrider blade is in the foreground.

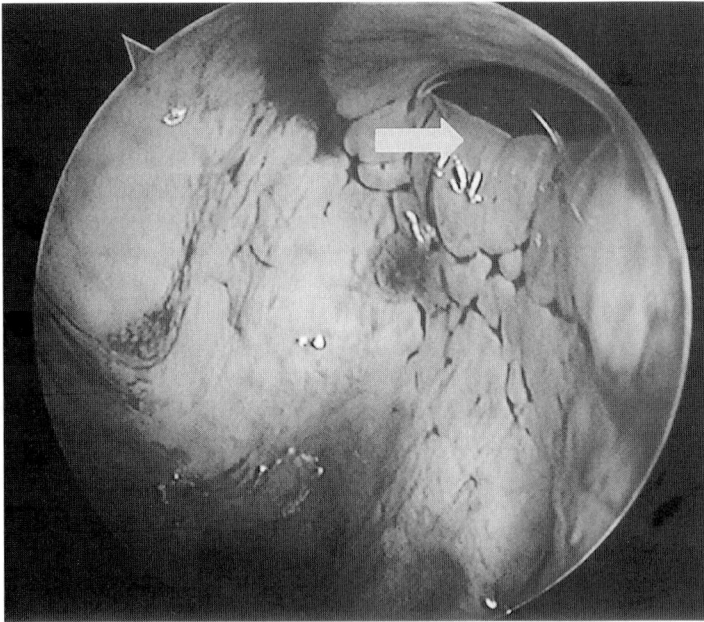

FIGURE 3.3. Opening of the nasolacrimal duct into the inferior meatus. The arrow identifies the opening of the nasolacrimal duct.

the valve of Hasner. The location of the nasolacrimal ostium is usually in the anterior portion of the inferior meatus at the lateral wall. It has also been described as high as the attachment of the turbinate.

The middle turbinate is a projection of the ethmoid bone that overhangs the complex anatomy of the middle meatus (Figure 3.4). This space is of vital importance in the drainage of the paranasal sinuses. The anterior attachment of the middle turbinate runs almost vertically and then bends to horizontal through the posterior portion. Under the high anterior portion is the highest part of the middle meatus known as the frontal recess. The frontal recess receives drainage from the frontal sinus superiorly. From the frontal recess, the middle meatus runs inferiorly and posteriorly. It is bordered by the face of the ethmoid sinus and the ethmoid bulla posteriorly. On the lateral wall, the uncinate process is a fold that projects posteriorly into the middle meatus. The natural ostium of the maxillary sinus lies below the inferior portion of the uncinate process. Scarring in the area of the middle meatus can be an iatrogenic cause of chronic sinus disease if the drainage pathways are blocked after manipulation and subsequent narrowing. This is particularly true for the frontal recess and chronic frontal sinusitis.

The most anterior part of the middle meatus corresponds to the location of the medial wall of the lacrimal sac. The sac can be fairly reliably

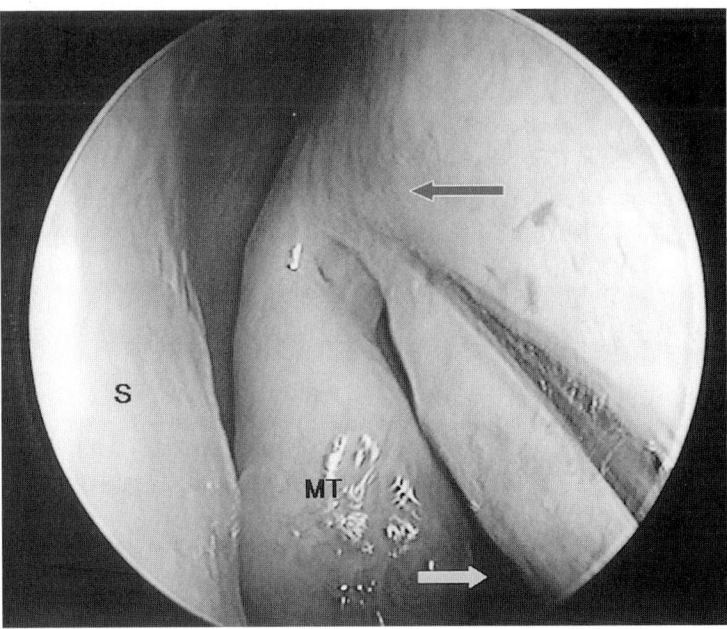

FIGURE 3.4. The middle meatus, injection of local anesthesia. The yellow arrow identifies the middle meatus. (MT) identifies the middle turbinate. The red arrow identifies the attachment of the middle turbinate, near the location of the lacrimal sac. (S) identifies the nasal septum.

located just anterior and inferior to the anterior attachment of the middle turbinate. The nasolacrimal duct courses within the bony nasolacrimal canal which runs inferiorly and slightly posteriorly and laterally between the lateral nasal wall and the maxillary sinus. The nasolacrimal duct can continue as the same diameter as the lacrimal sac, but generally narrows as it runs inferiorly. Whereas the nasolacrimal duct is intimately attached to the surrounding periosteum, the lacrimal sac is more loosely associated with its surrounding periosteum. As previously described, the nasolacrimal duct drains into the inferior meatus via its ostium.

The blood supply to the lateral nasal cavity posteriorly is largely from the sphenopalatine branch of the internal maxillary artery. The anterior and posterior ethmoid arteries from the internal carotid circulation supply more anterior and superior portions of the nasal cavity. The vestibule is largely supplied by branches of the facial nerve from the external carotid circulation.

Evaluation of the Nasal Cavity

Anterior Rhinoscopy

The most anterior portion of the nose, the nasal vestibule, can be easily evaluated with a light and direct vision. A nasal speculum will facilitate the examination by allowing the lateral retraction of the nasal ala. Alternatively, this can be accomplished with a handheld otoscope. In evaluation of the anterior nasal cavity, the physician should look for epistaxis, polyps, granulomas, skin malignancies, or benign lesions. A benign granuloma or hemangioma can bleed as easily as a malignancy. Consider biopsy or referral for biopsy for any suspicious lesion.

Nasal Endoscopy

Fiberoptic nasal endoscopes are valued tools in the evaluation of the nasal cavity. Both rigid and flexible endoscopes provide for thorough evaluation. The experienced examiner can proceed gently without the aid of a topical anesthetic, such as 4% lidocaine. The use of a topical decongestant, however, is advisable to aid in visualization and patient comfort.

With nasal endoscopy, the examiner can identify the presence of benign and malignant tumors, nasal polyps (Figure 3.5), septal deviation, and turbinate hypertrophy. Indeed, the completion of an endoscopic examination in the office is a good practice run for the use of a scope in the operating room and can help increase the comfort of the surgeon with the instrument as well as familiarize the surgeon with the anatomy.

Frequently, a 0°, 2.7-mm, rigid nasal endoscope is used. A wider, 4-mm endoscope will resist damage but will be more difficult to use in the nasal cavity. A flexible fiberoptic nasopharyngoscope may be more easily directed to the posterior nasal cavity; however, it cannot be used with one hand to allow manipulation of suction or forceps to remove

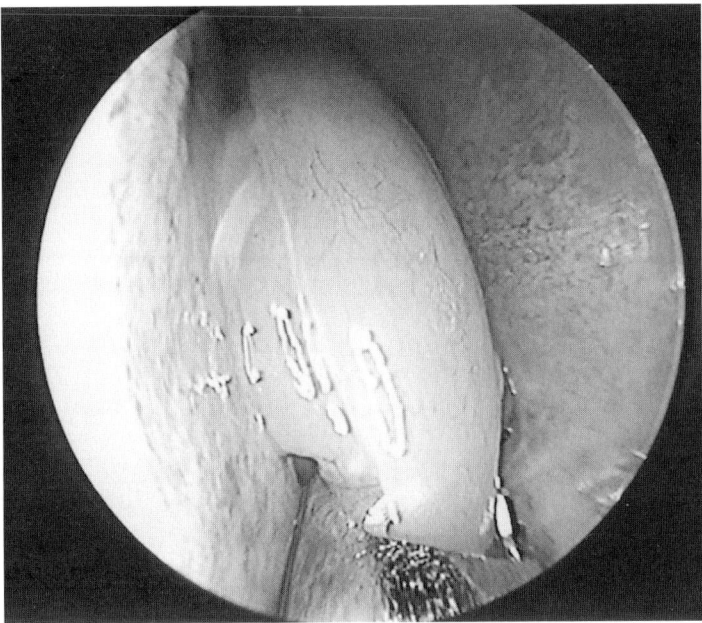

FIGURE 3.5. Benign nasal polyps: extensive nasal polyps in the nasal cavity.

debris. Caution must be used in the care and examination with nasal endoscopes. The optical fibers can break easily if the endoscope is dropped, and repairs and replacement are costly. Multiple articles describe the care and cleaning of endoscopic equipment and suppliers of these technologies are quite helpful in teaching about their upkeep.

Imaging Studies

Computer tomography in the coronal plane is an excellent modality in evaluation of the nasal cavity. Septal deformity, turbinate hypertrophy, and masses can all be evaluated. Computer-aided imaging systems used in neurosurgery, skull base surgery, and sinus surgery can be of assistance. The systems allow for real-time correlation of patient anatomy to computed tomography anatomy in the operating room. They can, however, increase operative time and may not be of much additional help for routine cases. Their utility may lie more in cases of severely abnormal anatomy, such as revision cases or in the setting of an anatomy-altering mass.

References

1. Mercandetti M, Mirante JP. Powered endonasal dacryocystorhinostomy. In: Krouse JH, Christmas DA, eds. Powered Endoscopic Sinus Surgery. Philadelphia: Williams & Wilkins; 1997:137–144.

2. Mercandetti M, Mirante JP. Endoscopic dacryocystorhinostomy. Facial Plast Surg Clin North Am 1997;5(2):195–202.
3. Christmas DA, Mirante JP, Yanagisawa E. Middle meatal obstruction following endoscopic dacryocystorhinostomy. Ear Nose Throat J 2002;81: 431–432.
4. Yanagisawa E, Mirante JP, Christmas DA. Endoscopic view of a hemostatic technique for endoscopic sinus surgery. Ear Nose Throat J 2003;2:749–750.

Section 2

Diagnosis

4

Congenital Etiologies of Lacrimal System Obstructions

William R. Katowitz and James A. Katowitz

The etiologies of congenital nasolacrimal duct obstruction can be separated into those affecting the upper system (puncta, canaliculi, common canaliculus) and those involving the lower system (lacrimal sac and nasolacrimal duct). The causes can range from abnormal embryogenesis with failure of dehiscence of embryonic membranes to tumors or strictures that curtail the normal development of the nasolacrimal apparatus. It has long been held that the most common site of obstruction is at the opening of the nasolacrimal duct into the inferior meatus. This was supported by Sevel,[1] who showed that 60%–70% of the fetuses in his series did not have a patent opening between the nasolacrimal duct and the inferior meatus; rather, there was a mucosal and epithelial membrane responsible for this obstruction. Given that this membrane most often canalizes within a month after birth, thereby allowing normal tear outflow, one can appreciate the delicate balance between embryogenesis and anatomic dysfunction.

Development of the nasolacrimal system begins at approximately the 6-week stage of embryonic development. An epithelial layer of ectodermal tissue is entrapped as a core between the lateral (fronto-nasal) and maxillary process (Figure 4.1). Sevel describes developmental anomalies of the nasolacrimal system as either a failure in complete separation of this epithelial core from the surface ectoderm or noncomplete patency of the apparatus attributed to failure of canalization. This ectodermal core projects into the upper and lower lids as a bifurcation at the medial canthus to form the canaliculi and puncta. Incomplete formation, misdirection, accessory budding, and deformation from amniotic bands can contribute to a developmental obstruction of the nasolacrimal system. A third process described by Duke-Elder[2] is complete absence of the nasolacrimal passage caused by a nonunion or clefting of the nasal and maxillary processes during embryogenesis. This rare developmental anomaly has been seen in cyclopia, cryptophthalmos, or from amniotic band pressure necrosis.

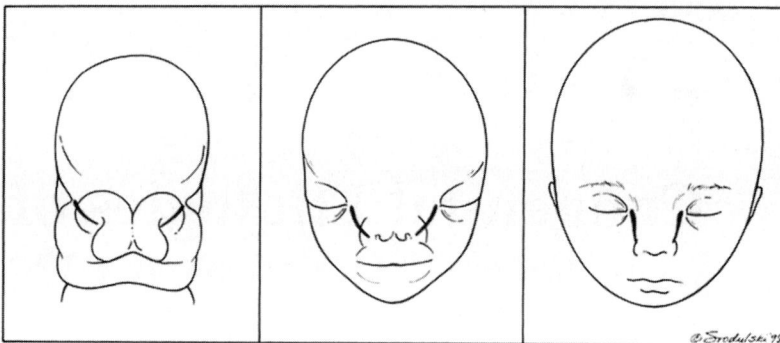

FIGURE 4.1. Development of the nasolacrimal system begins at approximately the 6-week stage of embryonic development. An epithelial layer of ectodermal tissue is entrapped as a core between the lateral (frontonasal) and maxillary process.

Congenital Obstructions of the Upper Nasolacrimal System

Abnormalities of the Puncta

Many anomalies of the puncta have been described. Atresia or agenesis of the lacrimal puncta is not uncommon. When this occurs, a veil or membrane consisting of conjunctiva and canalicular epithelium occludes the punctal orifice. This membrane may be present within the punctal orifice or may lie over the punctum as a veil and appear only as a small dimple in the lid margin.

Congenital absence of the punctum is less common but can be attributed to failure or incomplete outbudding of the nasolacrimal core (Figure 4.2). Duke-Elder[2] (1964) cited examples from the literature of an autonomic dominant pattern of inheritance for an absence of puncta. The EEC syndrome (ectrodactyly–ectodermal dysplasia–clefting syndrome) is also associated with absent puncta, as well as the Levy-Hollister syndrome (lacrimo-dento-digital syndrome).[3]

The presence of epiphora must be investigated to distinguish actual nasolacrimal duct obstructions from other nonobstructive functional abnormalities. Congenital lid malpositions such as congenital entropion or ectropion, telecanthus, hypertelorism, and lid colobomas can cause poor punctum to globe apposition and may explain symptoms of tearing in an infant. Abnormalities of the lashes can also cause tearing in the newborn. In addition, an inadequate lid pumping mechanism can be seen in congenital paresis of the orbicularis muscle caused by seventh nerve palsies. Such etiologies must

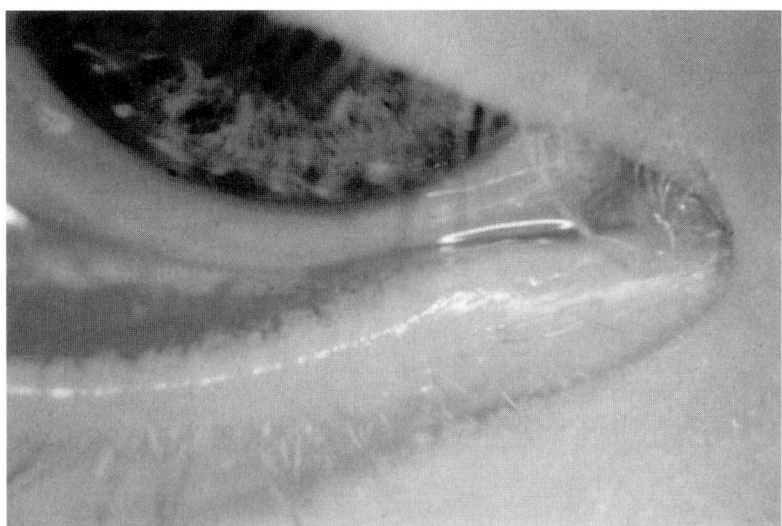

FIGURE 4.2. Congenital absence of the punctum is less common but can be attributed to failure or incomplete outbudding of the nasolacrimal core.

be distinguished from actual obstructions as a cause of tearing in the infant.

Abnormalities of the Canalicular System

Anomalies of the canaliculi may include developmental abnormalities such as canalicular atresia or absence of the canalicular system altogether. The latter is attributed to anomalous development of the epithelial core.[1] Canalicular atresia can be classified as proximal, mid-canalicular, or distal.

Supernumerary (Anlage) Ducts

Accessory channels may exist and communicate with the skin ending in the canalicular system, the lacrimal sac, or even the lacrimal duct. These lacrimal anlage ducts or lacrimal fistulae may result from additional extensions of the embryonic epithelial cord or as outpouchings from the developing canaliculi. The openings of these ducts may be on the skin below the punctum, at the lid margin, or at the medial aspect of the lower lid crease (Figure 4.3).

Dacryoliths

Stones are known to cause acquired nasolacrimal duct obstructions but have not been reported in congenital cases of nasolacrimal duct obstruction.

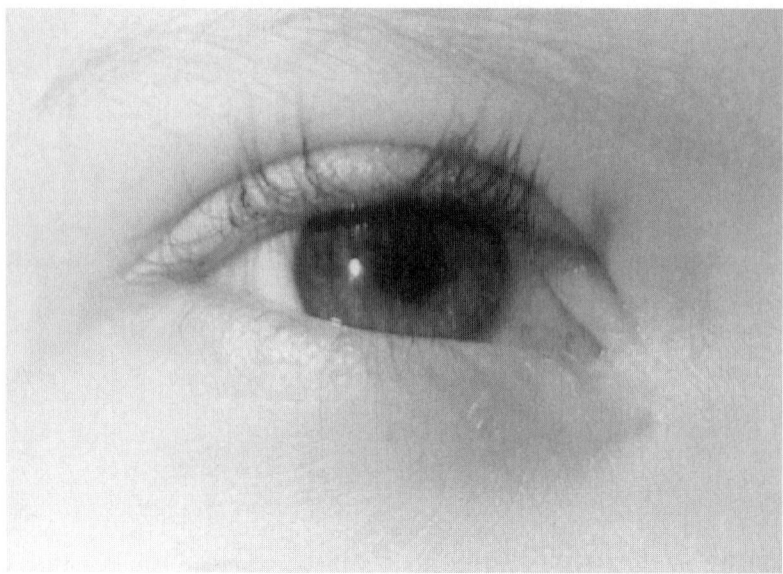

FIGURE 4.3. Accessory channels may exist and communicate with the skin ending in the canalicular system, the lacrimal sac, or even the lacrimal duct. The openings of these ducts may be on the skin below the punctum, at the lid margin, or at the medial aspect of the lower lid crease.

Congenital Obstructions of the Lower Nasolacrimal System

Sevel[1] has described two main causes of abnormal embryogenesis in the lacrimal sac and duct as attributed to incomplete or abnormal separation of the epithelial core or attributed to abnormal canalization.

Congenital Fistula of the Lacrimal Sac

Anlage ducts involving the upper system have already been discussed; however, abnormal canalization can lead to direct communications between the skin and lacrimal sac. Canalization begins at the fourth month of gestation and can be caused by a defect in the optic end of the naso-optic fissure.[4] An internal fistula between the lacrimal sac and nasal cavity may also occur, although this is not a cause of obstruction.

Congenital Dacryocystocele

When fluid is entrapped in a nonpatent nasolacrimal system, a neonate may present with a mass below the medial canthus representing cystic distention of the lacrimal sac (Figure 4.4). This entity may be attributable to entrapped mucous (mucocele) or amniotic fluid (amniotocele).

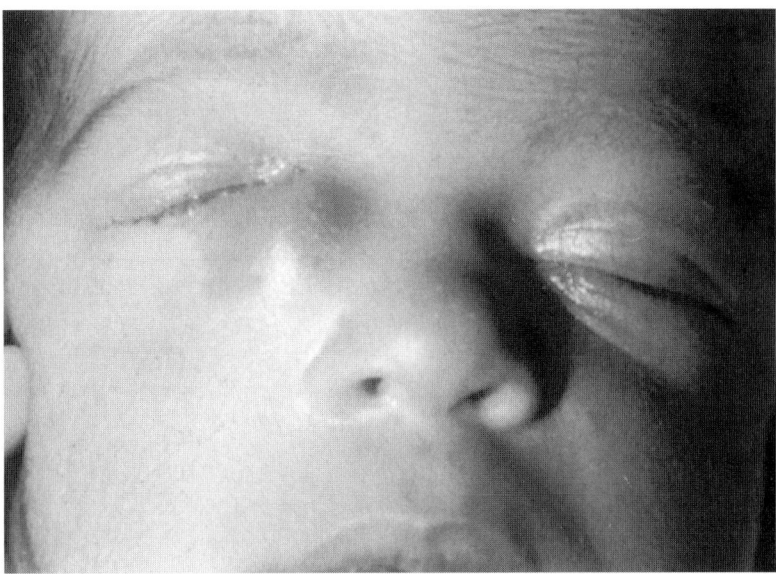

FIGURE 4.4. When fluid is entrapped in a nonpatent nasolacrimal system, a neonate may present with a mass below the medial canthus, representing cystic distention of the lacrimal sac. This entity may be caused by entrapped mucous (mucocele) or amniotic fluid (amniotocele).

One other rare cause for distention in the region of the lacrimal system is an encephalocele, although its usual location above the medial canthal tendon, as well as associated pulsations, helps to distinguish it from benign fluid collections. Other causes of a mass in the medial canthus can be a hemangioma or dermoid. Tumors of the lacrimal sac are rare in the pediatric age group. The presence of a bluish discoloration and confirmation with imaging studies, ultrasonography, or nasal endoscopy can aid in diagnosis. Dacryocystoceles can be large enough to extend into the nasal cavity and have been reported to cause respiratory distress.[5]

Congenital Dacryocystitis

Inflammation of the nonpatent nasolacrimal system can occur in the setting of a dacryocystocele or simply a nonpatent nasolacrimal duct. Neonates classically present with tearing followed by a muco-purulent discharge without the presence of an inflamed mass below the medial canthus. When bacteria actually infect the lacrimal sac and edema at the common opening prevents decompression of the sac contents, an acute dacryocystitis can occur (Figure 4.5). The most common causative organisms have been reported as gram-positive cocci Streptococcus pneumoniae, Staphylococcus, and gram-negative Enterobacteriaceae.[6]

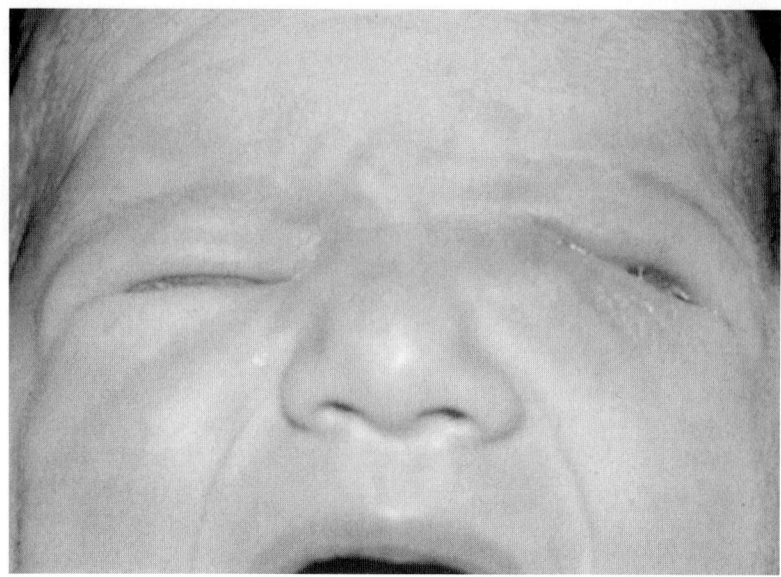

FIGURE 4.5. When bacteria actually infect the lacrimal sac, and edema at the common opening prevents decompression of the sac contents, an acute dacryocystitis can occur.

Dacryostenosis

The most common etiology of congenital nasolacrimal obstruction is a persistent membrane covering the nasolacrimal ostium at the valve of Hasner. Failure of dehiscence of this epithelial membrane creates a blockage or valve-like fold over what is normally the valve of Hasner. Using serial histologic sections, Cassady[7] in 1952 examined the nasolacrimal duct of 15 full-term stillborn infants and reported the presence of this membrane in 13 of the subjects (87%). Sevel[1] described this membrane histologically as attenuated nasal mucosa and stretched epithelium from the nasolacrimal duct lining. A membranous obstruction of the nasolacrimal duct represented 73% of the cases treated by Kushner[8] in his 1982 report. He described this clinically as lack of resistance during probing until entering the lower portion of the system, followed by reaching a point of obstruction that could be easily perforated when advancing the probe.

Although the majority of obstructions at the lower end of the nasolacrimal duct occur at the valve of Hasner, the location of the distal end of the duct can vary.[9] This can be appreciated clinically if one encounters an unusual pathway that does not respond to simple perforation when probing the distal end of the duct. In this instance, nasal endoscopic examination may be of value. If one cannot safely pass a probe at the time of examination, however, then consideration should be given to further diagnostic imaging such as dacryocystography or magnetic resonance imaging with contrast injection. More definitive surgical intervention such as a dacryocystorhinostomy may be required based on information obtained from these studies.

Facial Clefts

Congenital facial clefts can disrupt the nasolacrimal system in the newborn. These can involve the soft tissue of the face and extend into the bony structures. Tessier devised a clock-face system to describe the craniofacial clefting syndromes. According to the Tessier classification system, clefts 2, 3, and 4, located in the lower medial canthal and nasolacrimal region, are associated with congenital nasolacrimal abnormalities. The cause of these clefts can be attributed to external or internal forces. Amniotic bands formed in utero from amniotic sac rupture can wrap across the developing fetus, thus causing strictures and pressure necrosis. If these bands are swallowed in utero by the developing fetus they may specifically constrict across the face. There are many reports in the literature of various internal influences on clefting syndromes, from genetic causes to exposures to intrauterine infectious or pharmacologic agents (Figure 4.6).[10–12]

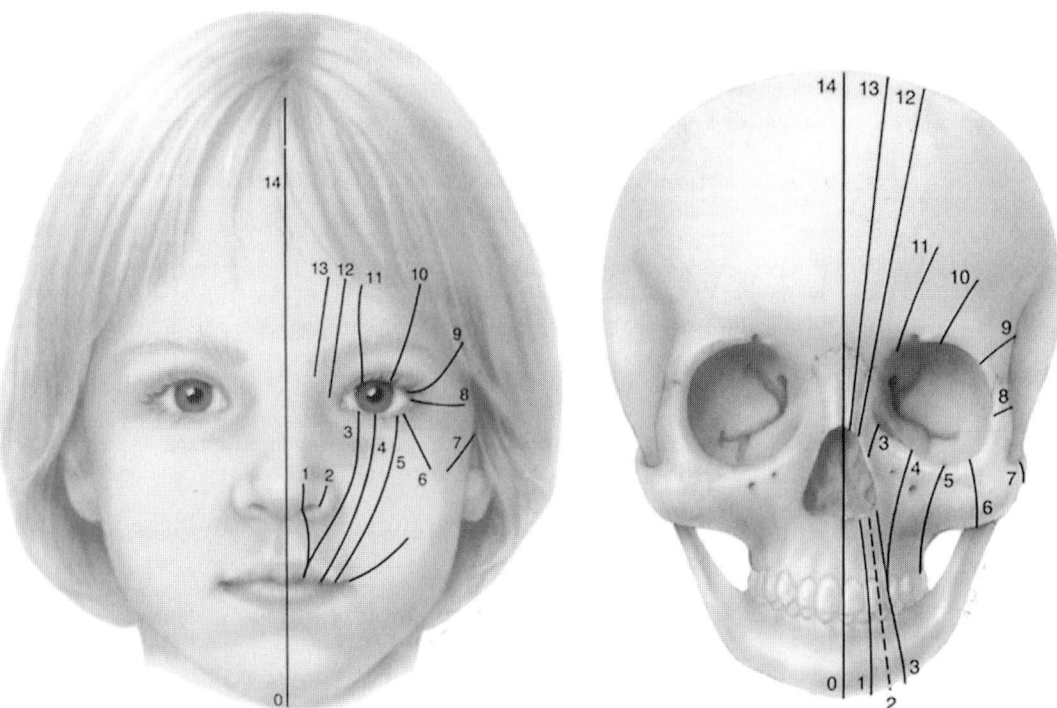

FIGURE 4.6. Congenital facial clefts can disrupt the nasolacrimal system in the newborn. These can involve the soft tissue of the face and extend into the bony structures. Tessier devised a clock-face system to describe the craniofacial clefting syndromes.

Conclusion

The etiologies of nasolacrimal outflow obstruction are multifactorial. They can be the result of external forces causing clefts in the outflow pathway or of pressure causing occlusion of the system, as seen with nasal cysts or masses. Genetic factors may have a role in the embryogenesis of syndromic entities that are associated with epiphora. Obstruction to outflow must be distinguished from other causes of tearing such as lid malpositions, abnormal or misdirected lashes, or a poor lacrimal pump mechanism. An understanding of the various etiologies can help in better appreciating the anatomic sites of dysfunction and in the selection of the most appropriate medical and surgical solutions.

References

1. Sevel D. Developmental and congenital abnormalities of the nasolacrimal apparatus. J Pediatr Ophthalmol Strab 1981;18(5):13–19.
2. Duke-Elder S. Congenital deformities. Part 2. In: Duke-Elder S, ed. System of Ophthalmology. Vol 3. St. Louis: CV Mosby; 1964:923–940.
3. Low JE, Johnson MA, Katowitz JA. Management of pediatric upper system problems: punctal and canalicular surgery. In: Katowitz JA, ed. Pediatric Oculoplastic Surgery. New York: Springer-Verlag; 2002:337–346.
4. Hurwitz JJ. Embryology of the lacrimal drainage system. In: Hurwitz JJ, ed. The Lacrimal System. Philadelphia: Lippincott-Raven; 1996:9–13.
5. Grin TR, Mertz JS, Stass-Isern M. Congenital nasolacrimal duct cysts in dacryocystocele. Ophthalmology 1991;98(8):1238–1242.
6. Huber-Spitzy V, Steinkogler FJ, Haselberger C. The pathogen spectrum in neonatal dacryocystitis. Klin Monatsbl Augenheilkd 1987;190(5):445–446.
7. Cassady JV. Developmental anatomy of nasolacrimal duct. Arch Ophthalmol 1952;47:141–158.
8. Kushner BJ. Congenital nasolacrimal system obstruction. Arch Ophthalmol 1982;100:597–600.
9. Jones JT, Wobig JL. Congenital anomalies of the lacrimal system. Surgery of the eyelids and lacrimal system. Birmingham: Aesculapius; 1976: 157–163.
10. Fries PD, Katowitz JA. Congenital craniofacial anomalies of ophthalmic importance. Surv Ophthalmol 1990;35(2):87–117.
11. Piest KL. Embryology and anatomy of the developing face. In: Katowitz JA, ed. Pediatric Oculoplastic Surgery. New York: Springer-Verlag; 2002:11–29.
12. Jockin YJ, Katowitz JA, Fries PD, Hertle RW. Congenital craniofacial deformities: ophthalmic considerations. In: Katowitz JA, ed. Pediatric Oculoplastic Surgery. New York: Springer-Verlag; 2002:533–558.

5

Acquired Etiologies of Lacrimal System Obstructions

Daniel P. Schaefer

Acquired obstructions of the lacrimal excretory outflow system will produce the symptoms of epiphora, mucopurulent discharge, pain, dacryocystitis, and even cellulitis, prompting the patient to seek the ophthalmologist for evaluation and treatment. Impaired tear outflow may be functional, structural, or both. The causes may be primary – those resulting from inflammation of unknown causes that lead to occlusive fibrosis—or secondary, resulting from infections, inflammation, trauma, malignancies, toxicity, or mechanical causes. Secondary acquired dacryostenosis and obstruction may result from many causes, both common and obscure. Occasionally, the precise pathogenesis of nasolacrimal duct obstruction will, despite years of investigations, be elusive.

To properly evaluate and appropriately treat the patient, the ophthalmologist must have knowledge and comprehension of the lacrimal anatomy, the lacrimal apparatus, pathophysiology, ocular and nasal relationships, ophthalmic and systemic disease process, as well as the topical and systemic medications that can affect the nasolacrimal duct system. One must be able to assess if the cause is secondary to outflow anomalies, hypersecretion or reflex secretion, pseudoepiphora, eyelid malposition abnormalities, trichiasis, foreign bodies and conjunctival concretions, keratitis, tear film deficiencies or instability, dry eye syndromes, ocular surface abnormalities, irritation or tumors affecting the trigeminal nerve, allergy, medications, or environmental factors. Abnormalities of the lacrimal pump function can result from involutional changes, eyelid laxity, facial nerve paralysis, or floppy eyelid syndrome, all of which displace the punctum from the lacrimal lake. If the cause is secondary to obstruction of the nasolacrimal duct system, the ophthalmologist must be able to determine where the anomaly is and what the cause is, in order to provide the best treatment possible for the patient.

Tearing is a common complaint, and a complete workup is multifaceted and requires a detailed history as well as a comprehensive ophthalmic examination with special emphasis on the anterior segment, lacrimal system, and nasal cavity. The cause of tearing can be secondary to hypersecretion, lacrimation, or impairment of drainage. The patient should be questioned regarding the following: unilateral versus bilateral vision; subjective symptoms of foreign body sensation, burning; constant versus intermittent problems; allergies; prior use of medications; prior probing; sinus disease and/or surgeries; prior trauma, midfacial trauma, nasal fractures; radiation treatment to the periocular or paranasal sinus area; ocular diseases; ocular or periocular surgeries; prior episodes of lacrimal sac inflammation or infection; discharge; clear, or bloody tears.

Inspection of the eyelids and lashes may reveal signs of blepharitis, concretion, cyst, molluscum contagiosum, chalazion, ectropion, entropion, trichiasis, lid laxity, lagophthalmos, poor blinking mechanism which may be secondary to seventh cranial nerve paralysis, poor lacrimal pump function, and overriding of the upper and lower lids. A notch on the lid margin secondary to trauma or surgery may allow tears to flow out of the tear pool onto the face. The punctum should be evaluated for size, stenosis or occlusion, its position, movement, and for possible obstruction by the conjunctiva, the plica semilunaris, an enlarged caruncle, conjunctivochalasis, or hyperplasia. A badly slit punctum or canaliculus may also be a source of chronic epiphora. Palpation with pressure over the lacrimal sac may produce a reflux of mucoid or mucopurulent material through the canalicular system and punctum if the common canaliculus and valve of Rosenmüller are patent.

Examination of the nose should be performed to rule out the possibility of intranasal tumors, allergic rhinitis, polyposis, or turbinate impaction or other possible obstructions of the distal end of the nasolacrimal duct.

Symptoms of epiphora can reflect excess tearing, or hypersecretion of tears, caused by the reflex arcs initiated by such processes as keratoconjunctivitis sicca, keratitis, allergies, or uveitis. In some patients, the clinical examination is unremarkable and the cause of epiphora remains unclear, a functional block.

Unilateral tearing is suggestive of a lacrimal outflow problem because of either obstruction or poor function of the tear pump caused by weakness of the orbicularis muscle, seventh cranial nerve palsy, or lower lid laxity. Also to be considered in unilateral tearing is the possibility of intracranial processes, such as an acoustic neuroma, which can compress the lacrimal innervation pathway in the brain and result in decreased tear production and unilateral dry eye symptoms and signs, including epiphora. Lymphoma, adenoid cystic carcinoma, or other tumors of the lacrimal gland can infiltrate the gland and/or its innervation, causing decreased tear production on one side, with epiphora. However, bilateral outflow abnormalities can occur and result in bilateral tearing.

Symptomatic tearing can result when a normal lacrimal drainage system is overwhelmed by hypersecretion, or when a drainage system is anatomically comprised and unable to handle normal tear production. Epiphora is determined by a balance between tear production and tear drainage and not by the absolute function or dysfunction of either.

Nasolacrimal duct occlusion is more common in the middle-aged woman, is often of unknown etiology, and may present with or without dacryocystitis. This higher prevalence of primary acquired nasolacrimal duct obstruction in women may be secondary to their narrower nasolacrimal ducts, and, or the possible hormonal effects on its mucosa leading to obstruction. There is an increased incidence of dacryocystitis in females (71.3%).[1]

Cicatricial nasolacrimal duct drainage obstruction has been reported to result from various medical therapies, both topical and systemic medications, radiation, systemic chemotherapy, and bone marrow transplantation.

Patients with Down's syndrome have been noted to develop a dacryostenosis, more frequently caused by anatomic abnormalities, canalicular stenosis, and atresia. Punctal atresia and canalicular obstruction are also more common in patients with midface abnormalities.

Bartley modified the Linberg and McCormick etiologic classification system for "primary acquired nasolacrimal duct obstruction" (PANDO), and published an expanded classification for "secondary acquired lacrimal drainage obstruction" (SALDO). The etiologies causes of SALDO were divided into five categories: infectious, inflammatory, neoplastic, traumatic, and mechanical[2] (Table 5.1).

Location of Stenosis or Occlusion

Punctum and/or Vertical Canaliculi

Acquired stenosis or occlusion of the punctum and canaliculi may be caused by a variety of conditions, including inflammatory conditions, infections, trachoma, cicatrizing diseases of the conjunctiva, that are secondary to the toxic effect of topical or systemic medications, especially systemic chemotherapeutic medications, masses in the area of the punctum, surgery, burns, trauma, long-standing ectropion or lid malposition, aging changes, blepharitis, trauma, tumors, or iatrogenic response.

Punctal stenosis is more common in postmenopausal women, probably secondary to hormonal changes. Chronic blepharitis causes inflammatory and cicatricial changes resulting in inflammatory membrane formation, conjunctival epithelial overgrowth, and keratinization of the walls of the punctum. Membranous stenosis at the internal punctum is the most common location for canalicular stenosis. Involutional changes of these tissues, atrophy, and dense fibrous stricture of the punctum cause it to be less resilient and the orbicularis muscle fibers to become atonic and stenotic.

Conjunctivochalasis, excess conjunctiva that occludes the inferior punctum, is often overlooked. In mild cases, it may cause tearing because of tear film instability; in moderate cases, it may cause

TABLE 5.1. Causes of secondary acquired nasolacrimal duct obstruction.

Neoplastic
  Primary
  Secondary
  Metastatic
1. Primary neoplasms
   a. Adenocarcinoma
   b. Adenoid cystic carcinoma
   c. Angiofibroma
   d. Angiosarcoma
   e. Cavernous hemangioma
   f. Cyst
   g. Dermoid cyst
   h. Fibroma
   i. Fibrous histiocytoma
   j. Glomus tumor
   k. Granular cell tumors
   l. Hemangioendothelioma
   m. Hemangiopericytoma
   n. Leukemia
   o. Lymphoma
   p. Lymphoplasmacytic infiltrate
   q. Melanoma
   r. Mucoepidermoid carcinoma
   s. Neurilemoma
   t. Neurofibroma
   u. Oncocytic adenocarcinoma
   v. Oncocytic adenoma
   w. Oncocytoma
   x. Papilloma and inverted papillomas
   y. Plasmacytoma
   z. Pleomorphic adenoma
   aa. Pyogenic granuloma
   bb. Squamous cell carcinoma
   cc. Transitional cell carcinoma
2. Secondary involvement by neoplasm
   a. Adenoid cystic carcinoma
   b. Amyloid
   c. Basal cell carcinoma
   d. Capillary hemangioma
   e. Esthesioneuroblastoma
   f. Fibrosarcoma
   g. Fibrous dysplasia
   h. Intraosseous cavernous hemangioma
   i. Leukemia
   j. Lymphoma
   k. Maxillary and ethmoid sinus tumors
   l. Midline granuloma
   m. Mucoepidermoid carcinoma
   n. Mycosis fungoides
   o. Neurofibroma
   p. Osteoma
   q. Papilloma
       i. Conjunctival
       ii. Inverted (schneiderian)
   r. Rhabdomyosarcoma
   s. Sebaceous gland carcinoma
   t. Squamous cell carcinoma
3. Metastatic
   a. Breast carcinoma
   b. Melanoma
   c. Prostate carcinoma

TABLE 5.1. *Continued*

Inflammations
1. Endogenous
    a. Wegener's granulomatosis and other forms of vasculitis
    b. Sarcoidosis and sarcoid granuloma
    c. Cicatricial pemphigoid
    d. Stevens-Johnson syndrome (erythema multiforme)
    e. Sinus histiocytosis
    f. Orbital inflammatory syndrome (pseudotumor)
    g. Kawasaki's disease (mucocutaneous lymph node syndrome)
    h. Porphyria cutanea tarda
    i. Epidermodysplasia verruciformis, ichthyosis, scleroderma
    j. Idiopathic punctal stenosis
    k. Benign squamous metaplasia
    l. Sjögren's syndrome
    m. Lichen planus
2. Exogenous
    a. Eyedrops
        i. Antiviral agents
            1. Idoxuridine
            2. Vidarabine
            3. Trifluridine
            4. Acyclovir

        ii. Antiglaucoma medications
            1. Demecarium
            2. Echothiophate
            3. Isoflurophate
            4. Furmethide
            5. Neostigmine
            6. Physostigmine
            7. Epinephrine
        iii. Silver nitrate, silver protein, colloidal silver
        iv. Thiotepa
    b. Radiation therapy
    c. Fluorouracil (systemic)
    d. Graft-versus-host disease
    e. Pyogenic granuloma
    f. Foreign body granuloma
    g. Allergy
        i. Ocular
        ii. Nasal
    h. Burns
        i. Thermal
        ii. Chemical
    i. Chronic sinus disease
Infections
1. Bacterial
    a. *Actinomyces* sp.
        (1) *A. israelii*
        (2) *A. meyeri*
    b. *Propionibacterium propionicum* (*Arachnia propionica*)
    c. *Fusobacterium* sp.
    d. *Bacteroides* sp.
    e. *Mycobacterium* sp.
        (1) *M. fortuitum*
        (2) *M. leprae*
        (3) *M. tuberculosis*
    f. *Chlamydia trachomatis*
    g. *Nocardia asteroides*
    h. *Enterobacter cloacae*
    i. *Aeromonas hydrophila*
    j. *Treponema pallidum*

TABLE 5.1. *Continued*

k. *Staphylococcus aureus*
l. *Staphylococcus epidermidis*
m. *Pseudomonas aeruginosa*
n. *Proteus mirabilis*
o. *Haemophilus influenzae*
p. *Peptostreptococcus*
q. *Streptococcus viridans*
r. Gamma streptococcus
s. Diphtheroids
t. *Klebsiella*
u. *Moraxella*
v. Mononucleosis
w. *S. pneumoniae*
x. *Escherichia coli*
y. *N. gonorrhea*
z. *N. catarrhalis*
aa. Trachoma
bb. Leprosy
cc. Tuberculosis

2. Viral
   a. Herpes simplex virus
   b. Herpes zoster virus
       i. Varicella
   c. Smallpox
   d. Adenovirus
   e. Vaccinia virus
   f. Epstein-Barr virus
   g. Human papillomavirus

3. Fungal
   a. *Aspergillus* sp.
       i. *A. fumigatus*
       ii. *A. niger*
   b. *Candida* sp.
       i. *C. albicans*
       ii. *C. parapsilosis*
   c. *Pityrosporum* sp.
       a. *P. orbiculare*
       b. *P. pachydermatis*

   d. *Rhinosporidium seeberi*
   e. *Sporothrix schenckii*
   f. *Streptomyces somaliensis*
   g. *Trichophyton rubrum*
   h. Cephalosporiosis
   i. Blastomycosis
   j. Cryptococcosis

4. Parasitic
   a. *Ascaris lumbricoides*
   b. *Distoma felineum*
   c. Myiasis

Traumatic
   1. Iatrogenic
      a. Punctal occlusion for dry eyes
      b. After nasolacrimal duct probing with or without silicone intubation
      c. After canalicular repair with pigtail probe
      d. After dacryocystorhinostomy
      e. After conjunctivodacryocystorhinostomy
      f. After transantral orbital decompression
      g. After sinus surgery (conventional or endoscopic)
      h. After rhinoplasty, rhinotomy, or other nasal surgery
      i. After craniofacial surgery

TABLE 5.1. *Continued*

2. Noniatrogenic
   a. Laceration of canaliculus
   b. Laceration of lacrimal sac
   c. Fractures involving nasolacrimal duct nasoethmoid fractures, midfacial trauma

Mechanical
1. Internal
   a. Dacryolith
      i. Idiopathic
      ii. Eyelash nidus
      iii. Epinephrine cast
      iv. Quinacrine deposits
   b. Migrated or retained medical device
      1. Punctal plug
      2. Veirs rod
      3. Fragment of nasolacrimal probe
      4. Modified myringotomy tube
      5. Remnants of silicone tubing
   c. Pellet (BB)
   d. Canalicular cysts
   e. Blood
2. External
   a. Kissing puncta
   b. Conjunctivochalasis; enlargement of the plica, semilunaris, and/or caruncle
   c. Mucocele
   d. Migrated or malpositioned orbital floor or medial wall implants after repair of orbital floor or medial wall fractures
   e. Paget's disease
   f. Osteopetrosis
   g. Rhinolith or other nasal foreign bodies
   h. Suture stent after esophagocolostomy
   i. Exudative rhinitis
   j. Acute intranasal inflammation
   k. Nasal mucosal edema
   l. Lymphoid hyperplasia of the nasal cavity
   m. Nasal malformations
   n. Nasal polyps or polyposis
   o. Systemic syndromes or dysmorphism that involve abnormalities of facial development (clefting or malposition of the orbits or midface)
   p. Intranasal tumors
   q. Impacted turbinate
   r. Intranasal tumors

Source: Modified from Linberg JV, McCormick SA. Primary acquired nasolacrimal duct obstruction: a clinicopathologic report and biopsy technique. Ophthalmology 1986; 93:1055–1062; and Bartley.[2,9]

obstruction of the puncta, and in severe cases, it may cause foreign body sensation and irritation that result from ocular surface exposure.

Obstruction may occur within either the upper or lower canaliculus or in the common canaliculus. Causes of acquired canalicular obstruction include trauma and toxicity from medications (5-fluorouracil, idoxuridine, phospholine iodide, eserine, etc.).

Canalicular obstructions may be caused by chlamydial infections (trachoma), viruses (herpes zoster, herpes simplex, chickenpox, and smallpox), bacteria, or cicatrizing diseases (Stevens-Johnson syndrome or pemphigoid).

Canalicular cyst presents as a bluish lump or a cyst-like swelling. These cysts may arise after an episode of canaliculitis with an ecstatic canalicular diverticulum, an encysted abscess, or chronic canaliculitis.

Lacrimal Pump

The lacrimal pump is the mechanism that assists the tears in their travels from the tear pool through the nasolacrimal duct system into the interior meatus of the nose. The action of the pretarsal and preseptal orbicularis oculi produces the forces that drive the lacrimal pump.

Patients with tearing whose nasolacrimal duct systems are patent to syringing may have an incomplete anatomic obstruction or nonfunctional segments of the lacrimal passage from prior episodes of dacryocystitis, or an anatomically normal nasolacrimal duct system, but a physiologic dysfunction of the eyelids, punctum, lacrimal pump, or a lacrimal sac that drains poorly.

Lacrimal Sac and Duct

The mucosal lining of the nasolacrimal sac and duct excretes a range of mucin materials, which may aid in the flow of tears and provide a defense against microbes. Researchers have identified mRNA for a variety of mucins in human lacrimal sacs and ducts.[3]

Inflammation, trauma, or congenital defect in the drainage system may cause epiphora, dacryostenosis, and dacryocystitis. Inflammation originating at the eye, conjunctival sac, diverticula of the lacrimal system, or from the nose, infections or diseases of the nasal mucous membrane or sinuses can induce swelling of the lacrimal system's mucous membranes, resulting in narrowing or occlusion of the nasolacrimal system from the epithelial changes and fibrosis of the lamina propria.[4] The various mechanisms that cause inflammation result in a secondary fibrosis that causes a narrowing of the nasolacrimal duct system, and eventually, occlusion by scar tissue. The lacrimal sac and duct undergo similar changes, as the pseudostratified, ciliated, columnar epithelium undergoes squamous metaplasia and hyperplasia with loss of goblet cells, and ulceration. The underlying mucosa develops a secondary fibrosis. Basement membrane thickening may develop in the nasal mucosa but not in the lacrimal sac. The inflammation may cause a fibrosis of the lacrimal sac and the internal common punctum, which may result in obstruction and, in postoperative cases, to failure of dacryocystorhinostomies.[5]

Several valves are present in the nasolacrimal duct system to prevent the retrograde flow of tears. The most important valve clinically is the valve of Hasner, located at the entrance of the nasolacrimal duct into the inferior meatus, and frequently responsible for congenital nasolacrimal duct obstruction. The valve of Rosenmüller is found at the junction of the common canaliculus into the lacrimal sac. This valve prevents retrograde flow of fluid from the sac into the canaliculi and fornix. In episodes of dacryocystitis, this valve may swell closed even more tightly. Tears and the infection cannot drain out of the sac into the nose, or to the fornix. The valve of Rosenmüller is not a true valve, but an angulated entrance of the common canaliculus into the sac, functioning as a valve.

Descending inflammation from the eye or ascending inflammation from the nasal cavity may initiate swelling of the mucous membranes of the nasolacrimal duct system, remodeling of the helical arrangement of connective tissue fibers, malfunctions in the subepithelial cavernous body with reactive hyperemia, and temporary occlusion of the nasolacrimal duct system. The submucosa is very vascular, cavernous in structure, and rich in lymphatics, so that a slight infection, once established, will settle. The constriction of the tissue within the bony canal makes it obligatory that any swelling will lead to blockage. The submucosa of the nasolacrimal duct system surrounded by bone contains arterioles with sphincters and cavernous vessel complexes, which can cause swelling and approximation of the lumen according to the blood flow. Repeated episodes of dacryocystitis will result in permanent changes of the epithelial and subepithelial tissues; loss of goblet and epithelial cells, which are important in the tear outflow mechanism; fibrosis of the helical system of connective tissue fibers; and reduction and destruction of the vascular plexus, leading to a malfunction of the tear flow mechanism – all of which result in a vicious circle.[6] These structural epithelial and subepithelial changes may lead either to a total fibrous closure of the lumen of the nasolacrimal duct system or to a nonfunctional segment that may cause chronic epiphora and discharge, but be patent to irrigation.

Dacryocystitis has various causes, but the common end result is complete obstruction of the nasolacrimal duct, resulting in stasis of tear flow, leading to secondary infections, which may progress to mucocele, pyocele-mucocele, chronic conjunctivitis, preseptal and orbital cellulitis, and abscess formation if left untreated, or if inadequately treated. Gram-positive bacteria are the most common cause, but gram-negative organisms should be suspected in patients with diabetes or who are immunocompromised.

The lacrimal sac can be involved by inflammation, the most common being nongranulomatous inflammation, granulomatous inflammation, granulation tissue, lymphocytic infiltrate, inflammation and ulcerations, and sarcoidosis. The epithelial lesions that involve the lacrimal sac are inverted papilloma, papilloma, transitional cell carcinoma, oncocytoma, granular cell tumor, carcinoma, and adenocarcinoma. The nonepithelial lesions are lymphoma, lymphoplasmacytic infiltrate, plasmacytoma, and chronic lymphocytic leukemic. Infections that involve the lacrimal sac can be secondary to fungus, *Actinomyces*, and bacteria. The lacrimal sac can also be affected by dacryoliths, scarring, foreign bodies, pyogenic granulomas, amyloid, orbital and midfacial fractures, blood, trauma, and papillary hyperplasia.

Lacrimal diverticula, outpouchings of the canaliculi or the lacrimal sac, are rare but may cause intermittent or permanent swelling near the lacrimal sac. Most arise from the lateral sac wall, because this area is only covered by the periorbita, offering little resistance to distention of the sac. They may be congenital, inflammatory, result from prior dacryocystitis, or be traumatic in origin. This communication may be open or act as a one-way valve, becoming symptomatic, and may cause epiphora, swelling, and/or dacryocystitis-like symptoms. Dacryoliths may form inside the diverticulum.

Obstruction of the intraosseous segment of the nasolacrimal duct may be secondary to trauma, chronic sinus disease, granulomatous disease (Wegener's granulomatosis, sarcoidosis, and lethal midline granuloma), dacryocystitis, or involutional stenosis. Involutional stenosis is probably the most common cause, seen more frequently in older women.

Obstruction of the Nasal Portion of the Nasolacrimal Duct

Mechanical obstruction is frequently found with enlargement or flattening of the inferior turbinate, which may almost obliterate the anterior part of the meatus and may cause a local rhinitis. A deviated septum may compress the inferior turbinate against the lateral nasal wall.

Inflammatory conditions, chronic nasal catarrh, acute and suppurative infections, may spread into the inferior portion of the nasolacrimal duct, resulting in obstruction. Atrophic and destructive conditions of the nasal mucosa may create a patulous ostium permitting extension of the disease process upward and allowing the direct entrance of infective secretion into the duct on blowing the nose.

Congestive and hypertrophic conditions of the mucosa, vasomotor or inflammatory, may cause obstruction at or in the inferior portion of the nasolacrimal duct, as well as a nasal polyp or neoplasm. Dacryocystitis has also been reported after packing of the nose.

Intranasal pathology may affect the nasolacrimal duct. Intranasal scarring with inferior turbinate adhesions that occur from trauma, radiation therapy, surgical procedures, or nasal mucosal hypertrophy from allergic rhinitis may cause obstruction of the duct.

Etiologic Causes

Infectious

The infectious causes of PANDO may be secondary to bacteria, viruses, fungi, and parasites. Generalized infections are occasionally responsible for the onset of dacryocystitis, as seen with the occurrence of inflammation during the course of influenza, scarlet fever, diphtheria, chickenpox, smallpox, and tuberculosis.

The occurrence of acute dacryocystitis is dependent on the entry of a virulent strain of an organism into the stagnant contents of a lacrimal sac where the nasolacrimal duct is obstructed. Chronic dacryocystitis may be primary or secondary to an anatomic abnormality that has led to tear flow stasis. Obstructed lacrimal duct systems are colonized by increased numbers of pathogenic microorganisms. Some cases of PANDO may be secondary to unrecognized low-grade dacryocystitis. The organisms in the lacrimal sac may contribute to inflammation and scarring and therefore to the obstruction and then dacryocystitis. The microbiology of acute dacryocystitis has been reported to be frequently secondary to species of staphylococcus, streptococcus, pneumococcus, and *Staphylococcus pyogenes*, with mixed infections being common. The most frequently cultured organisms were *S. epidermidis* and *S. aureus*. The common gram-negative rods include *Pseudomonas aeruginosa*, *Proteus mirabilis*, *Enterobacter cloacae*, and *Haemophilus influenzae*. Frequently, in these studies, cultures were interpreted from the cul-de-sac or from cases of chronic dacryocystitis and therefore may not have accurately identified the causative organism. Studies have shown that there is not a significant correlation between organisms cultured from the lacrimal sac to those obtained from the conjunctiva and/or nose; therefore, the preoperative conjunctival and/or nose cultures do not accurately predict the causative organism of the dacryocystitis.[7]

The viruses of primary herpes simplex, herpes zoster, chickenpox, smallpox, vaccinia, epidemic keratoconjunctivitis, and Epstein-Barr viruses may cause inflammatory and cicatricial changes of the canaliculi, resulting in varying degrees of obstruction or occlusion. These infections can extend beyond the stratified squamous epithelium to involve the elastic tissue of the substantia propria rather than the canalicular epithelium alone, or because of the adherence of the raw surfaces caused by inflammation of the mucous membranes, resulting in stenosis. Bacterial infections do not frequently affect the elastic layer. During the first few weeks of these viral infections, the mucosal epithelium is edematous, causing a stenosis that will still be able to be probed. The cicatrization that occurs over the next several weeks to months generally causes an obstruction that involves the mid-zone or distal portions of the superior and inferior canaliculi, but occasionally may cause punctal occlusion. Early recognition, probing, and intubation when indicated can prevent permanent canalicular obstruction and the need for a conjunctivodacryocystorhinostomy.

Infectious mononucleosis, mumps, Nicolas-Favre lymphogranulomatosis, trachoma, Stevens-Johnson syndrome, and pemphigus may cause dacryostenosis.

Dacryocystitis has been reported to result from infections with several species of mycobacteria: *Mycobacterium fortuitum*, *M. leprae*, and *M. tuberculosis*.

Chlamydia trachomatis has been reported to cause punctal occlusion, canalicular scarring, and nasolacrimal duct obstruction.

Other bacteria associated with lacrimal drainage obstruction include *Nocardia asteroides*, *E. cloacae*, *Aeromonas hydrophila*, *Treponema pallidum*, and *S. aureus*.

Fungi generally occlude the lacrimal drainage system by the formation of stone or cast. *Aspergillus fumigatus*, *A. niger*, *Candida albicans*, *C. parapsilosis*, *Pityrosporum orbiculare*, *P. pachydermatis*, *S. somaliensis*, *Actinomyces*, and *Trichophyton rubrum* may cause lacrimal stones or casts.

Parasitic obstruction is unusual, but has been reported with the nematode *Ascaris lumbricoides*. The worm gains entrance to the nasolacrimal system through the valve of Hasner and then emerges from the punctum.

Verruca vulgaris and viruses may cause a bloody epiphora when they involve the punctum or canaliculus.

Nocardia, sporotrichosis, rhinosporidiosis, cephalosporiosis, *Pseudomonas*, *Candida*, *Aspergillus*, which is commonly associated with other bacteria, *H. influenzae*, *Treponema vincentii*, *Rhinosporidium seeberi*, *Sporothrix* fungus, as well as *Treponema*, and tuberculosis, have been reported to cause dacryocystitis.

Actinomyces, previously named *Streptothrix israelii*, an obligate parasite whose only host is humans, causes a canalicular obstruction and inflammation. *Actinomyces israelii* is a gram-positive aerotolerant rod with true branching, which causes inflammation rather than a blockage of the lacrimal duct. Most cases of canaliculitis are unilateral. *Actinomyces* organisms are sensitive to penicillin, but topical antibiotic therapy is usually ineffective without mechanical expression or surgical removal of the canalicular stones.

Dacryoliths are typically yellow or white, "sulfur granules" and are frequently secondary to *Actinomyces* organisms, but may occasionally be seen in infections secondary to *Nocardia*, *Streptomyces*, and *Staphylococcus*. Shed epithelial cells, amorphous debris, and lipids with or without calcium can form casts within the lacrimal sac, which can lead to obstruction. In addition to the above, casts have been reported to form from the oxidation products of long-term topical epinephrine use.

Canaliculitis

Canaliculitis may be caused by a variety of bacterial, viral, chlamydial, or mycotic organisms. *A. israelii* is a filamentous gram-positive rod that is reported as one of the most common causes. *Propionibacterium propionicum* – formerly *Arachnia propionica* – is gram-positive and has a branching, rod-shaped morphology. It is facultatively anaerobic; carbon dioxide is not necessary for growth, unlike with *Actinomyces*. *Fusobacterium*, *A. israelii*, and *Bacteroides* have also been cultured from cases of canaliculitis.

A. Meyeri is principally found in the periodontal sulcus, is an uncommon pathogen, is nonfilamentous, branching, may be difficult to demonstrate, and can cause canaliculitis.

Fungi generally occlude the lacrimal drainage system by the formation of stone or cast, which can be seen with *A. fumigatus*, *A. niger*,

C. albicans, C. parapsilosis, P. orbiculare, P. pachydermatis, S. somaliensis, Actinomyces, and *T. rubrum.*

Inflammatory

Inflammation caused by numerous diseases may cause narrowing or obstruction of the nasolacrimal system.

Endogenous Origin

Granulomatous diseases can occasionally produce a mass within the lacrimal sac, as seen with extraorbital manifestations of idiopathic orbital inflammatory syndrome (idiopathic inflammatory pseudotumor) and sarcoidosis. In patients with sarcoidosis, and the other inflammatory diseases, initially successful dacryocystorhinostomy has an increased incidence of late failure caused by the progression of the inflammation in the nasal and lacrimal sac mucosa.

Wegener's granulomatosis, a vasculitis that classically involves the triad of the upper respiratory tract, the lungs, and the kidneys, may cause obstruction of the nasolacrimal system. Nasolacrimal obstruction is typically associated with advanced nasal disease, late in the disease process. This obstruction is frequently secondary to contiguous nasal disease, but may also be secondary to a vasculitis of the lacrimal sac mucosa. Treatment of the nasolacrimal obstruction should be deferred until the inflammation is quiescent, if possible. Other forms of vasculitis may cause similar obstructions of the nasolacrimal duct system.

Cicatricial pemphigoid and Stevens-Johnson syndrome may cause nasolacrimal obstruction with advanced disease.

Sinus histiocytosis, a benign disease of unknown etiology, which may be related to an allergy or an immunologic abnormality of histiocytes, Kawasaki's disease (mucocutaneous lymph node syndrome), thyroid disease, and Sjögren's syndrome may cause nasolacrimal obstruction.

Punctal stenosis may occasionally occur spontaneously. The punctum may become stenotic with cicatricial diseases affecting the eyelid margin. Chronic punctal eversion may also result in stenosis of the puncta. Obstruction of the proximal sac or common canaliculus has been reported with epidermodysplasia verruciformis, ichthyosis, scleroderma, and the sclerodermoid variant of porphyria cutanea tarda. Lower lid ectropion, which often has an inflammatory or cicatricial component, and may be associated systemic diseases, has been reported occasionally to be associated with dacryostenosis.[8]

Lichen planus, an immune-mediated skin and mucosal disease similar to pemphigoid, may cause lacrimal stenosis and obstruction. There is a cell-mediated reaction at the level of the epithelial basement membrane. This may also cause a cicatrizing conjunctivitis with shortening of the fornices, symblepharon formation, and a keratitis.

Exogenous Factors

It is important to remove all remnants of silicone tubing from the lacrimal system to prevent secondary obstruction caused by inflammatory masses, because the mucosal surfaces are prone to the development of granulation tissue, pyogenic granuloma and true granulomas, and nongranulomatous reactions to the silicone tube may occasionally occur.

Ocular and periocular disorders, such as atopic disease, sinus and nasal inflammations, exudative rhinitis, and allergies, may develop into nasolacrimal stenosis and obstruction.

Allergic conjunctivitis in patients who chronically rub their eyes can cause an intermittent allergic obstruction at the level of the puncta, canaliculus or lacrimal sac, which may progress to a permanent occlusion.

Tumors (Neoplastic)

The insidious nature of lacrimal sac tumors may present as dacryostenosis or dacryocystitis. The mass is usually above the medial canthal tendon. The position of the medial canthal tendon does not frequently allow distention of the sac by fluid, or distention from dacryocystitis superior to the tendon. A tumor within the sac can create a mass effect above the tendon. Therefore, any distention of the lacrimal sac superior to the medial canthal tendon should be considered to be a tumor until proven otherwise. The dacryocystitis symptoms produced may differ from other causes of dacryocystitis, in that the irrigation fluid may pass into the nose or blood may reflux from the punctum, other factors may be telangiectasia and regional lymphadenopathy. Intermittent epiphora, sanguineous discharge, or an irreducible mass should always lead one to suspect a lacrimal sac tumor.

Approximately 45% of lacrimal sac tumors are benign and 55% are malignant. There have been cases reported in which the initial symptoms of epiphora, or dacryocystitis were found at surgery to be secondary to tumors. Squamous cell papillomas and carcinomas are the most common. Many papillomas initially grow in an inverted pattern into the lacrimal sac wall and therefore are often incompletely excised. Recurrence and malignant degeneration can occur.

Primary tumors of the nasolacrimal duct system are uncommon, but can arise from within the puncta, canaliculi, lacrimal sac, nasolacrimal duct, or about its entrance into the nasal cavity, at the valve of Hasner. The epithelial tumors account for 75% of the lacrimal sac tumors, and the nonepithelial tumors for 25%, which include mesenchymal tumors, melanoma, malignant lymphomas, and leukemia, particularly in older patients with chronic lymphocytic leukemia. Secondary tumors and metastatic lesions can infiltrate or compress the nasolacrimal system, resulting in symptoms of dacryostenosis and dacryocystitis that are much more common than primary tumors. The secondary tumors include adenoid cystic carcinoma, basal cell carcinoma, capillary hemangioma, esthesioneuroblastoma, fibrous dysplasia, fibrosarcoma, intraosseous cavernous hemangioma, leukemia, lymphoma, lymphomatous diseases, mucoepidermoid carcinoma, osteomas, conjunctival papillomas, inverted papillomas, sebaceous gland carcinoma, squamous cell carcinoma, and rhabdomyosarcoma.

The most common primary tumors of the nasolacrimal system of epithelial origin are papillomas and squamous cell carcinomas. Less frequent ones are adenoid cystic carcinoma, angiofibroma, angiosarcoma, cavernous hemangioma, dermoid cyst, fibroma, fibrous histiocytoma, hemangioendothelioma, hemangiopericytoma, lacrimal sac cyst, lymphoma, melanoma, mucoepidermoid carcinoma, neurofibroma, neurilemoma, oncocytic adenoma, oncocytic adenocarcinoma, pleomorphic adenoma, dermatofibrosarcoma protuberans, neurilemoma, adenocanthoma, and more often involve the lacrimal sac. Schwannoma, fibrous histiocytoma, leukemia, and granulocytic sarcoma may infiltrate the lacrimal sac.

The most common neoplasms of the lacrimal sac are epithelial tumors. The most common benign epithelial tumor is a papilloma. Papillomas exhibit epithelial papillomatosis and acanthosis, and an inflammatory papilloma exhibits granulomatous tissue. Inverted papillomas can arise *de novo* in the lacrimal sac or more frequently from an extension of the lateral aspect of the nasal cavity or maxillary sinus. The lesion is not malignant but has a high recurrence rate. Metaplastic transformation to squamous cell carcinoma occurs in 10%–15% of cases, and therefore should be treated as a malignant lesion. The other forms of lacrimal sac epithelial carcinomas are less common. These include adenocarcinoma and epidermoid carcinoma. Mucoepidermoid carcinoma is a very aggressive cancer but is also rare.

The surrounding vascular plexus, which is in a system of collagen bundles, elastic, and reticular fibers arranged in a helical pattern, and the mucosa of the nasolacrimal duct system may be an area where leukemic or lymphomatous tumors may form primary or metastatically from hematologic spread because of their mucosal-associated lymphoid tissue; and frequently occur the tumors more in the middle-aged or elderly. Epiphora will often be the first complaint, before a mass develops or dacryocystitis occurs, and the system may remain patent to probing and irrigation. These lesions usually respond to local irradiation, stenting of the nasolacrimal duct system, and/or chemotherapy.

Lymphoproliferative diseases may involve the nasolacrimal system leading to epiphora, acute or chronic dacryocystitis. They are the second most common type of tumor causing nasolacrimal obstruction. Lymphomas are more frequent than benign lymphoproliferative lesions. Lymphosarcomas, reticulum cell carcinomas, and Hodgkin's disease have been reported to occur in the lacrimal sac.

The most frequent secondary tumors are eyelid lesions, particularly basal cell carcinoma, then squamous cell carcinoma, and less frequently, sebaceous cell carcinoma, which can involve the medial canthal region and the nasolacrimal duct system or can cause pressure and compression and the resultant dacryostenosis and dacryocystitis. The most frequent maxillary sinus lesion is squamous cell carcinoma. The most common lesions arising from the nasopharynx are lymphomatous and squamous cell carcinomas. Metastatic disease as a cause of dacryostenosis and/or dacryocystitis is very rare; lymphoma is the most common, but cases secondary to prostate carcinoma, breast carcinoma, and malignant melanoma have been reported.[9]

Both benign and malignant tumors of mesenchymal elements, capillary and cavernous hemangiomas, and hemangiopericytomas have been reported to involve the lacrimal sac. Melanomas, neurilemoma, plexiform neuroma, and osteoma can involve the lacrimal sac both intrinsically and extrinsically. Fibromas, Kaposi's sarcoma, and other sarcomas can rarely involve the lacrimal sac.

Sinus tumors invade the orbit and nasolacrimal duct system and can be benign or malignant. The benign lesions include inverted papillomas, osteomas, juvenile angiofibromas, and neuroectodermal tumors. Inverted papilloma is the second most common lesion that invades the orbit after squamous cell carcinoma. Inverted papillomas can arise from the lateral nasal wall or the mucosa of the ethmoidal sinus. Mucoceles of the paranasal sinuses can invade the orbit and cause nasolacrimal obstruction. Squamous cell carcinoma, adenocarcinoma, adenoid cystic carcinoma, esthesioneuroblastoma, lymphoma, and melanoma can occur in the paranasal sinus and rare tumors of the odontogenic tumors, which include ameloblastoma and ameloblastic fibrosarcoma, as well as fibrosarcoma, chondrosarcoma, sinus glioblastomas multiforme, and mucoepidermoid carcinoma and may cause dacryostenosis. The most frequent sinus tumor is squamous cell carcinoma of the maxillary sinus, then lymphomas, adenocarcinoma, adenoid cystic carcinoma, transitional cell carcinoma, olfactory neuroblastoma, osteoblastoma, and malignant histiocytosis.

When neoplasms are excised in the medial canthal area, complete resection must be performed and histopathologically controlled (frozen borders or Mohs technique). This includes any portion of the nasolacrimal system involved. The canaliculi may be marsupialized, but dacryocystorhinostomy or canaliculodacryocystorhinostomy should be delayed for 5 or more years to ensure that there are no recurrences and to decrease the morbidity and mortality.

Traumatic

Thermal or chemical burns may cause inflammation, dacryostenosis, and obstruction. Blunt trauma or lacerations usually damage the canaliculus, the lacrimal sac, or the nasolacrimal duct. The dense fibrous tissue of the tarsus is much stronger than the medial canalicular portion of the eyelid; therefore, any tractional force along the eyelid margin can result in avulsion of the medial eyelid with canalicular involvement. All canalicular lacerations should be repaired within 1 day of the injury, to prevent scarring and epithelialization of the wound.

Midfacial trauma and the resultant facial fractures frequently involve the bone about the lacrimal sac fossa, and/or nasolacrimal ducts, leading to obstruction of the nasolacrimal system. Fractures involving the distal portions of the nasolacrimal duct include the midface fractures of naso-orbital, LeFort II, and LeFort III fractures. It is always important to consider and evaluate the patient for involvement of the nasolacrimal duct with these types of fractures rather than waiting for the patient to present with epiphora and/or dacryocystitis. Even if lacrimal irrigation is easy and disappearance of fluorescein dye normal, only lacrimal duct probing can identify and define the extent of injury in these cases, because the fluid may pass into the nose through bony and membranous defects. Direct repair of these injuries is not possible, but stent placement will help to promote patency. Prophylactic intubation with silicone tubing should be considered to prevent this occlusion when indicated. Bony fractures may also initiate an inflammatory and cicatrizing reaction that may result in nasolacrimal duct obstructions shortly after or years after the injury.

Iatrogenic Obstruction

Dacryostenosis and obstruction may result from many procedures, such as repeated and traumatic probing of the canalicular system. Poor technique in the probing of the nasolacrimal ducts may cause the creation of a false passage and subsequent scarring of the lacrimal drainage system.

The pigtail probe has frequently been reported to cause iatrogenic damage to the nasolacrimal duct system, and many consider it to be a potentially harmful device. There have been reported cases of treatment of a single canalicular laceration, or congenital agenesis of only one punctum/canaliculus with the pigtail probe that resulted in obstruction of both canaliculi, which will then commit the patient to a conjunctivodacryocystorhinostomy.

Cheese wiring of silicone intubation tubes through the puncta, as well as nasal migration with complete healing of the eroded puncta and canaliculus, can occur. The erosion of the punctocanaliculi may also be the result of chronic irritation by the tubes, or tubes that were placed under tension. The tubes may be colonized with bacteria, including atypical *Mycobacterium*.

Punctal occlusion, which is frequently performed for the treatment of dry eye syndrome, keratoconjunctivitis sicca, may subsequently cause epiphora in a few patients, and may less frequently cause dacryocystitis. Partial or complete dacryostenosis, pyogenic granulomas, intracanalicular migration, and canaliculitis have been reported after the placement of permanent punctal plugs.

Collared punctal plugs are designed to be removable, but there have been rare cases of these plugs fracturing during removal, with migration of the remainder of the plug into the lacrimal system. The intracanalicular plugs have been noted to cause pyogenic granulomas, indicating that they are associated with an inflammatory process that disrupts the normal cellular functions and can cause a fibrosis and reactive mass. They have also been hypothesized to facilitate the overgrowth of bacteria and a chronic canaliculitis that can result in canalicular obstruction which may erode through the canalicular mucosa, resulting in synechia, symptomatic lacrimal stenosis, or even the formation of fistula.[10]

Intracanalicular plugs used for the treatment of dry eye syndrome, which are implanted in the horizontal canaliculus, may be difficult to remove and may be associated with significant lacrimal complications. It may be difficult to irrigate these intracanalicular plugs through the nasolacrimal system. Irrigation does not reliably flush these intracanalicular plugs from the nasolacrimal system. The collarless intracanalicular plugs theoretically can be flushed through the nasolacrimal system but are not recovered from the nose. Therefore, successful removal cannot be objectively documented. Their retention may act as a nidus for infection, inflammation, epiphora, canaliculitis, and eventually obstruction of the nasolacrimal duct system, with dacryocystitis. Distal migration of the plugs may require complicated canalicular surgery, dacryocystorhinostomy, or conjunctivodacryocystorhinostomy.

Herrick plugs may cause irreversible chronic adverse reactions with persistent inflammation and epiphora. They may cause destruction of the normal canalicular architecture, proliferative tissue reaction, pericanalicular fibrosis, granulomatous tissue, pyogenic granuloma, giant cells reaction, canaliculitis, dacryocystitis, and lymphocytic infiltration. This reaction will cause chronic epiphora and canaliculitis.

Dacryostenosis may occur after a dacryocystorhinostomy as a result of new or persistent stenosis at the common internal punctum or of an improperly fashioned osteotomy. Dacryocystorhinostomy failure may be the result of retained stenting material. Migrated medial or orbital floor implants, or poorly placed or secured medial or orbital floor implants, may cause an external compression or occlusion of the nasolacrimal sac and/or duct.

Transantral orbital decompression has been reported to cause obstruction of the nasolacrimal duct system, possible secondary to delayed scarring around the nasoantral window. Dacryostenosis and obstruction has been reported as a complication of nasal operations, paranasal sinus surgery, both endoscopic and conventional external procedures, and craniofacial procedures.

Nasoantral window procedures are generally placed at the most anterior–inferior portion of the maxillary sinus. If they are placed too high or too posterior, or if the nasolacrimal duct is in an anomalous position, damage to the duct may occur. The Ogura procedure of orbital decompression that removes the medial and floor of the orbital, through an antrostomy, may also cause damage to the lacrimal duct.

Mechanical

Mechanical compression or blockage of the nasolacrimal duct system can result from external compression or occlusion of the system from an intraluminal foreign body, hematoma, or stone. Direct occlusion or external compression may impede or block the canaliculi or nasolacrimal duct.

The most common cause of internal mechanical obstruction is dacryoliths. Some are secondary to fungal infections, but frequently the cause is indeterminate. There are cases reported in which an eyelash served as a nidus for formation of the dacryoliths. Others have postulated that metabolic factors such as high calcium and phosphate levels within an obstructed lacrimal system may contribute to the formation of dacryoliths. Various medications, epinephrine, and quinacrine have been reported to contribute to the formation of casts of the nasolacrimal ducts.

The foreign bodies that may cause internal mechanical obstruction are generally migrated or retained medical devices, such as punctal plugs, or incompletely removed silicone tubing. Rarely, intranasal bleeding can cause a hematoma of the lacrimal sac and duct.

External factors may cause a mechanical obstruction of the lacrimal system. Opposing superior and inferior puncti may cause a proximal obstruction, as in ptosis. Redundancy of the bulbar conjunctiva, conjunctivochalasis, may cause a mechanical obstruction, epiphora, or foreign body sensation. Excision of an ellipse of the redundant conjunctiva is often curative.

Masses arising from the paranasal sinuses, nasal polyps, mucoceles, mucopyoceles, nasal mucosal edema, lymphoid hyperplasia of the nasal cavity, exudative rhinitis, or tumors may cause an external compress of the lacrimal sac or duct. Nasal mucosal edema and mucopurulent exudates may lead to obstruction of the nasolacrimal duct at the intranasal ostium, valve of Hasner. Allergic, viral, or bacterial pharyngitis and rhinitis can produce sufficient nasal mucosal edema, lymphoid hyperplasia, and exudates to result in obstruction of the nasolacrimal duct and progression to a dacryocystitis.

Lacrimal sac cysts, dacryops, are congenital or traumatic in origin. They grow slowly, and may present as a painless epiphora or dacryocystitis.

Maxillary sinus cysts, antral mucoceles, retention cysts, pseudocysts, dentigerous cysts and keratocysts, ameloblastoma, ossifying fibroma, giant cell granuloma, and cholesteatoma, may rarely lead to nasolacrimal obstruction.

Nasal malformations, systemic syndromes, or dysmorphisms that involve abnormalities of facial development, such as clefting or malposition of the orbits or midface, can be associated with maldevelopment of the nasolacrimal duct system. Patients with the centurion syndrome have an anterior displacement of the medial canthal tendon, a prominent nasal bridge, and displacement of the punctum away from the tear pool, resulting in epiphora.

Paget's disease and osteopetrosis have been reported as causes of acquired nasolacrimal obstruction.[11] Sarcoid granuloma, oncocytoma, rhinoliths, and nasal foreign bodies in the inferior meatus can cause a mechanical obstruction of the nasolacrimal duct system at the valve of Hasner.

A retrospective study of 377 dacryocystorhinostomy specimens demonstrated nongranulomatous inflammation (321, 85.1%), granulomatous inflammation consistent with sarcoidosis (8, 2.1%), lymphoma (7, 1.9%), papilloma (4, 1.11%), lymphoplasmacytic infiltrate (4, 1.1%), transitional cell carcinoma (2, 0.5%), and single cases of adenocarcinoma, undifferentiated carcinoma, granular cell tumor, plasmacytoma, and leukemic infiltrate. Neoplasms resulting in chronic nasolacrimal duct obstruction occurred in 4.6% of cases and were unsuspected before surgery in 2.1% of patients.[12]

Punctal eversion, ectropion, or facial palsy may also impair the lacrimal pump action.

Medications

Acquired dacryostenosis may result from the use of antiviral, antiglaucoma, or systemic chemotherapeutic medications. The most common cause of iatrogenic punctal or canalicular stenosis and occlusion is ophthalmic medications. Idoxuridine, vidarabine, trifluridine, acyclovir, demecarium, echothiophate, isoflurophate, adenine arabinoside, furmethide, floxuridine, fluorouracil, neostigmine, physostigmine, epinephrine, pilocarpine, quinacrine, silver preparations, and thiotepa, have been most frequently associated with dacryostenosis and occlusion.

Idoxuridine, trifluridine, and adenine arabinoside generally cause occlusion of the punctum, rather than the mid-zone of the canaliculi as seen from viral infections. The punctal stenosis that occurs from antiviral toxicity will frequently reverse on discontinuation of the medication early on. The antiglaucoma medication may cause a cicatricial conjunctivitis that may be similar to, and indistinguishable from, cicatricial pemphigoid.

Chronic topical epinephrine may affect the vascular plexus of the nasolacrimal duct system. This specialized vascular system permits opening and closing of the lumen of the lacrimal passage, effected by the bulging and subsiding of the vascular system, which can regulate tear outflow.[13] Frequent topical cyclopentolate hydrochloride has been reported to cause dacryostenosis.

The systemic use of some antineoplastic agents, such as 5-fluorouracil and docetaxel has been reported to cause punctal and canalicular stenosis and occlusion with epiphora.[14]

Systemic 5-fluorouracil, a pyrimidine analog that blocks the enzyme thymidylate synthetase and docetaxel can cause obstruction of the nasolacrimal system, punctal and canalicular stenosis and obstruction. 5-fluorouracil may also cause lacrimation, conjunctivitis, blepharitis, keratitis, blurred vision, pain, ankyloblepharon, and cicatricial ectropion. It may cause an inflammatory response in mucosal membranes, as evident by conjunctivitis, as well as oral and gastrointestinal inflammation. The inflammation and fibrosis of the lacrimal drainage system causes extensive fibrous adhesions that obstruct the canaliculi and lacrimal sac.[15] These drugs and similar ones cause damage to the mucosal lining, which occasionally may cause permanent damage to the lacrimal system.

Docetaxel is an effective chemotherapeutic agent for advanced breast cancer and other common malignancies in the antineoplastic class of taxanes. Epiphora and permanent canalicular stenosis can occur in up to 50% of patients receiving weekly docetaxel and to a lower percentage in patients receiving docetaxel every 3 weeks. Chronic inflammation and extensive fibrotic changes have been demonstrated in the stroma of the lacrimal sac and the nasal mucosa. In advanced cases, this occlusion is not reversible. The mechanism of canalicular stenosis may be secondary to secretion of docetaxel in the tear film and fibrosis of the canaliculi from direct contact, or the mucous membrane lining of the puncta and canaliculi develop a fibrosis secondary to the systemic effects of the drug, similar to the widespread edema and fibrosis seen elsewhere in the body. Patients receiving docetaxel should be screened for epiphora and canalicular stenosis, and should receive treatment in the form of silicone intubation to prevent the need for a conjunctivodacryocystorhinostomy.[16] With the newer regimens that use lower doses of the drug for shorter periods than in the past, lacrimal stenosis and occlusion should be less frequent.

Radiation

External radiation in the treatment of neoplasia can cause inflammation of the lacrimal drainage system, stenosis, and occlusion. The reported dose in the literature has varied greatly, and it has been reported to occur in a case receiving as little as 1,800 rad (cGy). Other reports state that the lacrimal passages are relatively immune to radiation therapy until significantly higher doses are delivered. It has been hypothesized that the epiphora probably results from a combination of anatomic lacrimal obstruction, conjunctival epithelial alterations, damage to conjunctival epithelial cells, and damage to conjunctival goblet cells and glands. It is recommended that intubation be considered in patients undergoing radiation for medial canthal tumors. Topical corticosteroids may also be useful in preventing punctal stenosis.[17]

Cobalt and iridium brachytherapy have been reported to cause severe dermatitis and lacrimal drainage stenosis. Lovato et al.[17] reported a prospective study in which 11 of 12 patients that had prophylactic nasolacrimal intubation with silicone tubing maintained lacrimal duct patency, whereas 10 of 12 patients who did not receive prophylactic silicone intubation developed punctal occlusion after helium ion therapy for uveal melanoma.

Radioiodine ablation, I^{131} therapy for thyroid carcinoma at cumulative activities of 150 mCi of I^{131} or more, may produce clinically significant nasolacrimal drainage system obstructions in 4.6% of patients. The areas of obstruction involved the nasolacrimal duct, common canaliculus, and rarely, the superior and inferior canaliculi. The mechanism of the dacryostenosis may be a contribution of local toxicity from direct radiation injury from the passive flow of radioactive tears and/or active uptake and concentration of I^{131} in the nasolacrimal drainage tissues from the blood by the sodium/iodide symporter, the same iodine uptake mechanism used by the thyroid gland. This increased incidence of dacryostenosis and obstruction is likely to be dose-related. Symptomatic patients should receive early evaluation and treatment, possibly with silicone tube placement, because once complete obstruction has developed, it has proven to be difficult to manage.[18]

It is hoped that these classification systems will be useful in the evaluation and treatment of nasolacrimal disorders. Determination of the location of the stenosis or occlusion, and the etiologic classification system presented above, provide a useful mechanism in the formulation of a differential diagnosis and help to develop the appropriate evaluation and treatment plan for each individual patient. These divisions may not be completely isolated; there will be cases that overlap; and there are some diseases and/or clinical situations that have not been included in this review.

References

1. Burns JA, Cahill KV. Modified Kinosian dacryocystorhinostomy: a review of 122 cases. Ophthalmic Surg 1985;16:710–716.
2. Bartley GB. Acquired lacrimal obstruction: an etiologic classification system, case report, and a review of the literature. Part 1. Ophthal Plast Reconstr Surg 1992;8(4):237–242.
3. Paulsen F, Corfield AP, Hinz M, et al. Characterization of mucins in human lacrimal sac and nasolacrimal duct. Invest Ophthalmol Vis Sci 2003;44(5):1807–1813.
4. Paulsen FP, Thale AB, Maune S, Tillman BN. New insights into the pathophysiology of primary acquired dacryostenosis. Ophthalmology 2001;108(12):2329–2336.
5. Mauriello JA, Palydowycz S, DeLuca J. Clinicopathologic study of lacrimal sac and nasal mucosa in 44 patients with complete acquired nasolacrimal duct obstruction. Ophthal Plast Reconstr Surg 1992;8(1):13–21.
6. Paulsen FP, Thale AB, Maune S, Tillman BN. New insights into the pathophysiology of primary acquired dacryostenosis. Ophthalmology 2001;108(12):2329–2336.
7. Blicker JA, Buffam FV. Lacrimal sac, conjunctival, and nasal culture results in dacryocystorhinostomy patients. Ophthal Plast Reconstr Surg 1993;9(1):43–46.
8. Bartley GB. Acquired lacrimal drainage obstruction: an etiologic classification system, case reports, and a review of the literature. Part 2. Ophthal Plast Reconstr Surg 1992;8(4):243–249.
9. Bartley GB. Acquired lacrimal drainage obstruction: an etiologic classification system, case report, and a review of the literature. Part 3. Ophthal Plast Reconstr Surg 1993;9(1):11–26.
10. White WL, Bartley GB, Hawes MJ, et al. Iatrogenic complications related to the use of Herrick Lacrimal Plugs. Ophthalmology 2001;108(10):1835–1837.
11. Bartley GB. Acquired lacrimal drainage obstruction: an etiologic classification system, case report, and a review of the literature. Part 3. Ophthal Plast Reconstr Surg 1993;9(1):11–26.
12. Anderson NG, Wojno TH, Grossniklaus HE. Clinicopathologic findings from lacrimal sac biopsy specimens obtained during dacryocystorhinostomy. Ophthal Plast Reconstr Surg 2003;19:173–176.
13. Paulsen FP, Thale AB, Maune S, Tillman BN. New insights into the pathophysiology of primary acquired dacryostenosis. Ophthalmology 2001;108(12):2329–2336.

14. Esmaeli B, Valero V, Ahmadi MA, Booser D. Canalicular stenosis secondary to docetaxel (taxotere): a newly recognized side effect. Ophthalmology 2001;108:994–995.
15. Esmaeli B, Burnstine MA, Ahmadi MA, Prieto VG. Docetaxel-induced histologic changes in the lacrimal sac and nasal mucosa. Ophthal Plast Reconstr Surg 2003;19(4):305–308.
16. Esmaeli B, Valero V, Ahmadi MA, Booser D. Canalicular stenosis secondary to docetaxel (taxotere): a newly recognized side effect. Ophthalmology 2001;108:994–995.
17. Lovato AA, Char DH, Castro JR, Kroll SM. The effect of silicone nasolacrimal intubation on epiphora after helium ion irradiation of uveal melanomas. Am J Ophthalmol 1989;108:431–434.
18. Burns JA, Morgenstern KE, Cahill KV, et al. Nasolacrimal obstruction secondary to I[131] therapy. Ophthal Plast Reconstr Surg 2004;20:126–129.

6

Evaluation of the Tearing Patient

Joshua Amato and Morris E. Hartstein

Patients with insufficient lacrimal drainage may present to the oph-thalmologist with a complaint of tearing. This tearing may be unilateral or bilateral, intermittent or constant, isolated or associated with other ocular symptoms. Tearing may cause blurred vision, problems with contact lens wear, or annoyance with tears flowing down the cheek. Patients may also complain of a buildup of mucopurulent material in the medial canthus, leading to mattering of the eyes.

To correctly identify and treat the cause of tearing, it is helpful to first differentiate between hyperlacrimation (tear overproduction) and epiphora (decreased tear outflow).

Hyperlacrimation may be attributable to a variety of causes and must be ruled out before addressing any potential outflow problems. Causes of hyperlacrimation, listed in Table 6.1, include the general categories of supranuclear and infranuclear etiologies, reflex lacrimation, and direct lacrimal gland stimulation.[1–3]

Epiphora may be caused by problems at any point along the lacrimal outflow apparatus: punctum, canaliculus, lacrimal sac, lacrimal pump, nasolacrimal duct, and the valve of Hasner at the nasal opening of the nasolacrimal duct. Specific problems involving these areas are listed in Table 6.2.

History

When evaluating any patient presenting with a complaint of tearing, one should begin with a simple history and a clear understanding of the presenting complaint (Figure 6.1). Does the patient complain of "watery eyes" or of tears actually flowing down the cheek? One should inquire about the severity, duration, and frequency of the tearing, as well as any association with certain activities or conditions. The patient's ocular history, such as previous eye surgery, trauma, or topical medications used may provide clues to arriving at a diagnosis. Any associated symptoms that may assist in the diagnosis should also be elucidated. For instance, many older people with macular degeneration

TABLE 6.1. Causes of hyperlacrimation.

Supranuclear etiologies
  Emotional distress
  Central nervous system disorders

Infranuclear etiologies
  Aberrant regeneration
  Cerebellopontine angle tumors

Reflex lacrimation
  Keratoconjunctivitis
  Tear film abnormality

Direct lacrimal gland stimulation
  Inflammation
  Tumor

complain of "watery eyes," referring to the visual distortion they experience.

A patient who complains of chronic or intermittent irritation or who describes a burning or gritty feeling would likely have a tear film abnormality, such as meibomian gland dysfunction or keratoconjunctivitis sicca. A complaint of severe itching or a seasonal nature of the symptoms would suggest an allergic component. Presence of crusting or mucus may suggest meibomian gland dysfunction, allergy, or blepharitis. Purulence should cause one to consider nasolacrimal obstruction

TABLE 6.2. Causes of epiphora.

Punctal abnormalities
  Stenosis
  Ectropion

Lacrimal pump dysfunction
  Orbicularis oculi weakness
  Eyelid laxity
  Eyelid retraction

Canalicular stenosis
  Trauma
  Canaliculitis
  Topical medications
  Chemotherapeutic agents
  Herpetic disease

Lacrimal sac pathology
  Dacryocystitis
  Dacryoliths (Figure 6.4)
  Neoplastic

Nasolacrimal duct obstruction
  Involution
  Traumatic
  Neoplastic

Nasal disease
  Allergy
  Sinusitis
  Neoplastic

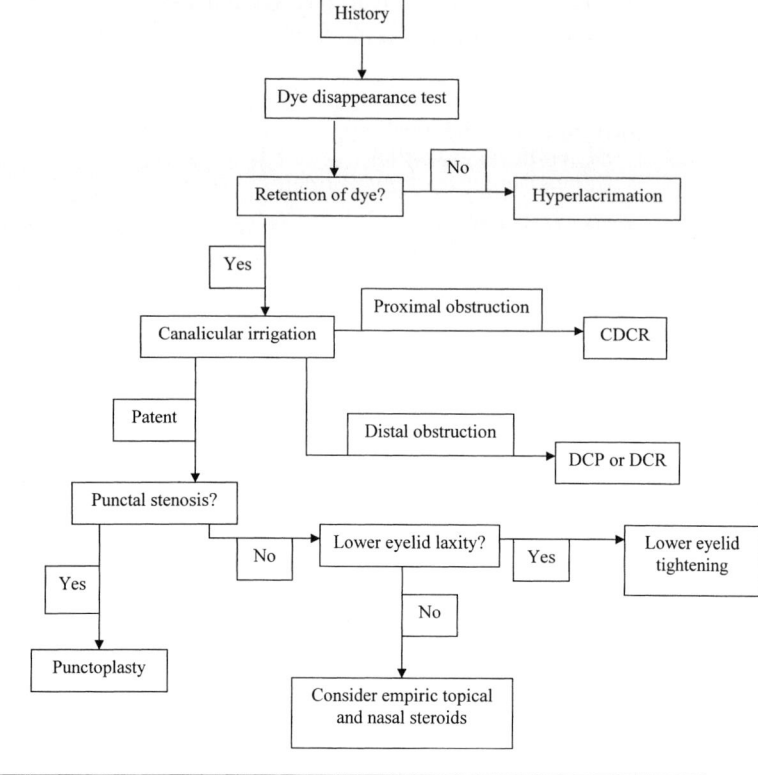

CDCR = Conjunctivodacryocystorhinostomy
DCP = Dacrocystoplasty
DCR = Dacryocystorhinostomy

FIGURE 6.1. General approach to evaluation of a patient with excess tearing.

with dacryocystitis or conjunctivitis, whereas tearing in the presence
of pain may suggest a dacryolith as the etiology.

Unilateral tearing would more likely be caused by a local irritant or
lacrimal obstruction, although these conditions can occur in a bilateral
manner. Bilateral tearing would be more consistent with allergy or a
tear film abnormality. Punctal malposition or a dysfunctional lacrimal
pump could present either unilaterally or bilaterally, depending on the
etiology.

Ocular trauma can lead to tear film abnormalities, eyelid malposition, or lacrimal outflow obstruction. Chronic use of topical medications, such as pilocarpine, phospholine iodide, and idoxuridine, can
result in punctal or canalicular stenosis.

Clinical Examination

The evaluation should begin by examining the eyelids and periocular
structures. Any irregularity, swelling, or evidence of trauma should be
noted. Close attention should be given to the medial canthal region for

focal swelling or erythema overlying the nasolacrimal sac, which would suggest dacryocystitis. In addition, any facial adenopathy should be noted, which may herald an undiagnosed head and neck malignancy.

One should assess for lid position and proper apposition against the globe. Inferior scleral show, lid retraction, entropion, or ectropion should be noted. Lid tone can be assessed with the distraction test, whereby the lower lid is pulled away from the globe. A normal distance for this test is less than 8 mm. Resiliency can be assessed with the snapback test, in which the lower lid is pulled downward and let go, allowing the lid to snap back against the globe in the normal eye (Figure 6.2). Abnormalities on any of these tests would suggest lacrimal pump dysfunction as an etiology. Orbicularis strength should be evaluated as well, because it also contributes to lacrimal pump function. One should ask the patient to gently close the lids and observe for lagophthalmos, which may lead to keratopathy-induced tearing.

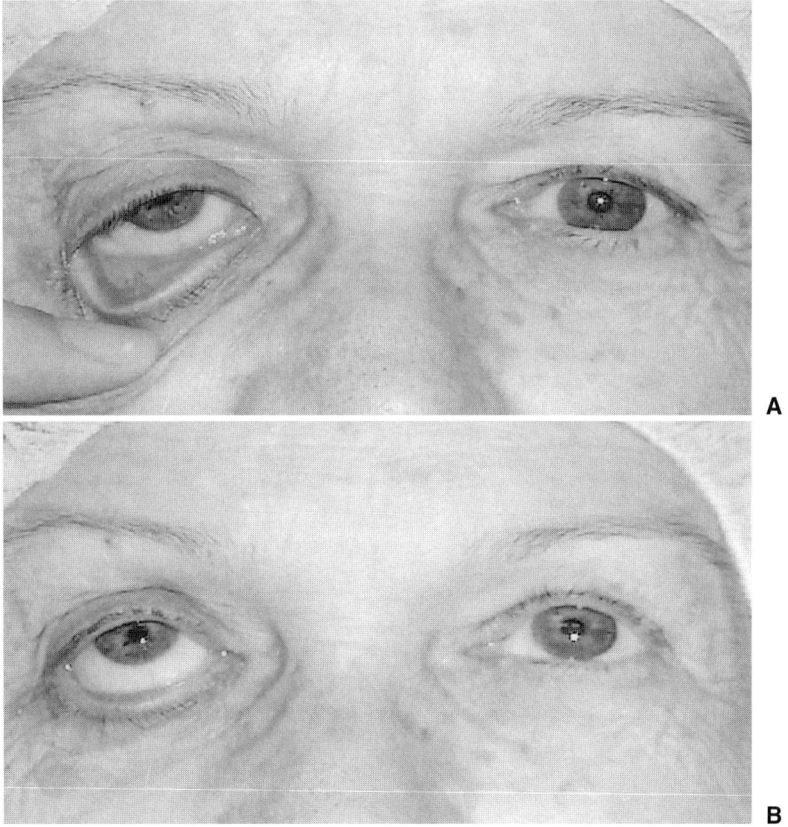

A

B

FIGURE 6.2. Snapback test. After inferior traction is applied to the lower lid **(A)**, it does not properly snap back against the globe when released **(B)** in this patient with lid laxity.

At the slit lamp, one should evaluate the puncta for patency and proper apposition against the globe. The lids should be further evaluated for meibomian gland inspissations and stigmata of blepharitis, and the quality and adequacy of the tear film should be noted. One should examine for trichiasis and associated keratopathy. Other corneal irregularities, defects, or keratitis, as well as conjunctival injection or a papillary reaction should be noted.

Schirmer I testing to measure total tear production can be performed by placing a filter paper strip around the lower lid margin and checking the length of wetting of the strip after 5 minutes. Alternatively, a reading at 1 minute can be multiplied by 3 as estimation. Normal wetting is greater than 10–15mm. Schirmer II testing, which involves stimulation of the nasal mucosa after placing similar strips on the lids, can be used to further evaluate the reflex arc for tear production. Basal secretory rate can then be tested by reapplying the strips after applying an anesthetic to suppress reflex tearing. Normal basal rate is greater than 10–15mm.

Fluorescein should be instilled in each cul-de-sac, and the cornea and conjunctiva again examined for punctate staining, which may suggest a dry eye syndrome or other surface disease. One should also measure the tear breakup time by observing the time to disruption of the tear film after the patient blinks. If this time is less than 10 seconds, the patient may have a relative deficiency of the mucin layer of the tear film.

The dye disappearance test is a very simple and useful tool. With the fluorescein already present, one can assess for a decrease or asymmetry in tear drainage by observing the amount of fluorescein remaining in each eye after about 5 minutes. A decrease in fluorescein clearance is nonspecific and is likely secondary to an anatomic or functional drainage abnormality (Figure 6.3). Although high false-positive rates exist with dye retention in the tear film, clearance of the dye makes nasolacrimal dysfunction very unlikely.

The Jones I or primary dye test involves an attempt to recover fluorescein from the nasal opening of the nasolacrimal duct just beneath the inferior turbinate. Lack of dye retrieval at 5 minutes, a negative test, heralds a nonspecific drainage abnormality and the Jones II or second-

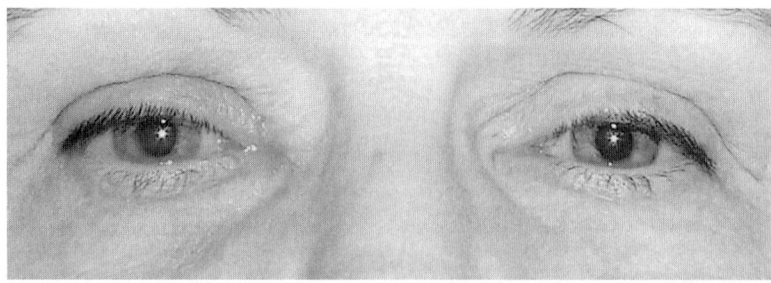

FIGURE 6.3. Dye disappearance test. Fluorescein clears more slowly in the right eye of this patient.

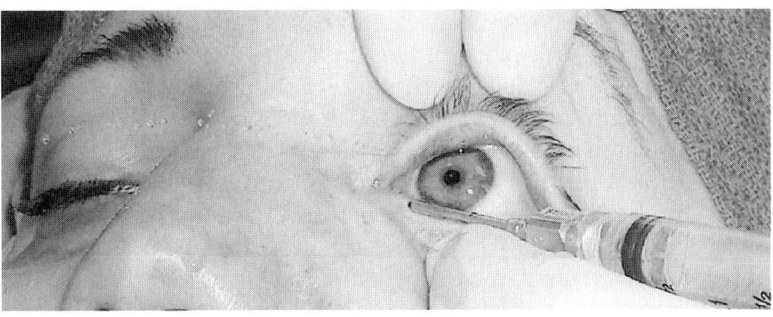

FIGURE 6.4. Canalicular irrigation. Saline is seen to reflux through the upper punctum when injected into the lower canaliculus in this patient with nasolacrimal duct obstruction.

ary dye test should be performed. This is done by injecting saline through the canalicular system at increased physiologic pressures after removal of any fluorescein remaining in the cul-de-sac. If no irrigant is retrieved from the nasal end, the patient has a nasolacrimal obstruction. Recovery of irrigant without fluorescein suggests that the patient has a functional obstruction proximal to the nasolacrimal sac, whereas the recovery of fluorescein suggests an obstruction distal to the sac allowing dye to pool there. Jones testing provides a significant number of false-positive and false-negative results and therefore is not routinely used.

One should use a nasal speculum to examine the nares for any mucosal swelling, tumors, or other anatomic abnormality in the vicinity of the inferior turbinate. Patients with allergy or sinusitis may develop mucosal thickening severe enough to occlude the nasolacrimal duct opening beneath the inferior turbinate. These patients may respond well to nasal steroids and antiallergy eye drops. Patients with a history of trauma or previous nasal surgery may have a deviated septum, which could narrow the opening as well.

Irrigation is the gold standard of nasolacrimal testing and can yield information to help determine if there is outflow obstruction. After an anesthetic drop is instilled, a punctal dilator is used to create a larger opening for a #23 lacrimal cannula or disposable anterior chamber cannula. Using a 3-cc syringe, saline is injected through this cannula, which is advanced through each canaliculus (Figure 6.4). A 3-cc syringe is preferred because a 10-cc syringe provides too much resistance to appreciate partial obstruction, whereas a 1-cc syringe provides too little resistance. If saline cannot be passed or refluxes through the same punctum entered, the patient has an obstruction of the canaliculus tested. This result is usually associated with moderate discomfort. If saline refluxes through the opposite punctum, the patient has an obstruction distal to the common canaliculus or nasolacrimal sac (Figure 6.5). If saline passes without difficulty into the patient's nose and throat, the nasolacrimal system is anatomically patent. A patient can have a partial obstruction that allows some saline to pass into the throat with a degree of resistance noted during the procedure. If irrigation demonstrates adequate outflow in the presence of a positive dye disappearance test or delay of irrigant reaching the nose, a functional abnormality may be present. This situation may be the result of a dilated nasolacrimal sac and/or lacrimal pump failure.

One can additionally use the lacrimal cannula, or alternatively a lacrimal probe, to advance nasally within the canaliculus toward the nasolacrimal sac and lacrimal fossa. If reflux occurred but the cannula can be advanced freely to encounter a hard stop against the bony wall of the lacrimal fossa, then a more distal obstruction should be suspected. However, if the cannula cannot reach bone and seems to get caught up on soft tissue to encounter only a soft stop, then obstruction within the canaliculus tested or common canaliculus would be present. In the latter case, the medial canthus can be seen to drag nasally as the cannula pushes against the soft tissue complex as opposed to passing through it.

General Approach

Evaluation of the tearing patient begins with a history to elucidate the nature of the patient's complaint and obtain additional clues to the etiology. One should determine if the patient has true epiphora, using the dye disappearance test and observing the tear meniscus. Any causes of hyperlacrimation, such as keratitis or tear film abnormality, should be ruled out or treated. The outflow system should then be evaluated with irrigation. If obstruction is encountered, dacryocystoplasty, dacryocystorhinostomy, or conjunctivodacryocystorhinostomy should be considered as indicated for the site and degree of obstruction. If anatomically patent, one should consider treatment of rhinitis, repair of punctal stenosis, or horizontal lid tightening as indicated. Additionally, imaging studies may be used when the diagnosis is uncertain or when tumefaction is suspected.

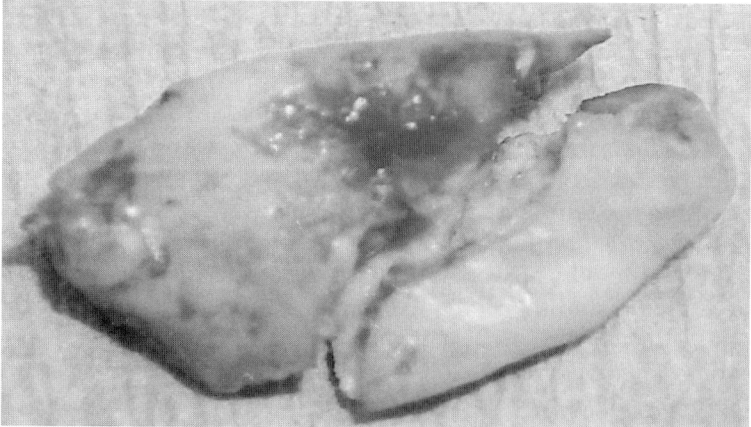

FIGURE 6.5. Dacryoliths removed from a patient with tearing and pain.

   As the evaluation is performed, it should be remembered that patients may have multiple causes of their tearing. The tearing patient with blepharitis may also have a partial nasolacrimal duct obstruction. One needs to determine whether the patient's tearing is primarily the result of ocular surface disease or outflow obstruction. Only after performing the complete examination can one decide on the best course for management. If the etiology is unclear, conservative treatment is usually recommended before surgical intervention.

References

1. Hurwitz JJ. The Lacrimal System. Philadelphia: Lippincott-Raven; 1996.
2. McCord CD. Oculoplastic Surgery. 3rd ed. New York: Raven Press; 1995.
3. Hartstein ME. The Complete Guide to the Evaluation and Management of the Tearing Patient. American Academy of Ophthalmology Annual Meeting. Dallas, TX. October 2000.

7

Imaging and Clinical Evaluation of the Lacrimal Drainage System

Jonathan J. Dutton and Jeffrey J. White

The lacrimal drainage system is an intricate mucous membrane-lined conduit, the function of which depends on a complex interplay of anatomy and physiology. Appropriate drainage of tears depends on several factors, including the volume of tear production, eyelid position, normal pump mechanisms, anatomic status of the drainage passages, gravity, and nasal air convection currents. The patient with symptomatic epiphora may have a normal anatomic system overwhelmed by an oversecretion syndrome, or a drainage system that is anatomically compromised and therefore unable to handle normal tear production. Conversely, patients may have partial or complete blockage of the nasolacrimal system but experience no symptoms or have symptoms of dry eye if tear production is significantly reduced. The clinical picture of bothersome epiphora thus depends on the balance of tear production and tear drainage, not on the absolute function of either one.

The etiologies of lacrimal drainage dysfunction can be divided into two categories, anatomic and physiologic. Anatomic obstruction refers to a gross structural abnormality of the nasolacrimal system. This can be a complete obstruction, such as punctal occlusion, canalicular blockage, or nasolacrimal duct fibrosis. The causes of partial obstruction include punctal or canalicular stenosis, inflammatory narrowing of the duct, or mechanical obstruction within the lacrimal sac, such as tumors or stones. Physiologic etiologies result from failure of functional mechanisms despite normal anatomy. These types of dysfunction may result from anatomic deformity, such as punctal eversion or other eyelid malposition, or from lacrimal pump inadequacy from poor orbicularis tone or eyelid laxity.[1] Determining the type of dysfunction and the exact location of the anatomic blockage with physical examination and ancillary testing are essential if appropriate therapy is to be offered.

The clinical evaluation of gross lacrimal function is usually not difficult and the diagnosis of epiphora can oftentimes be made largely on history alone. However, determination of the etiology of epiphora may be more difficult and often requires a variety of diagnostic procedures.

There is no single test that will pinpoint the anatomic site or physiologic basis for an imbalance between tear production and tear drainage. A host of clinical tests have been described, many of which must be used together to diagnose specific disease processes correctly. In this chapter, we briefly describe the most important tests and imaging techniques and discuss the clinical significance of each.

Clinical Diagnostic Tests

The following diagnostic tests have been devised to evaluate the tear production and lacrimal drainage systems. These tests include some simple clinical procedures that should be a routine part of every evaluation, as well as more complex radiographic and echographic examinations that are used in selected patients. In most cases of epiphora, several tests must be used to determine the specific etiology and to plan appropriate therapy.

Clinical History

Clinical history is one of the most important aspects in the evaluation of the patient with symptomatic epiphora, yet it is frequently glossed over or completely overlooked. Taking an adequate history can occasionally localize the site of obstruction and in most cases will allow the surgeon to decide which tests are appropriate. Epiphora in a child with a history of tearing since birth is almost always the result of a blockage at Hasner's membrane, whereas acquired epiphora in a child may have a very different etiology, such as canalicular obstruction. It is important to elicit a history of prior facial trauma or intranasal cautery, because this should prompt evaluation of the bony nasolacrimal canal. Prior use of ophthalmic medications (i.e., phospholine iodide), certain systemic chemotherapeutic agents, or orbital irradiation should lead the clinician to suspect canalicular obstruction. Previous sinus surgery, particularly intranasal antrostomy or ethmoidectomy should alert the surgeon to potential direct duct injury. History of a rapidly growing mass or bleeding from the puncta should raise the suspicion for the presence of malignancy. Intermittent epiphora can be related to early inflammation of the membranous duct or from allergic rhinitis. Recurrent episodes of dacryocystitis may suggest lower nasolacrimal duct obstruction but may lead to stenosis of the proximal system as well. Taking a thorough history as part of the routine evaluation will make further investigation considerably more efficient.

External Examination

Evaluation of epiphora begins with a careful examination of the external ocular surface and eyelid structures for causes of hypersecretion or for mechanical obstruction of drainage. Conjunctival or corneal irritation, either inflammatory or mechanical, may cause hypersecretion with resultant epiphora, even in the presence of a normally functioning drainage system. Blepharitis and allergic conjunctivitis will often trigger increased lacrimation. Eyelid malpositions such as entropion, with or without trichiasis, can produce corneal irritation and secondary reflex tearing. Lid laxity from aging or facial nerve palsy may lead to exposure keratitis and reflex epiphora. Lid laxity may also result in a weakened orbicularis pump mechanism or punctal eversion. The tear drainage system may be impaired by occlusion of the punctal opening from conjunctivochalasis or tight eyelid fissures with punctal opposition. Mass lesions in the medial canthal region may also mechanically obstruct tear drainage. Careful palpation of the lacrimal sac will reveal the presence of a sac mucocele, and pressure behind the anterior lacrimal crest may produce reflux of mucopurulent material suggestive of lower system obstruction. Examination of the nasal vestibule must be made, because hypertrophic mucosa or nasal polyps can obstruct the nasolacrimal ostium. Such findings during external examination will direct the clinician toward further specific diagnostic tests.

Schirmer Tests

In 1903, Schirmer described this technique for evaluation of tear production. Since that time, the Schirmer tests have become an important clinical tool for the diagnosis of dry eye and hypersecretion syndromes. The Schirmer I test is used to evaluate gross tear production. It is usually performed without topical anesthetic. A strip of #41 Whatman filter paper, 50mm long and 5mm wide, is folded 5mm from one end, and the small folded end is placed into the inferior conjunctival fornix at the junction of the lateral and middle thirds of the lower eyelid. The amount of wetting on the filter paper is measured at 5 minutes. The test should be performed in subdued lighting, and both eyes must be tested simultaneously. This test measures the aqueous component of the tear film and does not distinguish between basic and reflex tear production. It gives only a very crude estimate of true tear flow. The paper itself may stimulate reflex lacrimation. If the investigator is not careful to wipe the tear lake from the conjunctiva before inserting the paper strips, an excessive degree of wetting will be recorded. If the tear drainage system is functioning, a significant volume of tear flow passes into the puncta without being recorded. The fractional volume lost is in proportion to the adequacy of the drainage system and may be significantly more than the volume recorded. Normal values for the Schirmer I test range from 10 to 30mm at 5 minutes, with values more than 25mm typical of patients younger than age 30 and values 10mm or less in those older than age 60.

If the Schirmer I test is abnormal, the test may be modified to separate the reflex component from basic secretion. A drop of topical anesthetic is instilled into the eye and the test is repeated. This test must be performed in the dark, because light can stimulate reflex tearing. Any combination of basic and reflex tearing may be found in patients with symptomatic dry eye or epiphora, and the volume of aqueous flow alone is not a complete indication of tear function.

When the Schirmer I test results are below normal, the Schirmer II test will give some indication of stressed reflex capability. Topical anesthetic is used in the eye, and the nasal mucosa is stimulated mechanically with a cotton swab or chemically with ammonium chloride. The amount by which the Schirmer II test exceeds basic production represents stressed reflex secretion.

Rose Bengal Staining

Rose bengal is a chloride-substituted iodinated fluorescein dye that stains devitalized epithelial cells. Increased conjunctival staining is a sensitive indicator of inadequate tear function, regardless of gross aqueous tear flow determined by the Schirmer test. In the patient with epiphora and significant staining, reflex hypersecretion and inadequacy of tear physiology should be suspected.

Tear Breakup Time

Stability of the normal tear film depends on its basal mucin layer, which increases the hydrophilic quality of epithelial cells, allowing uniform wetting of the corneal surface. When this mucin component is reduced, the tear film will bead up on the relatively more hydrophobic corneal surface. The tear breakup time is a simple clinical test for evaluation of this component of tear function. One drop of fluorescein is placed in the eye and the patient is instructed to blink once. Viewing the corneal surface under slit-lamp magnification with cobalt blue illumination, the observer notes at what time dry spots appear in the tear film. Normal tear breakup time is between 15 and 30 seconds. A tear breakup time of less than 10 seconds indicates a probable mucin deficiency, which may result not only in the symptoms of dry eye syndrome but in reflex hypersecretion of the aqueous component and epiphora.

Dye Disappearance Test

The dye disappearance test is usually performed as part of the primary Jones dye test (Jones I test). It is a rudimentary measurement of the rate of tear flow out of the conjunctival sac. One drop of 2% fluorescein is placed in the lower conjunctival fornix and the amount remaining at 5 minutes is graded on a 0 to 4+ scale, with 0 representing no dye remaining and 4+ representing all the dye remaining. The test is most meaningful when both sides are compared simultaneously. Little or no fluorescein remaining in the conjunctival sac (a positive test) indicates probable normal drainage outflow, whereas most or all of the dye remaining (negative test) indicates partial or complete obstruction, or pump failure. Care must be taken to note any lid overflow. Also, a significant amount of dye may disappear in the presence of a large dilated sac mucocele and distal obstruction. The test cannot distinguish between physiologic and anatomic causes of drainage dysfunction, nor can it localize the site of mechanical blockage. The dye disappearance test has been shown to be positive in 95% of asymptomatic normal individuals and may be more sensitive than the primary Jones test.[2] Unlike the latter, it does not seem to be dependent on gross tear flow as measured by the Schirmer test.

Primary Jones Dye Test

In 1961, Jones described a simple test of lacrimal drainage function that has become one of the most frequently used procedures in the evaluation of epiphora. The primary Jones dye test (Jones I) is a true functional test and should be performed in as nearly physiologic conditions as possible. The patient should be in an upright position, and should blink normally. Topical anesthesia is not used, although the clinician may anesthetize the nasal mucosa for comfort. Two percent fluorescein is instilled into the conjunctival sac and a fine cotton-tipped applicator is passed beneath the inferior turbinate to the level of the nasolacrimal ostium after 2 minutes and again after 5 minutes. The test is positive if dye is recovered, and indicates patent anatomy and adequate physiologic function. However, the dye may be very difficult to retrieve and therefore there is a high false-negative rate with this test. Transit time for the dye to reach the nose is quite variable and shows a significant correlation with the Schirmer test. Even in eyes without epiphora, passage of dye into the nose may take considerably longer than the 5 minutes allowed for the test. Testing conditions may alter results because transit time is influenced by factors such as blink rate, gravity, and fluorescein volume. Although a positive test strongly suggests a normal system, it does not completely rule out physiologic dysfunction or mild anatomic obstruction. More significantly, a negative test alone does not necessarily indicate abnormal drainage.

The fluorescein appearance test, described by Flach,[3] is a modification of the primary Jones dye test. It is designed to avoid the difficulty and variability involved in recovering dye from the inferior meatus. Two percent fluorescein is placed in the conjunctival sac and the oropharynx is examined with ultraviolet light, beginning at 5 minutes and continuing up to 1 hour if necessary. With this technique, 90% of normal individuals are said to show oropharyngeal fluorescence within 30 minutes, and 100% within 60 minutes. This procedure is best used as a supplement to a negative primary Jones test and can be performed 20–30 minutes later. Because of the persistence of fluorescence, only one eye can be tested by this technique during a single office visit.

In 1973, Hornblass[4] elaborated on a variation of the primary Jones dye test originally mentioned by Lipsius.[5] In this version, 0.4 mL of 1% sterile solution of sodium saccharin is instilled into the conjunctival sac and the patient is asked to report when he or she tastes the solution. Hornblass found a mean transit time to the nose of 3.5 minutes, with

65% of normal individuals reporting a positive test within 6 minutes, and 90% reporting positive results within 15 minutes. Transit times in excess of 15 minutes suggest partial nasolacrimal duct obstruction. The test depends on a subjective response from the patient, and before the solution can be tasted, it must pass into the pharynx, where threshold taste sensitivity is quite variable. Lipsius noted that 3% of normal individuals were incapable of tasting saccharin.

Secondary Jones Dye Test

A negative primary Jones dye test suggests delayed transit time through the lacrimal drainage system but it does not differentiate physiologic dysfunction from anatomic obstruction. The secondary Jones dye test (Jones II) evaluates anatomic patency of the system in such cases. Residual fluorescein is flushed from the conjunctival sac and a topical anesthetic is instilled. The patient sits with head tilted forward while clear saline is irrigated into one canaliculus through a cannula. The patient is instructed to blow or spit any fluid that passes into the nose or pharynx onto a clean tissue. The presence of any fluid in the nose indicates gross anatomic patency of the nasolacrimal passages. In this situation, complete obstruction is not present because saline did traverse the system under pressure. Recovery of dye-stained saline demonstrates normal punctal and canalicular anatomy, because the dye must have passed freely into the sac during the previous Jones I test. Such a result is compatible with a partial anatomic block at the level of the lower sac or duct. Recovery of clear saline without fluorescein suggests punctal or canalicular stenosis, with failure of dye from the primary Jones test to enter the lacrimal sac. If fluid does not reach the nose at all but regurgitates from the opposite punctum, a high-grade obstruction is likely. Regurgitation of dye-stained fluid suggests blockage at the level of the lower sac or duct, with residual dye in the sac being flushed out by the irrigation. Very rarely, a dilated canalicular mucocele may retain sufficient dye to produce similar results. Regurgitation of clear saline from the opposite punctum suggests obstruction at the level of the distal common canaliculus or upper sac with no residual dye from the primary Jones test. When clear saline regurgitates from the same punctum that is being irrigated without flow from the opposite punctum, a proximal obstruction in that canaliculus is likely.

During the irrigation of saline, distension of the lacrimal sac to palpation confirms the presence of lower nasolacrimal duct obstruction. Under such conditions, a palpable sac without fluid passing into the nose suggests complete nasolacrimal duct blockage, whereas a palpable sac with fluid passing into the nose implies a partial obstruction. However, a sac that is contracted and fibrotic because of chronic inflammation may not dilate under these conditions.

The secondary Jones dye test evaluates anatomic patency under increased hydrostatic pressure. When positive, it does not differentiate between epiphora caused by physiologic dysfunction and epiphora resulting from partial anatomic obstruction. When a primary Jones test is positive, the secondary Jones test should always be positive and is therefore unnecessary. With a negative primary test, a positive secondary test would be consistent with physiologic or partial anatomic dysfunction, but would rule out complete blockage. Negative results on both the primary and secondary tests confirm high-grade obstruction.

Probing

When the secondary Jones test indicates canalicular obstruction, the canaliculus in question should be probed gently to the lacrimal sac with a small Bowman probe. The punctum may first be dilated by pulling the lid laterally to prevent canalicular kinking and inserting a pointed dilator. The distance of the stenosis or blockage from the punctum is noted in millimeters by measuring directly on the probe. In most individuals, a short common canaliculus is present 6–9 mm from the puncta. The canalicular system should not be probed without prior indication of possible obstruction because of the risk of inadvertent injury and subsequent fibrosis.

Diagnostic Imaging Techniques

Diagnostic Ultrasonography

The techniques of A- and B-mode ultrasonography provide a simple, noninvasive method of evaluating gross anatomic abnormalities of the lacrimal drainage system (Figures 7.1A and B, and 7.2A and B). Physiologic dysfunction cannot be evaluated, nor can the precise site of anatomic obstruction be localized. However, a dilated lacrimal sac can easily be distinguished from one of normal dimensions. It is also possible to differentiate air from mucus or solid masses, making the identification of lacrimal sac neoplasms possible.[6]

With the B-mode probe oriented vertically, placed in the medial canthus, and aimed toward the lacrimal sac fossa, an oblique longitudinal cross-section of the lacrimal sac and upper duct is obtained. The canaliculi cannot usually be visualized unless they are dilated. The diameter of the sac and upper duct may be evaluated and the thickness of the walls can often be appreciated. Diverticula may also be identified and a variety of echogenic densities within the system, such as inflammatory membranes, tumors, and stones, can be detected. The position and size of a surgically created ostium (Figure 7.3) may also be imaged with this technique, although its patency cannot easily be evaluated.

For precise measurements of the sac and evaluation of the internal reflectivity of sac contents, A-mode scanning must be used. The probe is first oriented as for a periocular orbital study, but with the beam aimed just behind the anterior lacrimal crest toward the sac fossa. An oblique anterolateral–posteromedial cut of the sac is thus obtained. If

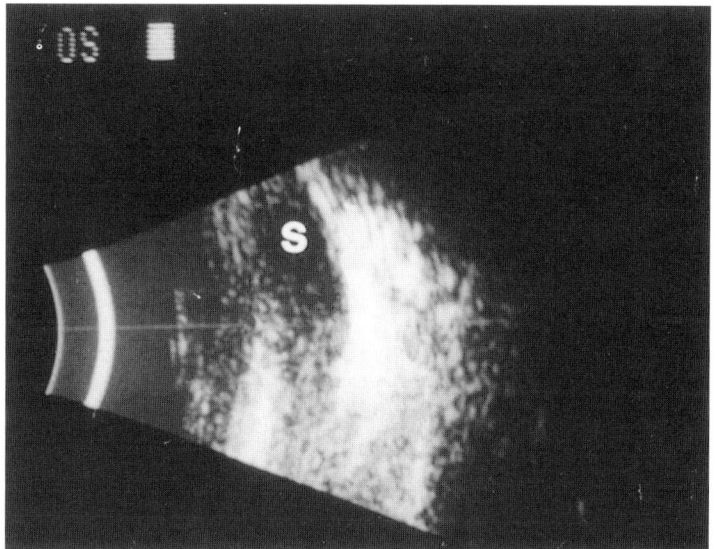

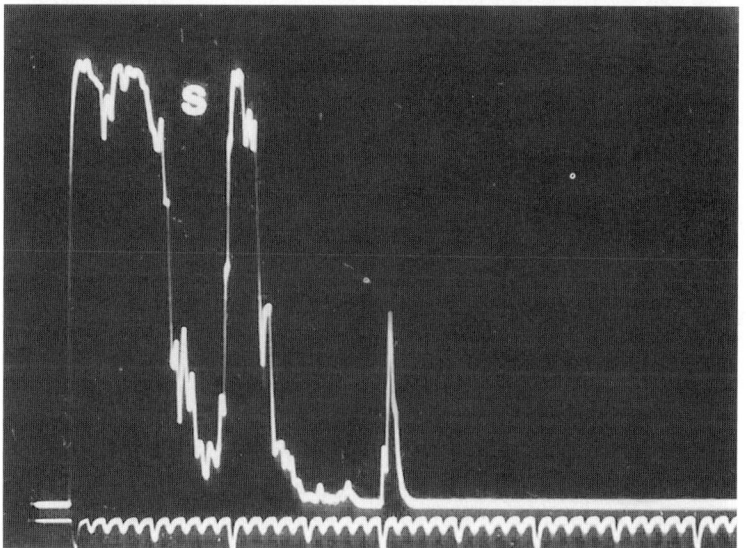

FIGURE 7.1. **(A)** B-scan ultrasound of a nasolacrimal system with a normal nasolacrimal sac (S). The anterior lacrimal crest can be visualized anteriorly and inferiorly and the lacrimal bone is seen posteriorly. **(B)** A-scan ultrasound of a normal nasolacrimal system. Nasolacrimal sac with low reflectivity (S) and sharply defined anterior and posterior walls. The smaller peak represents lacrimal bone.

the sac is filled with air, it appears as an echolucent defect bounded by sharply defined vertical anterior and posterior sac walls. Often, the presence of dilated diverticula can be detected. Mucus in the sac produces uniform, homogeneous, low-density internal echoes, and inflammatory exudates and membranes show stronger, more irregular echoes. Multiple high-density, irregular echoes with infiltration of the sac walls suggest a sac tumor. A transocular A-mode image of the sac is obtained with the probe held above the lateral canthus and directed toward the lacrimal sac fossa. This technique gives an approximate horizontal cross-section of the sac. The average dimensions of the sac in normal individuals are 2.5mm (SD = 0.95mm) in horizontal diameter and 4.0mm (SD = 1.49mm) in anteroposterior extent.[7] A sac more than 4.5mm wide or 7.0mm deep should be considered abnormally dilated.

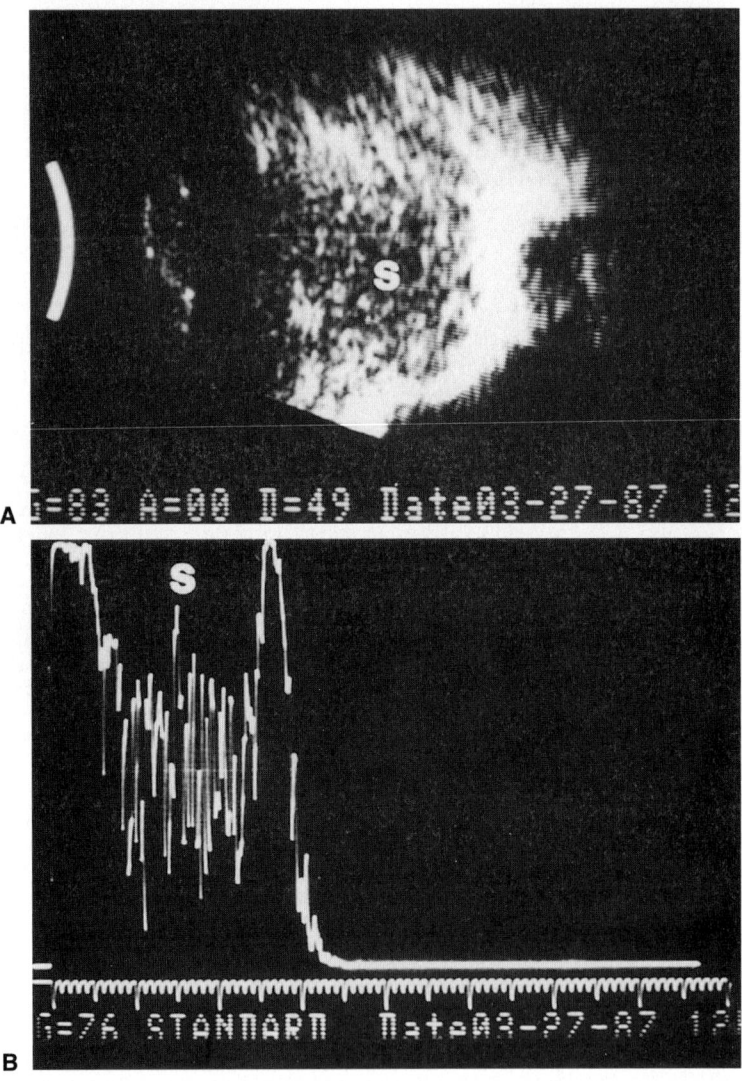

FIGURE 7.2. (A) B-scan ultrasound of a patient with acute dacryocystitis demonstrating a massively enlarged nasolacrimal sac (S) and thickened anterior and posterior walls. (B) A-scan ultrasound of the same patient as in part A showing dilated nasolacrimal sac (S) with irregular, medium reflectivity indicating the presence of mucopurulent exudates.

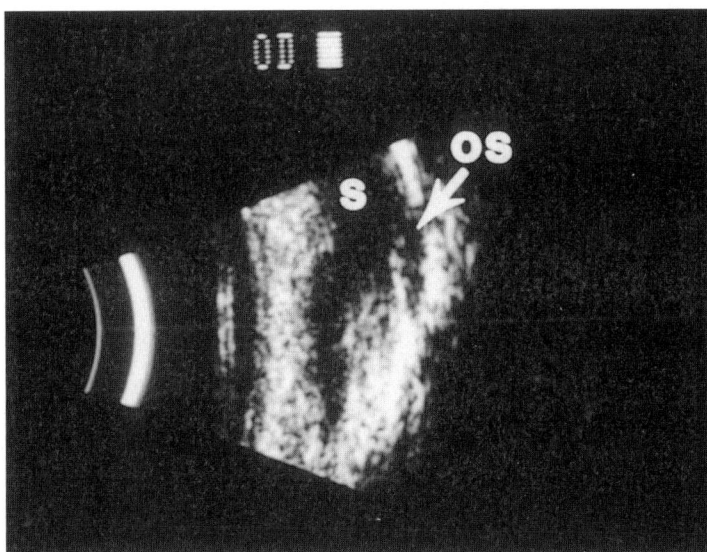

FIGURE 7.3. Postdacryocystorhinostomy B-scan ultrasonography showing the surgically created lacrimal–nasal ostium (OS). The lacrimal sac (S) is somewhat dilated because of soft tissue closure of the ostium.

Contrast Dacryocystography

The first attempt to visualize the lacrimal drainage system radiographically was made by Ewing in 1909. He used bismuth paste for retrograde filling of the nasolacrimal duct. Such early attempts proved unsatisfactory, and the technique was used infrequently until the introduction of better aqueous contrast media such as Sinografin and Angiografin, and especially the low-viscosity iodized oils such as Pantopaque, Ethiodol, and ultrafluid Lipiodol. In a standard dacryocystography (DCG) study, the canaliculi are intubated with intravenous catheters and contrast material is injected into the lower canaliculus on each side, and films are taken immediately in Caldwell's posteroanterior frontal projection and in both lateral projections. Repeat films are obtained at 5 and 15 minutes and upright films may be taken to evaluate the effects of gravity on lacrimal drainage. DCG can also be combined with computed tomography (CT) or magnetic resonance imaging (MRI) to give further information on the nasolacrimal system.

In 1968, Iba and Hanafee[8] described the technique of distension DCG, first used by Barrie Jones in 1959. Here, films are taken during injection of 0.5–1.0 mL of contrast material so that the lacrimal system is imaged in the distended state. Both sides are studied simultaneously and injection is accomplished through the placement of canalicular indwelling tapered Teflon catheters or intravenous catheter tubing. This method provides maximum visualization of the anatomic structure of the system and, because of the backpressure, gives good filling of the canaliculi. It is the best technique for demonstration of fistulae,

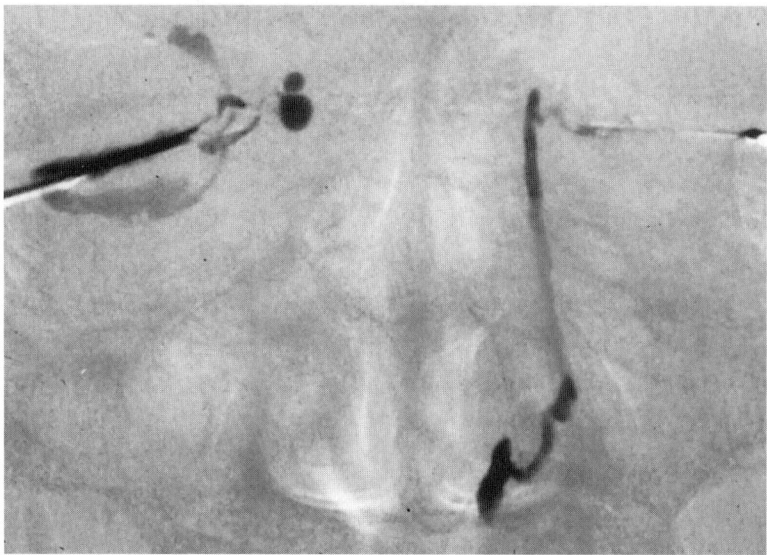

FIGURE 7.4. Digital subtraction contrast dacryocystogram. Patient with normal passage of contrast through the left nasolacrimal system and complete blockage of the right proximal nasolacrimal duct and mild dilation of the right nasolacrimal sac.

diverticula, supernumerary canaliculi, and the presence of stones and sac tumors. However, it does not reveal sac and duct dimensions under normal physiologic conditions. This test also requires either the ophthalmologist or a skilled technician to be in the radiology suite to inject the material and can lead to some patient discomfort.

Improved imaging can be obtained with a technique adopted from subtraction angiography (Figure 7.4) that eliminates confusing bony shadows. A scout film is taken before injecting contrast material and is used to produce bone-free images of the dacryocystogram. More sophisticated computer-assisted digital subtraction images can be produced using fluoroscopically controlled angiographic equipment and an image intensifier.[8,9]

The dacryocystogram of a normal lacrimal drainage system will usually show the canaliculi when less viscous aqueous contrast media are used. The sac appears as a smooth, straight, or gently curved passage with the concavity facing laterally. The anteroposterior dimension is wider than the transverse. There is usually a constriction at the sac–duct junction caused by the split fascia of the orbicularis muscle as it passes around the system. The duct widens at the level of the bony rim and its inner surface becomes more irregular because of the presence of mucosal folds. Such folds may be exceptionally well developed in younger children. Further constrictions are seen in the duct's midportion in the region of Hytle's and Taillefers' valves. Finally, in its lower third, the duct widens again. Visualization by DCG reveals considerable variations in the structure of the sac and duct among normal individuals. Atypical narrowing and widening of the sac and duct, as well as unusual angulations and diverticula, may all be seen in the absence of clinical symptoms.

A combination of subtraction, distension, and macrodacryocystography provides the best visualization of the anatomic structure of the lacrimal drainage system. This approach will provide accurate localization of any anatomic obstruction in the majority of cases. Imaging of the canaliculi with dye failing to pass into the sac or duct implies obstruction at the common canaliculus. Obstruction at the sac–duct junction usually results in a dilated sac with no dye reaching the duct or nose, even on late films. Obstruction at the level of the nasolacrimal duct will show dilatation of the sac, with dye in the duct, but not reaching the nose. A patent dacryocystorhinostomy ostium is easily demonstrated by passage of contrast into the nose at the level of the middle meatus. Demonstration of patent lacrimal passages by DCG in the face of epiphora suggests physiologic dysfunction or a mild incomplete anatomic block.

DCG is considered the gold standard for imaging of the nasolacrimal system, but it does not allow for imaging of the soft tissue or bony structures surrounding the nasolacrimal sac or duct. DCG can be combined with CT and MRI studies to obtain a complete picture of the nasolacrimal system and the surrounding anatomy.

Computed Tomography

In selected cases, CT of the lacrimal system can be extremely useful in the evaluation of epiphora. In axial scans through the lower orbit (Figure 7.5), the lacrimal sac fossa appears as a depression in the antero-

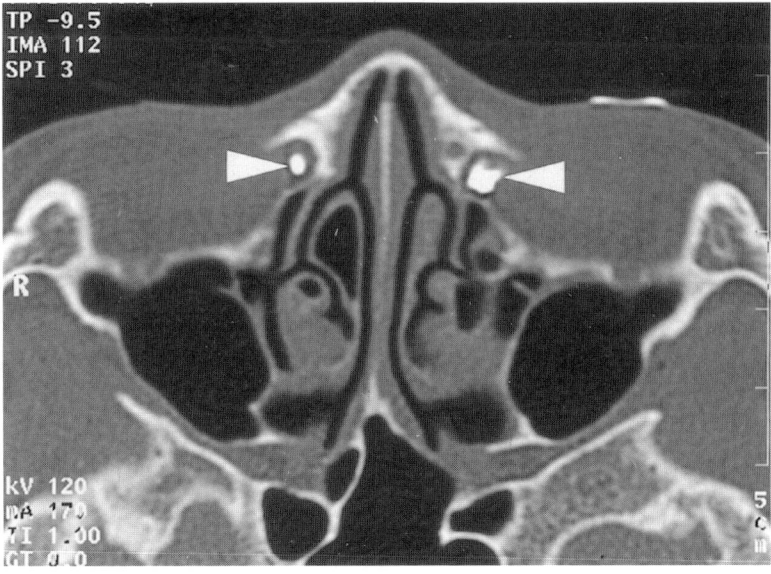

FIGURE 7.5. Axial CT–DCG demonstrating contrast-filled lacrimal sacs (arrowheads). The left system is dilated compared with the right. (Courtesy of Susan K. Freitag, MD, reprinted with permission from Lippincott, Williams & Wilkins ©2002.)

medial wall. In successively lower sections, the duct appears as a round to oval defect in the frontal process of the maxillary bone at the antero-medial corner of the antrum. The duct may be filled with air or fluid. As the duct is traced inferiorly, it can be seen to open beneath the inferior turbinate. Cross-sections of the system are seen in coronal reformatted images because the line of section is oriented downward and obliquely backward. Parasagittal reformatted images will reveal the entire length of the system in longitudinal section.

Although dilatation of the sac and dacryocystitis can be seen, these are more easily and inexpensively studied by other techniques. When epiphora follows trauma and subsequent clinical studies indicate nasolacrimal duct obstruction, CT may reveal orbital rim or maxillary fractures compressing the sac or duct. In cases of congenital lacrimal amniocele, CT will reveal the dilated duct, often associated with bony changes. It is essential to differentiate this soft, near-midline dilated sac from a meningocele. In most cases of suspected malignancy, especially if there is a history of bloody epiphora or pain, a CT scan may demonstrate soft tissue masses of the sac or adjacent paranasal sinuses. MRI is more sensitive for soft tissue abnormalities but does not image the bony structures well.

When combined with DCG, CT scan is excellent at identifying bony structures around the nasolacrimal system (Figures 7.6 and 7.7). By using modern spiral CT techniques with topical contrast material, the surgeon can accurately identify obstructions in the nasolacrimal system. This can be especially useful in patients who have had facial trauma, prior sinus or lacrimal surgery, or tumors of the medial canthus.[10] Newer techniques using spiral CT and three-dimensional reconstruction technology have improved the diagnostic accuracy for patients with partial obstructions of the nasolacrimal system by allowing the surgeon to view a three-dimensional image of the entire system from multiple projections.[11]

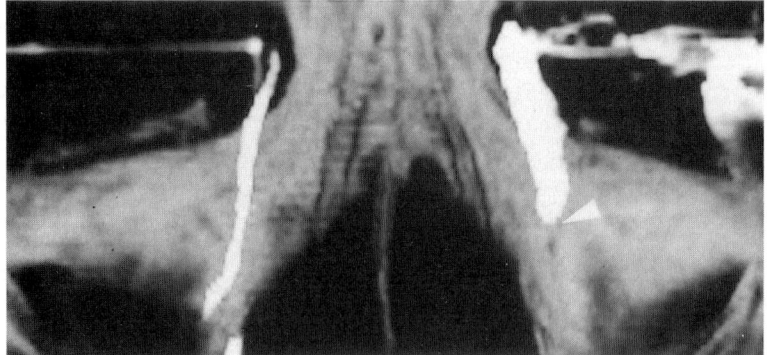

FIGURE 7.6. CT–DCG three-dimensional reconstruction in the left oblique projection confirms the left complete obstruction and proximal dilation. Right system is normal. (Courtesy of Susan K. Freitag, MD, reprinted with permission from Lippincott, Williams & Wilkins ©2002.)

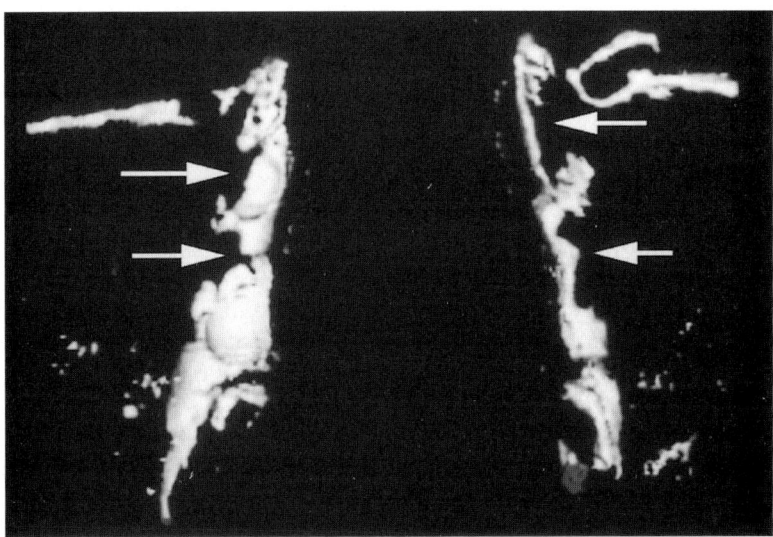

FIGURE 7.7. CT–DCG three-dimensional reconstruction demonstrates bilateral filling defects (arrows) in distorted and dilated lacrimal systems. (Courtesy of Susan K. Freitag, MD, reprinted with permission from Lippincott, Williams & Wilkins ©2002.)

There are some disadvantages to CT scan. As mentioned previously, it is not the best study for evaluating soft tissue masses of the nasolacrimal system. Also, in standard CT, the images are presented as a series of axial images and make identification of small obstructions difficult. Longitudinal and oblique images can be created, but this reconstruction results in decreased spatial resolution in the reformatted images. The exposure to ionizing radiation is also more than for standard DCG.

Magnetic Resonance Imaging

Since 1990, MRI has been used as an adjunctive diagnostic test in the evaluation of lacrimal system pathology that allows for excellent resolution of the nasolacrimal system.[12,13] When combined with a contrast agent, MRI offers several advantages over other imaging studies. Gadolinium can be given as a topical solution (Magnevist) diluted from 1:10 to 1:100 with normal saline, one drop to each eye per minute for 5 minutes. The patient should stay in an upright position until just before image acquisition. Because the lacrimal system is not cannulated, and therefore not under increased hydrostatic pressure, this study gives a picture of the functional status of the nasolacrimal system. There have been no reports of ocular complications from the administration of topical gadolinium and this obviates the need to risk damage to puncta from the direct instillation of contrast agents. Exposure to ionizing radiation is also avoided with this technique.

MRI allows very fine resolution of soft tissue structures within and surrounding the nasolacrimal system compared with dacryoscintigraphy, DCG, and even CT.[14,15] The superficial location of the nasolacrimal system facilitates imaging with small surface coils which can give a spatial resolution of $0.3 \times 0.3 \times 3$ mm or better.[16] Manipulation of signal intensities, repetition times, and tip angles, as well as the use of fat suppression algorithms, can oftentimes allow for differentiation of mucous or blood from solid neoplasms. Also, because of volumetric acquisition, magnetic resonance images can be viewed in any plane without degradation of the quality of images. This is a key advantage over CT–DCG which requires reformatting of images that are out of plane and results in degradation of image resolution. Coronal images are superior for determining the distal extent of contrast transit and axial images are excellent for examining the lumen of the nasolacrimal duct and intraductal pathology.

Although MRI can be a useful diagnostic study, it is an expensive study and therefore should not be used routinely. Other drawbacks include poor ability to image bony structures, and there can be artifact from the nearby ethmoidal air cells. MRI is also susceptible to movement artifact because of the relatively long acquisition times required.

Radionuclide Dacryoscintigraphy

The first use of radionuclide tracer to image the lacrimal drainage system employed radioactive ^{198}Au and measured the buildup of activity over the sac and duct. Rossomondo et al.[17] introduced the first modern nuclear imaging technique for the lacrimal drainage system. They instilled a drop of saline with [^{99m}Tc] sodium pertechnetate, and imaged the system with a gamma camera. In the first clinical evaluation of the technique, Carlton et al.[18] demonstrated its value in visualizing the lacrimal system, and in measuring some physiologic parameters of tear flow. In their study of 28 asymptomatic volunteers, they recorded a transit time for the nuclide of 4–43 seconds to the sac, and 4–323 seconds to the nose. There is a high degree of correlation between dacryoscintigraphy and contrast DCG; however, the former is more sensitive to incomplete blocks, especially in the upper system. Because dacryoscintigraphy is a physiologic test, it is also very sensitive in finding abnormalities in patients with physiologic nasolacrimal duct obstruction and can often localize the site of blockage.[19]

The technique often employed today uses [^{99m}Tc]pertechnetate in saline or technetium sulfur colloid delivered as a 10-μL drop to the lateral conjunctival sac by micropipette. The patient is advised to blink normally and the nasolacrimal system is imaged every 10 seconds for the first 2–3 minutes, and then late images are taken every 5 minutes for a total of 20 minutes (Figure 7.8). The specific activity of this dose is in the range of 50 to 150 μCi, and results in radiation exposure to the lens of less than 2% of that for a complete contrast dacryocystogram.

Dacryoscintigraphy does not provide the detailed anatomic visualization available with contrast DCG. In standard nuclear studies, the

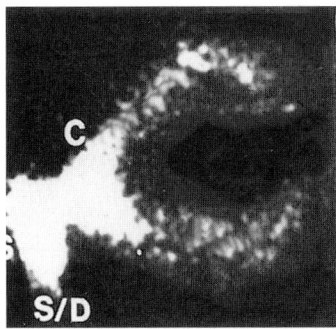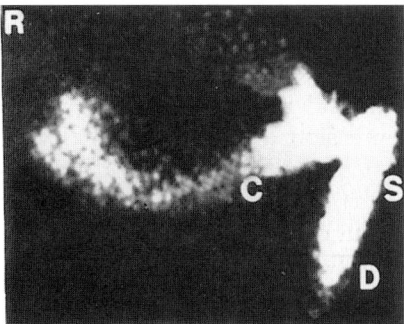

FIGURE 7.8. Dacryoscintigraphy in a patient with unilateral epiphora on the left side. The right lacrimal drainage system fills normally, with tracer concentrated in the canaliculi (C), sac (S), and duct (D). The left system shows no tracer below the sac–duct junction (S/D).

proximal canalicular system is usually poorly imaged unless it is dilated. The sac and duct are usually well outlined. Complete blocks in the sac or duct can be detected, although precise localization of the obstruction may be difficult. However, the procedure can yield considerable information concerning physiologic function. Generation of dynamic activity curves for specific regions of interest will demonstrate incomplete anatomic obstructions as well as a rather subtle degree of functional impairment.[20,21] This technique is most accurate and reproducible for the upper lacrimal system. Transit times become quite variable for the lower system, with 25–32% of asymptomatic individuals showing no tracer in the nose after 12 minutes. This is consistent with findings on the primary Jones dye test. By using more sophisticated rapid sequence display and computer interfacing for image optimization by contrast enhancement, background subtraction, and frame arithmetic, quantitative evaluation of tracer movement provides the most revealing interpretation of lacrimal function and tear flow dynamics currently available.

Other Diagnostic Techniques

Percutaneous Contrast Dacryocystography

The common canaliculus is a common site of obstruction seen on radiographic imaging in patients with epiphora. When such blockages are complete, routine DCG is not possible, and the concomitant presence of lower sac or duct pathology cannot be easily demonstrated unless echography is used to detect a dilated sac. In 1972, Putterman[22] described a technique of percutaneous injection of aqueous contrast material directly into the lacrimal sac to bypass the occluded common canaliculus. In his small series of four patients, there were no complications and results were good.

Chemiluminescence

The use of chemiluminescent materials is a nonradiologic technique for demonstrating the outline of the lacrimal drainage system and verifying its patency. The luminescent agents are dimethylphthalate and tertiary butyl alcohol activated by dibutylphthalate, which produce an intense cold light. This product is commercially used as a safety light. When these agents are injected into the lacrimal system, the glow is visible through the skin and clearly outlines the upper system. The lower duct is not readily demonstrated. The compounds are safe and nontoxic, if confined within the lacrimal system, but extravasation into tissues or onto the globe can produce severe complications of corneal scarring and vascularization, purulent infection, granuloma formation, and fibrosis.[23] Chemiluminescence has not yet been used extensively enough to evaluate its clinical effectiveness as an alternative or adjunct to other procedures.

Lacrimal Thermography

The canaliculi and lacrimal sac have been visualized by thermography, using an infrared scanner and color monitor with a resolution of $0.5°C$.[24] The lacrimal system is easily differentiated from surrounding tissues by irrigation with cold water, and decreased temperature in the nose demonstrates patency. A large dilated sac can be visualized, and persistent inflammation will produce increased temperature within the sac. The duct is not demonstrated with this method.

In a related technique, a mini-thermocouple probe has been used to detect temperature differences with the lacrimal sac. Increased temperatures are seen with vascularity and inflammation, and decreased temperatures with hemorrhage and mucocele formation. Nasolacrimal duct obstruction without associated inflammation shows no difference in temperature compared with the contralateral uninvolved side.

Nasolacrimal Endoscopy

Direct visualization of the lacrimal drainage system has been attempted with rigid and flexible endoscopes, however, results have been mixed and these techniques are not recommended. No clinical evaluation of these instruments has been presented, and their reliability in evaluating nasolacrimal obstruction remains to be demonstrated.

Interpretation of Diagnostic Tests

As is the case with many diagnostic tests in medicine, most of those described above required some subjective interpretation to determine the probable etiology of epiphora (Tables 7.1 and 7.2). Some knowledge of the variability in patient response, as well as of the reliability of the specific tests in suggesting pathology, is needed before meaningful conclusions can be drawn. The mere demonstration of lacrimal system pathology, either anatomic or physiologic, does not indicate lacrimal dysfunction. Patients with significant degrees of partial or even com-

TABLE 7.1. Interpretation of clinical tests in the evaluation of epiphora.

Dye disappearance test	Jones I	Jones II	Probing	Palpation	Diagnosis
Rapid	+	+	Normal	Normal	Probable oversecretion
+	+	+	Normal	Normal	Normal vs. functional
+	−	+	Normal	Normal	Normal vs. functional vs. mild NLD obstruction
+	−	+	Normal	Abnormal	Partial NLD obstruction with dilated sac
Slow	−	+	Normal	Normal	Mild NLD obstruction vs. functional
Slow or −	−	+	Normal	Abnormal	Partial NLD obstruction
−	−	−	Normal	Abnormal	Complete NLD obstruction
−	−	+	Stenotic	Normal	Partial canalicular obstruction
−	−	−	Stenotic	Abnormal	Combined NLD obstruction with canalicular obstruction
−	−	−	Blocked	Normal	Complete canalicular obstruction

NLD, nasolacrimal duct.

plete obstruction may be entirely asymptomatic as long as tear production and drainage balance are maintained.

Not every test mentioned here must be performed on each patient with epiphora. In most cases, a relatively simple clinical evaluation in the office will adequately demonstrate the cause of tearing and allow appropriate therapeutic decisions. Some cases, however, will present more difficult diagnostic challenges, particularly those with proximal system anatomic stenosis and physiologic dysfunctions. Here, more elaborate procedures, including radiographic studies, may be required.

In the face of a normal Schirmer test of basic and reflex tear response, the dye disappearance test can be a sensitive, though subjective, indicator of gross drainage. With a normally draining system, fluorescein

TABLE 7.2. Results of primary and secondary Jones tests and probable sites of lacrimal system obstruction.

Jones I	Jones II	Probable site of obstruction
+	+, Dye in nose	Patent system: normal vs. low-grade partial obstruction vs. functional (nonlocalizing)
−	+, Dye in nose	Partial NLD obstruction vs. functional
−	+, Saline in nose	Partial canalicular obstruction vs. functional
−	−, Regurgitation of dye from opposite punctum	Complete NLD obstruction
−	−, Regurgitation of saline from opposite punctum	Complete common canaliculus obstruction
−	−, Regurgitation of dye from same punctum	Complete opposite canalicular obstruction with NLD obstruction
−	−, Regurgitation of saline from same punctum	Complete canalicular obstruction

NLD, nasolacrimal duct.

should be almost gone within 5 minutes. Epiphora attributed to physiologic dysfunction or partial anatomic obstruction will show prolonged presence of dye in the conjunctival sac, whereas epiphora resulting from oversecretion syndrome with normal drainage should yield normal or even rapid disappearance of dye. It is important to realize that the rate of dye clearance through the lacrimal system is strongly influenced by the pressure head from above. Even in the presence of decreased drainage function, a large volume of fluorescein augmented by increased reflex tear secretion from conjunctival irritation may result in an artifactually rapid dye disappearance. It is therefore important to administer this test under conditions as nearly physiologic as possible, with the patient in an upright position, blinking normally, and receiving only one drop of fluorescein.

When the dye disappearance test is abnormal or the history strongly suggests inadequate drainage, the primary Jones dye test is usually performed next. In interpreting the results of this test, it is essential to keep in mind that in up to one-third of asymptomatic individuals, dye will not be recovered in the nose after 5 minutes. It is also important to remember that this test correlates well with the results of the Schirmer test and therefore with the volume of fluorescein placed into the conjunctival sac. Similar to the dye disappearance test, an artifactually positive Jones I test may result from volume overload even when epiphora is present under normal physiologic conditions. Variants of the Jones I test, such as the saccharin taste test, add little, and are difficult to interpret. When the primary Jones dye test is positive, one may conclude that the system is grossly patent, although minor stenoses and physiologic dysfunctions cannot be ruled out. When the test is negative, it is likely that significant anatomic or physiologic pathology exists, but this test alone is not sufficient to document this conclusion.

When the dye disappearance test is prolonged and the primary Jones dye test is negative, the probability of drainage dysfunction is greater than would be indicated by a negative primary Jones dye test alone. The secondary Jones dye test is then performed and, if negative, will demonstrate complete obstruction in the system. The results of the test will indicate the location of the block. When the secondary test is negative and saline irrigated through one punctum causes dye to regurgitate from the opposite punctum, then the dye must be left over from the primary Jones test. If only clear saline regurgitates from the opposite punctum, the block is probably at the common canaliculus. Probing should encounter an obstruction at the distal canaliculus 6–9 mm from the puncta. If an obstruction or stenosis is not found, the test should be repeated with care. However, if there is a lengthy delay between the primary and secondary tests, there may be too little dye remaining in the sac to stain the regurgitating fluid.

When the secondary Jones test is positive, a low-grade partial obstruction or stenosis may be present that can be overcome by increased hydrostatic pressure, or failure of the lacrimal pump mechanism may be responsible for the negative primary Jones test and delayed dye disappearance test. Recovery of clear saline alone in the nose suggests partial canalicular obstruction because no dye entered the sac during the primary test. Appearance of dye-stained saline in the nose demonstrates free flow of fluorescein to the sac during the primary test and therefore an open canalicular system. The partial block is probably present in the distal system at the lower sac or duct. Retrograde flow out of the canaliculi may be seen even with a partially open duct if injection pressures are more than 100 mm Hg. A negative primary Jones test and positive secondary test could also be compatible with intact canalicular capillary action, but with pump failure in propulsion through the lower system.

When hypersecretion syndrome has been ruled out and the dye disappearance test and primary and secondary Jones tests are all negative, a complete anatomic blockage is present somewhere along the nasolacrimal system. The results of the secondary Jones test will usually indicate if the block is proximal, requiring canalicular repair or bypass, or distal enough to be corrected with a dacryocystorhinostomy. If the results are equivocal, and there is a history of trauma, suspicion of tumor, recurrent epiphora after surgery, or persistent chronic dacryocystitis, then radiographic evaluation may be indicated to image the anatomic structure of the system and to pinpoint the site of obstruction. DCG clearly outlines the patent conduit of the lacrimal drainage system, but may not demonstrate low-grade stenoses that are easily opened when the distension technique is used. Variations in normal anatomy include widened or narrowed sac or duct, diverticulum, angulations of the system, or occlusions of one canaliculus, all of which may give false-positive indications of pathology. The test does not easily visualize the canalicular system without intubation distension and subtraction, and gives no information concerning physiologic function. Nevertheless, DCG gives the most reliable anatomic information about the sac and duct. In certain cases, the addition of CT or MRI in conjunction with DCG will add useful information on soft tissue and bony abnormalities within and surrounding the nasolacrimal system that can affect management and aid in planning a surgical approach.

When the primary Jones test is negative and the secondary test is positive, the surgeon must distinguish between physiologic dysfunction and partial anatomic obstruction. In the absence of obvious eyelid or punctal deformity or atonic orbicularis muscle, the problem is likely anatomic, and the secondary Jones test should indicate whether it is proximal or distal. Nevertheless, minor degrees of stenosis and functional failure caused by eyelid laxity, a dilated sac, a diverticulum, or a calculus cannot be differentiated with the above tests. DCG will usually demonstrate the presence of a stenotic segment.

If clinical and radiographic evaluation fails to show an anatomic blockage, physiologic dysfunction is probably responsible for the epiphora. Radionuclide dacryoscintigraphy is indicated here, especially when used with computer interfacing for qualitative evaluation of function. Subtle functional abnormalities may be uncovered, particularly in the proximal system. However, the physiology of lacrimal drainage is poorly understood. The function of Rosenmüller's and Hasner's valves is complex, their competency varies with age, and their patency is influenced by hydrostatic pressure and volume. The results of dacryoscintigraphy are influenced by head position, blinking, and volume overload. A significant number of asymptomatic individuals will show some dysfunction with this test, making interpretation in patients with epiphora more difficult.

In summary, most patients with epiphora can be evaluated adequately with a few relatively simple office procedures. A small number of cases will require more sophisticated studies to confirm the site of anatomic block or region of physiologic dysfunction. With the range of tests available, appropriate medical or surgical management can be determined in the vast majority of patients with tear production and drainage imbalance.

References

1. Vick VL, Holds JB, Hartstein ME, Massry GG. Tarsal strip procedure for the correction of tearing. Ophthal Plast Reconstr Surg 2004;20(1):37–39.
2. Zappia RJ, Milder B. Lacrimal drainage function. 2. The fluorescein dye disappearance test. Am J Ophthalmol 1972;74(1):160–162.
3. Flach A. The fluorescein appearance test for lacrimal obstruction. Ann Ophthalmol 1979;11(2):237–242.
4. Hornblass A. A simple taste test for lacrimal obstruction. Arch Ophthalmol 1973;90(6):435–436.
5. Lipsius EI. Sodium saccharin for testing the patency of the lacrimal passages. Am J Ophthalmol 1957;43(1):114–115.
6. Montanara A, Mannino G, Contestabile M. Macrodacryocystography and echography in diagnosis of disorders of the lacrimal pathways. Surv Ophthalmol 1983;28(1):33–41.
7. Malik SRK, Gupta AK, Chaterjee S, et al. Dacryocystography of normal and pathological lacrimal passages. Br J Ophthalmol 1969;53(3):174–179.
8. Iba GB, Hanafee WN. Distention dacryocystography. Radiology 1968;90(5):1020–1022.
9. Galloway JE, Kavic TA, Raflo GT. Digital subtraction macrodacryocystography. Ophthalmology 1984;91(8):956–962.
10. Ashenhurst M, Jaffer N, Hurwitz JJ, et al. Combined computed tomography and dacryocystography for complex lacrimal problems. Can J Ophthalmol 1991;26(1):27–31.
11. Freitag SK, Woog JJ, Kousoubris PD, et al. Helical computed tomographic dacryocystography with three-dimensional reconstruction: a new view of the lacrimal drainage system. Ophthal Plast Reconstr Surg 2002;18(2):121–132.
12. Karagulle T, Erden A, Erden I, et al. Nasolacrimal system: evaluation with gadolinium-enhanced MR dacryocystography with a three-dimensional fast spoiled gradient recalled technique. Eur Radiol 2002;12(9):2343–2348.
13. Goldberg RA, Heinz GW, Chiu L. Gadolinium magnetic resonance imaging dacryocystography. Am J Ophthalmol 1993;115(6):738–741.
14. Manfre L, de Maria M, Todaro E, et al. MR dacryocystography: comparison with dacryocystography and CT dacryocystography. Am J Neuroradiol 2000;21(6):1145–1150.

15. Kirchhof K, Hahnel S, Jansen O, et al. Gadolinium-enhanced magnetic resonance dacryocystography in patients with epiphora. J Comput Assist Tomogr 2000;24(2):327–331.
16. Rubin PA, Bilyk JR, Shore JW, et al. Magnetic resonance imaging of the lacrimal drainage system. Ophthalmology 1994;101(2):235–243.
17. Rossomondo RM, Carlton WH, Trueblood JH, et al. A new method of evaluating lacrimal drainage. Arch Ophthalmol 1972;88(5):523–525.
18. Carlton WH, Trueblood JH, Rossomondo RM. Clinical evaluation of microscintigraphy of the lacrimal drainage apparatus. J Nucl Med 1973; 14(2):89–92.
19. Wearne MJ, Pitts J, Frank J, et al. Comparison of dacryocystography and lacrimal scintigraphy in the diagnosis of functional nasolacrimal duct obstruction. Br J Ophthalmol 1999;83(9):1032–1035.
20. Amanat LA, Hilditch TE, Kwok CS, et al. Lacrimal scintigraphy. II. Its role in the diagnosis of epiphora. Br J Ophthalmol 1983;67(11):720–728.
21. Hilditch TE, Kwok CS, Amanat LA. Lacrimal scintigraphy. I. Compartmental analysis of data. Br J Ophthalmol 1983;67(11):713–719.
22. Putterman AM. Dacryocystography with occluded common canaliculus. Am J Ophthalmol 1973;76(6):1010–1012.
23. Vettese T, Hurwitz JJ. Toxicity of the chemiluminescent material Cyalume in anatomic assessment of the nasolacrimal system. Can J Ophthalmol 1983;18(3):131–135.
24. Raflo GT, Chart P, Hurwitz JJ. Thermographic evaluation of the human lacrimal drainage system. Ophthalmic Surg 1982;13(2):119–124.

Section 3

Management and Surgical Techniques

8

The Tear-Deficient Patient

Michael A. Lemp

In consideration of the patient presenting with symptoms of tearing, it might seem incongruous to add tear deficiency to a list of diagnostic possibilities. This is, however, an important aspect that must be considered in view of the prevalence of dry eye and the fact that some patients with dry eye can present with subjective symptoms simulating those of obstructive disease of the lacrimal drainage system.

Dry eye is a rubric used to describe a clinical condition caused by a variety of factors resulting in an alteration in the tear film associated with damage to the ocular surface. The term "dry eye" is used along with a number of synonyms for the same condition, also known as keratoconjunctivitis sicca, dry eye syndrome, lacrimal insufficiency state, and dysfunctional tear syndrome. It is characterized either by a decrease in the secretion of the lacrimal glands, an increase in evaporative tear loss, or both. In some cases, there is a hypersecretory response of the lacrimal glands to excessive evaporative tear loss leading to the clinical conclusion that there is no dry eye when, in fact, the clinician is observing a compensatory mechanism which is not associated with obstructive disease of the lacrimal outflow ducts.

Dry eye is an extremely common condition. Recent epidemiologic studies have reported that at least four million and up to perhaps nine million Americans have moderate to severe dry eye. It is estimated that more than 30 million Americans have some form or degree of dry eye. Dry eye is one of the most common conditions encountered in ophthalmic practice yet the diagnostic rate is low because of a relatively low index of suspicion and the lack of a single diagnostic test of high sensitivity and specificity.

The initiating factors in the pathogenesis of dry eye include: an autoimmune state, genetic predisposition, decrease in androgen levels and/or availability of aging glandular atrophy, and changes in apoptotic cellular death in the lacrimal and meibomian glands and the ocular surface. These factors lead to changes in the tear film composition and function which create an unstable tear film and damage to the ocular surface cells. The events operative in the tear film and the ocular surface comprise a zone of interaction in which hyperosmolarity of the tear film occupies a central role. Elevated tear osmolarity is the result of decreased lacrimal fluid secretion, excessive evaporative tear loss, or both. Hyperosmolarity leads to changes in the epithelial cells of the cornea and conjunctiva, initiating an inflammatory cascade. Inflammation of the ocular surface, in turn, causes a down-regulation of the sensory receptors which act as sentinels signaling to increase tear production in response to damage to the ocular surface. In addition, elevated tear osmolarity alters the function of the stabilizing tear mucins and adversely affects the interactions of the lipid layer of the tear film with other tear components, further destabilizing the tear film.

An unstable tear film is characterized by a rapid breakup after a blink. This has an adverse effect on the optical image presented to the retina, causing marked blurring of vision between blinks. This is a subtle finding, usually not well described by the patient and not apparent on standard visual acuity testing. Continued tear instability over a period of time leads to discernible damage to the ocular surface manifest as uptake of vital staining dyes, including fluorescein, rose bengal, and lissamine green. Usually, however, staining of the ocular surface is a late manifestation of dry eye.

Another peculiar feature of dry eye is that there is frequently dissociation between signs and symptoms; symptoms usually precede signs. Ocular discomfort is the hallmark of dry eye. Patients describe the discomfort as dryness, grittiness, stinging, foreign body sensation, sandiness, photophobia, blurred vision, or severe stabbing pain. These different descriptors reflect sensory input from a distressed ocular surface to the central nervous system, where integrative functions interpret the signals based on past experience and comparative sensations, resulting in the verbal choice of descriptor. A common but vague descriptor is that of ocular fatigue. This is probably attributable to an excessive blink rate seen in dry eye as a response to the rapid tear breakup between blinks in an attempt to reestablish a clear visual image.

Classification

In 1995, the Report of the NEI/Industry Workshop on Clinical Trials in Dry Eye produced a classification system for dry eye states (Figure 8.1).[1-3] This system recognizes two major classes of dry eye, an aqueous tear-deficient state and an evaporative dry eye state. There are a number of subtypes of each category such as Sjögren-associated dry eye and non-Sjögren dry eye. It is not completely clear whether these two categories represent distinct entities or rather different loci on a spectrum of severity.

The most common type of evaporative dry eye is that associated with meibomian gland dysfunction (MGD).[4,5] This is an extremely common form of dry eye that frequently coexists with aqueous tear deficiency. Common pathogenetic mechanisms have been identified, including androgen insufficiency. Studies have demonstrated that approximately

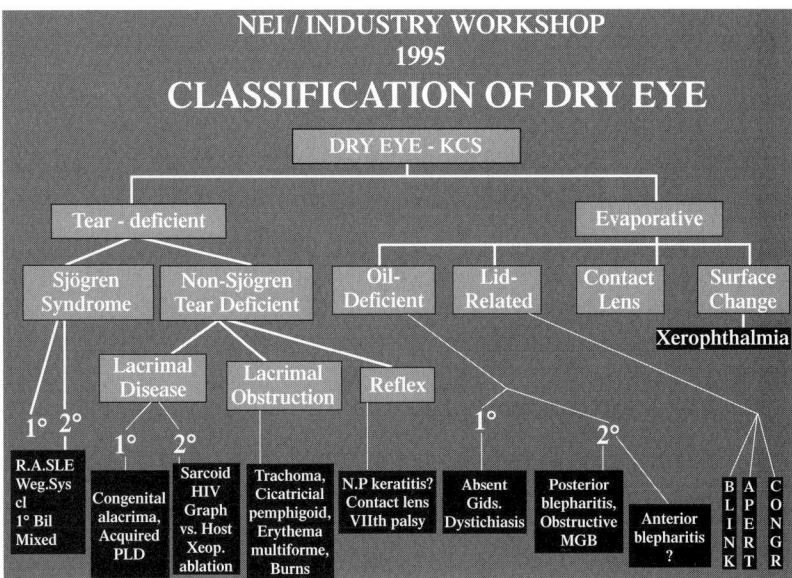

FIGURE 8.1. The National Eye Institute/Industry Classification of Dry Eye. (Adopted from Lemp.[1])

two-thirds of Sjögren's patients have MGD; other studies have shown that about two-thirds of patients presenting to a clinic with ocular irritation show evidence of MGD. This condition affects about 60% of people over the age of 50.

There is, however, not good agreement between signs of MGD and symptoms. Recent reports have identified qualitative changes in the secretion of the meibomian glands in patients with symptomatic MGD in which there is a decrease in two lipids thought to have a role in the anti-evaporative effects of the meibomian-derived outermost lipid layer of the tear film. In normal subjects, approximately 40% of tear volume is lost to evaporation; in MGD, this figure increases to 100%. When lacrimal gland function is still relatively unimpaired, a compensatory increase in aqueous tear secretion can be seen. This can give rise to normal results with Schirmer strip testing but this compensatory lacrimation cannot keep up with marked evaporative tear loss. Damage to the ocular surface results from desiccation, osmotic changes which lead to inflammation, an unstable tear film, and an alteration in the apoptotic cell loss from the surface.

Evaluation of the Possible Tear-Deficient Patient

In addition to the usual clinical examination of the eyelid position and movement and tests of tear drainage, there are several specific tests to determine the secretory state of tears and the health of the ocular surface. The tests described below are suitable for all patients; more extensive tests for patients with more suggestive symptoms and signs

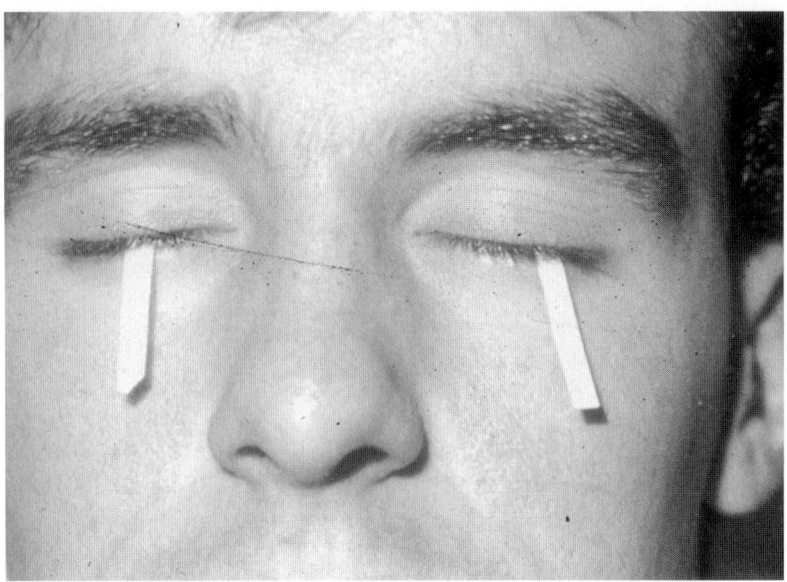

FIGURE 8.2. Schirmer strips in place at the lateral aspects of the lids with the lids closed.

are available and referral to a subspecialist in this area is recommended. The screening tests listed below fall within the scope of the ophthalmic plastic surgeon.

The Schirmer Test

This test (Figure 8.2) uses a special cellulose paper strip which is inserted over the lower lid margin at the junction of the middle and outer thirds. The strip is left in place for 5 minutes and the length of the strip wetted by tears is measured. This test is performed either with or without topical anesthetic in the eye. Anesthetizing the cornea and conjunctiva will result in a lower value but the use of topical drops does not eliminate sensory stimulation from the lashes or lid margins. The author prefers to perform the test without anesthesia and with the eyes closed because this will identify those patients with impaired ability to rapidly and reflexively secrete tears. In the case of the patient presenting with epiphora, however, a case can be made for performing the Schirmer test with anesthesia because this will be more likely to identify patients who are tear-deficient without the sensory input from the ocular surface. Results of Schirmer tests either with or without anesthetic that are 5 mm or less of wetting at 5 minutes (especially if serial testing is consistent) are suggestive of dry eye.

A variant of the Schirmer test is the phenol red test. In this test, a thin thread impregnated with an indicator dye, phenol red, is inserted over the temporal side of the lower lid. The length of the thread that is wetted by tears turns from yellow to bright orange because of exposure of the pH of the tears. After being in place for 15 seconds, it is withdrawn and measured. The test is performed without anesthesia. Whereas this test is widely used in Japan, it has not met with general acceptance in North America.

Ocular Surface Staining

Three vital dyes are in clinical use to detect damage to the ocular surface. A 1% fluorescein solution will stain epithelial disruptions in the cornea. This staining is visualized by shining a cobalt blue light onto the eye. This wavelength excites the fluorescein molecules which turn bluish-green (Figure 8.3). Rose bengal 1% solution (Figure 8.4) and lissamine green 1% are two dyes used to detect disruptions in the conjunctival surface. The former, rose bengal, is a red dye that can be irritating and tends to stain clothes. It stains areas of the conjunctival surface in which the protective mucin layer is missing. Because of concern for the irritative effects of rose bengal, clinical usage is shifting to lissamine green. Whereas rose bengal staining is evident almost immediately after application, lissamine green staining takes about 2 to 3 minutes to become apparent. The staining patterns are similar for both rose bengal and lissamine green. There are various grading systems, but any stain present suggests dry eye and warrants further investigation.

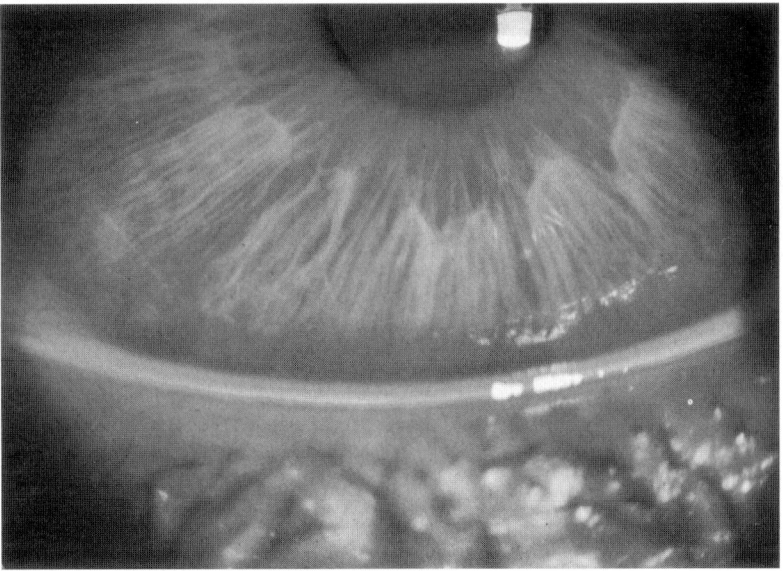

FIGURE 8.3. Marginal tear film stained with fluorescein as seen preparatory to inserting Schirmer strips for a fluorescein dilution test.

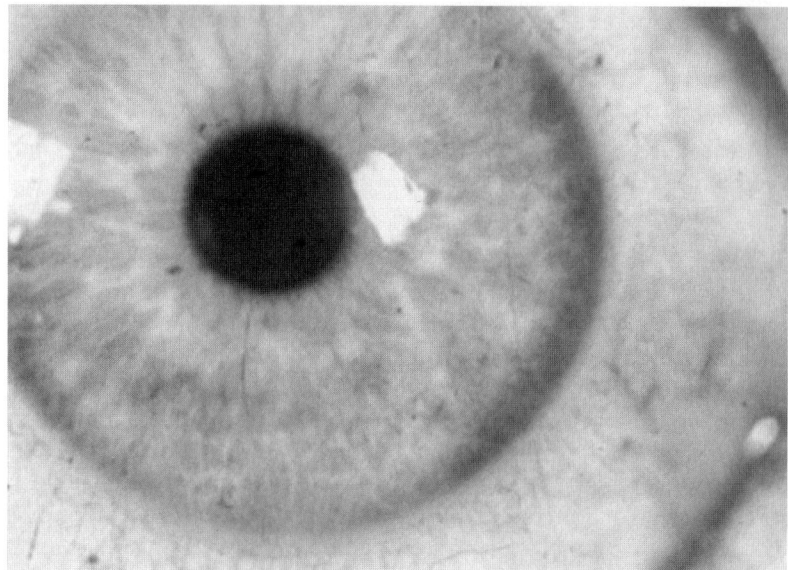

FIGURE 8.4. Rose bengal staining of the conjunctival and corneal surfaces in dry eye. Although staining can be seen on the corneal surface in this photograph, this dye is better visualized on the conjunctiva.

Fluorescein Clearance Test

A small standardized amount of 1% fluorescein solution is instilled into the cul-de-sac. Sequential 1-minute Schirmer tests are performed every 10 minutes. Reduced tear turnover (and thus decreased tear secretion) is demonstrated by persistent staining of the strips with fluorescein at approximately 30 minutes.

Tear Breakup Time

This test of tear film stability is characteristic of all forms of dry eye. A small amount of 1% sodium fluorescein is instilled into the tear film. The patient is asked to blink several times and stare straight ahead. The cobalt blue filter light of the slit lamp is used to scan the ocular surface while the patient keeps the eyes open (Figure 8.5). The time from the last complete blink to the appearance of the first randomly distributed breakup or dry spot is noted and is recorded in seconds. Values of less than 7 seconds are suggestive of dry eye.

MGD is very common (Figure 8.6). Although there is not a general consensus on how to diagnose this condition accurately, the examination must include an inspection of the lid margins, looking for increased vascularity, telangiectasias, and capping of the openings of the glands. These are signs of glandular dysfunction but are also seen as part of a general aging change. Critical to an assessment of glandular function is an assessment of the state of glandular secretion (meibum). By placing the index finger near the margin of the lower lid and applying mild

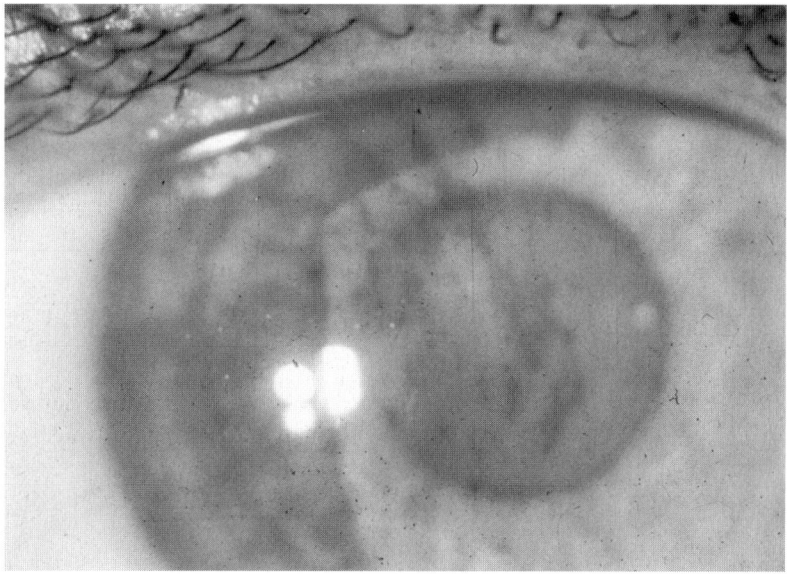

FIGURE 8.5. Dark spots represent breakup of the tear film as seen in standard tear breakup time test.

pressure, it is possible in normal subjects to express a small amount of clear liquid oil from about two-thirds of the glands. In MGD, it is more difficult or impossible to express oil and/or the quality of the oil is changed either to a turbid oil or frankly coagulated secretion with a toothpaste consistency. These changes are pathognomic for MGD.

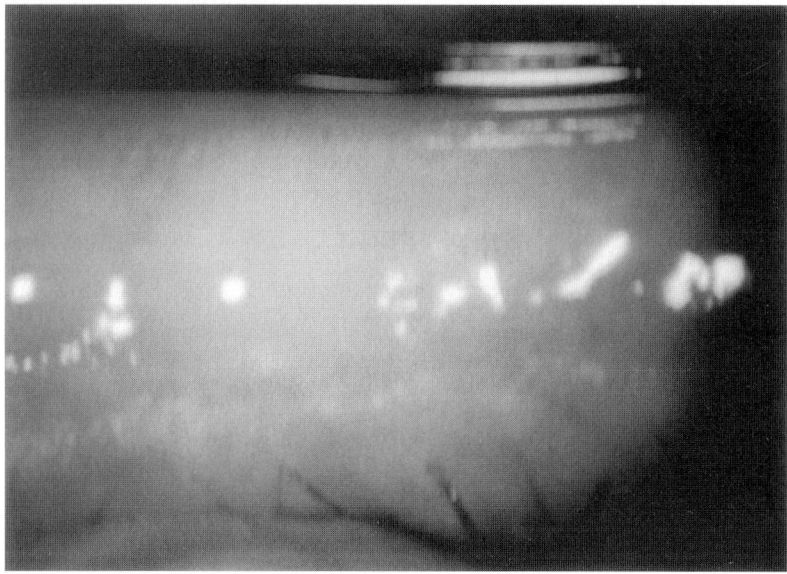

FIGURE 8.6. Turbid secretion of the meibomian glands after expression with finger. This finding is pathognomonic of MGD.

Additional tests are being evaluated for clinical utility. A new computer chip-based test for tear osmolarity, which is a global marker in dry eye, is still in development. The introduction of this test has the potential to render many of the previously described tests obsolete. Another novel approach to the diagnosis of dry eye involves a video-keratography system which records reflected concentric circular images in 1-second intervals. This test measures tear film instability. In this method, a diluted topical anesthetic is instilled and the patient directed to stare into the machine without blinking for 10 seconds. Rapid degradation of the images (in less than 3 seconds) is considered indicative of dry eye. The application of these technologies to general clinical practice is still in development.

In recent years, there has been increased interest in the use of questionnaires as a screening tool for dry eye syndrome. These tests measure symptoms that typically precede standard clinical signs and are probably markers for mild, intermittent dry eye. As mentioned earlier, there are a number of descriptors that patients use to explain their ocular discomfort. Some of these descriptors, such as itching, are not specific for dry eye but overlap with other conditions, such as allergic disease. Nonetheless, several questionnaires have been found to be useful in identifying patients with dry eye. Recent questionnaire design has included measures of quality-of-life attributes.

It is extremely important to make an assessment of tear function before contemplating lid or nasolacrimal surgery. In the latter case, failure to identify a compensatory tearing state will lead to poor results. In the former case, alteration of the lids with a widened interpalpebral fissure can precipitate the onset of a clinically symptomatic dry eye. Whereas the normal subject has several redundant mechanisms in place to assure a continuous flow of tears and normal levels of evaporative loss of tears, the normal structure and function of the lids is essential to maintain this finely regulated process. Patients who exhibit signs and symptoms of tear dysfunction are not equipped to adjust to alterations in the lid position. Surgery can precipitate an acute onset of symptoms ranging from mild ocular discomfort to severe debilitating pain and visual abnormalities. Recognition of predisposing abnormalities in tear function can prevent postoperative surprises for patient and surgeon alike.

The most common postoperative problem encountered after lid surgery is that of a widened interpalpebral fissure. As mentioned, this can greatly increase evaporative tear loss and precipitate the onset of symptoms. Although the magnitude of the increased lid opening might decrease as lid edema subsides and healing continues, early attention to massage of the lids and lid exercises can be of use. Protection of the ocular surface is of paramount importance and will alleviate symptoms.

Management of the Tear-Deficient Patient

Identifying the patient with dry eye and the one at risk for developing dry eye is essential to assure a successful outcome of lid surgery. Attention to the newly diagnosed dry eye patient with appropriate treatment to stabilize the tear film and heal the ocular surface can render patients who would otherwise be at high risk for postoperative problems into good candidates for surgery. In addition, patients experiencing symptoms of dry eye postoperatively will require treatment directed to the same ends.

Patients with severe dry eye and extensive ocular surface disease are poor candidates for elective lid surgery, which will increase the surface area of the exposed ocular surface. Patients who have staining of the cornea and conjunctiva despite intensive treatment; severe decreases in aqueous tear production; and persistent extensive meibomian gland disease are at higher risk for dry eye problems. If there is any doubt, consultation by a specialist is essential.

A standard laddered treatment plan for newly diagnosed cases of dry eye is presented. It is equally applicable to patients presenting with postoperative dry eye symptoms or signs.

First-Line Therapy

The use of an artificial tear product can replace missing aqueous tear volume and give considerable relief. These preparations usually consist of an electrolyte solution with a pH near normal and polymers that thicken the tear film and retard exit through the nasolacrimal ducts. The main limitation of artificial tears is their limited duration of action. Several newer products that have been introduced recently contain unique components that are directed to retarding evaporative tear loss or stabilizing the tear film.

Two products that contain an emulsion of oil in an aqueous carrier are thought to form a strengthened lipid layer covering the tears, thus retarding evaporative tear loss. Refresh Endura (Allergan) contains a microemulsion of castor oil and Soothe (Alimera Sciences) contains a metastable mineral oil emulsion. A different theory describes the action of Systane (Alcon) which contains HP guar and gum product with unusual gel-forming properties. When this solution encounters the pH of the tear film, it forms a gel and serves to create a more stable tear film with a longer-acting effect. The lipid-containing and gel-containing products should help to stabilize the tear film. They are available over-the-counter without a prescription.

Second-Line Therapy

Punctum Plugs

When treatment with artificial tear preparations is insufficient to ameliorate symptoms and restore ocular surface health, the next step is often to insert plugs into the canalicular spaces to prevent loss of tears through drainage. There are two major types of punctal plugs in use for the treatment of dry eye: absorbable and nonabsorbable. Absorbable plugs are made of collagen or synthetic material; they are intended for temporary use to determine whether punctal occlusion will improve symptoms or to manage a short-term condition. They are inserted into the puncta and will usually dissolve over several days.

In contrast, nonabsorbable plugs are composed of silicone or acrylic materials. These devices are intended for longer-duration treatment.

They vary in size and design but are intended to reside either within the canalicular passage or, in some cases, to migrate further down the nasolacrimal passage. By blocking the normal tear drainage, the tear film is thickened and improvement in signs and symptoms is frequently seen. These devices are in widespread use. They have been found to be of value in treating both temporary and long-term dry eye problems. Complications include occasional extrusion of the device, unwanted internal migration, epiphora, and infection associated with biofilm formation. Some of the newer designs can migrate further into the nasolacrimal duct. If necessary, removal can be challenging. A caveat to the use of plugs is the observation that in patients with clinically discernible inflammation of the ocular surface, the condition may actually worsen. Blocking the normal tear drainage reduces tear turnover, exposing the ocular surface to prolonged contact with proinflammatory cytokines in the tears and exacerbating inflammation of the surface.

Punctal plugs serve as a useful treatment for many patients with dry eye and are particularly useful in dry eye situations that may be temporary, such as postoperative periods.

Therapeutic Drugs
The first Food and Drug Administration–approved agent designed to treat underlying pathogenetic disease processes in dry eye is Restasis (Allergan). This formulation contains cyclosporin A 0.05% suspension, an immunomodulator, and anti-inflammatory agent. It is thought to suppress inflammation, thereby allowing healing of damaged glandular structures. It is instilled into the eye twice daily and improvement in signs and symptoms is typically expected within weeks to months. This delay in clinically apparent results reflects the time necessary for reparative processes to occur. Concomitant treatment with artificial tears and in some cases faster-acting anti-inflammatory medications is becoming common practice. In addition, there are a number of other therapeutic agents in varying stages of clinical development including mucin stimulants, other immunomodulating agents, topical androgen medications, and lacrimal gland stimulants. It is hoped that our clinical armamentarium will be substantially augmented in the next few years.

In severe cases of dry eye with extensive damage to the ocular surface that are unresponsive to treatment as outlined above, more stringent treatment modalities should be considered.

Autologous Serum
One technique uses autologous serum, in which the patient's own serum is collected, stored, and used as an eye drop. This treatment is inconvenient to implement and has an inherent risk of infection. However, it can be very helpful in managing severe cases.

Lateral Tarsorrhaphy
Another useful treatment in the management of severe ocular surface damage in dry eye is the use of a lateral tarsorrhaphy. The immobilization of the upper lid decreases abrasive lid forces. The continual apposition of the upper tarsal conjunctival surface to the damaged ocular surface allows for the diffusion of serum factors that supply many of

the nutritive components lacking in the tears of dry eye patients. A tarsorrhaphy can prove decisive in healing many patients with serious sight-threatening ocular surface damage. It has been noted that incomplete tarsorrhaphies (which do not completely close the lids) result in better clinical outcomes than complete tarsorrhaphies. It is hypothesized that the presence of an opening between the lids provides access to higher oxygen concentration than that available from the inner surface of the lids. The opening, moreover, affords a view of the ocular surface for clinical assessment.

In summary, dry eye is a common disease. Most cases are relatively mild and non–sight-threatening, and can be effectively managed. Attention to identifying patients at risk for developing clinically significant dry eye before surgery of the lids or nasolacrimal ducts can avoid unpleasant postoperative surprises for patient and surgeon alike. Postoperative management of dry eye symptoms can alleviate discomfort, improve vision, and improve the quality of life for patients.

References

1. Lemp M. Report of the National Eye Institute/Industry Workshop on Clinical Trials in Dry Eyes. CLAO J 1995;21:221–232.
2. Schaumberg DA, Sullivan DA, Dana MR. Epidemiology of dry eye syndrome. Adv Exp Med Biol 2002;506(pt B):989–998.
3. Stern ME, Beuerman RW, Fox RI, et al. The pathology of dry eye: the interaction between the ocular surface and lacrimal glands. Cornea 1998;17:584–589.
4. Stern ME, Pflugfelder SC. Inflammation in dry eye. Ocul Surf 2004;2:124–130.
5. Bron AJ, Tiffany JM. The contribution of meibomian dysfunction to dry eye. Ocul Surf 2004;2:149–164.

9

Surgery of the Punctum and Canaliculus

Jennifer S. Landy, Charles B. Slonim, and Jay Justin Older

Some diseases of the punctum and canaliculus can be treated medically, but many require surgical intervention. In this chapter, different surgical techniques involving the punctum and canaliculus are reviewed.[1-7]

Dilation, Probing, and Intubation

The lacrimal drainage system can be obstructed anywhere along its pathway. An obstruction can range from partial blockage or stenosis to complete atresia or anatomic absence of a structure. The anatomic details of the lacrimal system have been described in Chapter 1.

The most common indication for lacrimal probing is epiphora. Probing in children with congenital nasolacrimal obstruction is a delicate procedure. Probing can be performed in an office setting; however, the majority of ophthalmologists perform pediatric nasolacrimal probings in an ambulatory surgery setting with heavy sedation or general anesthesia. Adults can be probed in the office with only topical anesthesia and, occasionally, with a small amount of local or regional anesthetic blocks.

In preparation for the probing, a nasal decongestant/vasoconstrictor (e.g., oxymetazoline or 2.5% phenylephrine) should be placed in the nostril on the side of the probing. This can be accomplished by placing presoaked neurosurgical cottonoids or cotton-tipped applicators in the nose under the inferior turbinate in the region of the valve of Hasner. The surgeon allows a few minutes for the nasal mucosa to shrink. If the procedure is done in the office, a topical anesthetic drop should be instilled in the eye before probing. When attempting to probe, the surgeon should remember that the upper system begins vertically at each punctum followed by a 2-mm dilated vertical segment (the ampulla) followed by an 8-mm horizontal segment (the canaliculus).

Dilation

Punctal dilation can be performed first in order to safely introduce a lacrimal probe. The smallest-tipped punctal dilator is placed vertically for the 2-mm distance and is turned horizontally. The dilator is gently pushed medially to dilate the punctum. Too much force can cause a mucosal tear in the ampulla or the canaliculus.

Probing

A small Bowman probe, preferably a number "00" or "0," is inserted into the inferior or superior punctum. The probe is passed 2 mm vertically then medially and slightly superiorly while countertraction is held on the lid. Once the surgeon reaches the lacrimal sac, the lacrimal bone or a "hard stop" will be felt through the mucosa. The probe is rotated so that the tip points inferiorly, slightly laterally and slightly posteriorly before entering the nasolacrimal duct. To obtain proper orientation, the surgeon can align the top of the probe with the supraorbital notch or supraorbital foramen. The surgeon should avoid using significant force, although some resistance may be encountered. Use of excessive force could result in creation of a false passage. Resistance is typically encountered as the probe passes into the bony canal, and at the distal end of the duct as it passes through the obstructed valve of Hasner or rubs against the inferior turbinate. In children, the distance between the punctum and the floor of the nose is 20–25 mm and in adults it is 30–35 mm.

While inserting a nasal speculum into the nose, the surgeon directs a larger Bowman probe laterally under the inferior turbinate until the two probes touch and "metal-on-metal" is felt or heard. If there is difficulty identifying the lacrimal probe under the inferior turbinate, the inferior turbinate can be infractured using a periosteal elevator. When the procedure has been completed, fluorescein-tinted saline should be irrigated through the canaliculus and recovered from the nose using a suction tip to confirm patency of the system.

Intubation

Silicone intubation is used to provide a stent through the lacrimal apparatus in order to maintain patency. The stent is typically left in place for a predetermined amount of time. It is frequently performed in children who have had repeated probings. Other uses for silicone intubation are in primary cases in older children more than 12 months of age or when significant strictures are noted during primary probing. There are a number of commercially available silicone intubation systems.

The Crawford tubes have an olive-shaped tip on the ends of their two stainless steel probes to which the silicone tubing is attached. The tip is engaged by a retrieval hook and pulled out through the nose. The Crawford tubing is factory glued to metal probes and should not pull apart during intubation. The Crawford tubing sets come with and without an intraluminal 8-0 silk suture for tying the ends of the silicone tubing together.

The Ritleng probe is fashioned with a Prolene thread that lies between the silicone tube and a probe that is similarly engaged with a hook and pulled through the nose. There are a few probes (e.g., Guibor, Quickert-Dryden) that are removed from the nose either with the use of a grooved director or using a long narrow hemostat under direct visualization. These probes are either attached to or lie within the silicone tubing.

Retrieval of the metal probe from the nose can be aided by bending the probe 15 degrees at its distal third. The probe can be lubricated with an antibiotic ophthalmic ointment and passed vertically through the lower punctum into the lower canalicular system. The lower lid is pulled to avoid kinking of the canaliculus, and the probe is rotated 90 degrees so that it is in the horizontal plane. It is advanced nasally until it enters the lacrimal sac and the lacrimal bone and fossa are encountered. It is rotated 90 degrees vertically, angled 15 degrees posteriorly, and advanced down the nasolacrimal duct. The probe exits from under the inferior turbinate usually at the junction of the anterior and middle thirds of the undersurface of the turbinate. A retrieval hook is inserted laterally under the inferior turbinate with the hook tip preferably oriented vertically.

When metal-on-metal is heard or felt, the hook is rotated against the probe to engage the olive tip, if using the Crawford tubes. The probe is slowly retracted until the hook and olive tip are engaged. The hook is used to pull the probe out of the nose. After successful intubation of both canaliculi, the metal probes are removed from the ends of the tube and the silicone tubing is tied together in multiple knots to secure the silicone tube as a single loop within the nose. The tube can then be anchored to the lateral mucocutaneous junction inside the ala using a 6-0 Prolene suture (Ethicon, Somerville, NJ) or left unattached.

Punctoplasty

The most common condition requiring punctoplasty is punctal stenosis. A one-snip punctoplasty is successful in the majority of cases. Topical anesthesia (e.g., 4% lidocaine, tetracaine, proparacaine) on a cotton-tipped applicator applied directly to the punctum, or a local injection with 2% lidocaine infiltrated near the punctum can be used to obtain anesthesia. In cases where there is complete punctal stenosis or atresia, a sharp probe or needle may be used to initiate a small opening. This small opening should then be dilated and a lacrimal probe passed to assure a connection to the lumen of the canaliculus. In cases without complete stenosis, the punctum should also be dilated with a punctal dilator.

The punctum is secured by gently grasping the lid margin just lateral to the punctum with toothed forceps. Using Westcott scissors, the surgeon completes a one-snip punctoplasty on the posterior surface of the ampulla. The scissors are held perpendicular to the lid margin with one blade of the scissors inserted into the dilated punctum and ampulla while the other blade is left outside the ampulla on the conjunctival surface. A single vertical snip approximately

2–3mm long is made along the conjunctival surface in the vertical canaliculus. Once this is performed, gentle redilation of the puncto-plasty with a lubricated dilator will help ensure healing in a patent position.

Two-snip and three-snip punctoplasty procedures have been des-cribed. In the two-snip procedure, two connecting strips are made along the conjunctival side of the punctum and a triangular wedge is excised. This procedure, however, offers little advantage over the one-snip procedure. Three-snip procedures are advocated less often because of their potential for destruction to the lacrimal outflow appa-ratus. Essentially, two vertical snips are made along the punctum with a third horizontal snip connecting the two vertical snips at their base.

If stenosis recurs after punctoplasty, a repeat one-snip punctoplasty should be combined with silicone intubation.

Punctal Ectropion

Repairs of involutional, noncicatricial, punctal ectropia are performed to rotate the punctum posteriorly into the lacrimal lake. Local anesthe-sia, composed of 2% lidocaine with epinephrine 1:100,000 injected transconjunctivally into the medial aspect of the lower lid both lateral and inferior to the punctum, is required. Subcutaneous injection on the anterior surface of the ampulla is recommended. With the lower lid retracted outward, the conjunctiva is dried with a cotton-tipped applicator and a diamond pattern is marked with the apex 3–4mm below the punctum, measuring 4mm vertically and 6–8mm horizon-tally. To protect the canaliculus, a lacrimal probe can be inserted. The conjunctiva and subconjunctival tissue are excised. Double-armed 5-0 absorbable sutures are used to close the defect. The first needle is passed through conjunctiva and deep tissue above the spindle, exiting within the wound. The needle is then regrasped and passed full-thickness through the center of the wound and out through the skin. The other suture is then passed in a similar manner but through the lower edge of the wound. A single stitch is all that is required, although more sutures can be used, depending on the horizontal length of the spindle. As the sutures are tied externally on the skin without bolsters, the punctum should turn in toward the globe.

Canalicular Surgery

Lacerations

In canalicular lacerations, repair of a lacerated lower canaliculus is imperative for the prevention of chronic posttraumatic epiphora. The repair of upper canalicular lacerations, although not as critical for the prevention of posttraumatic epiphora, should be performed, if possible. Repair should be performed within the first 24–48 hours after injury, preferably within the first 24 hours. Regional blocks (e.g., infraorbital

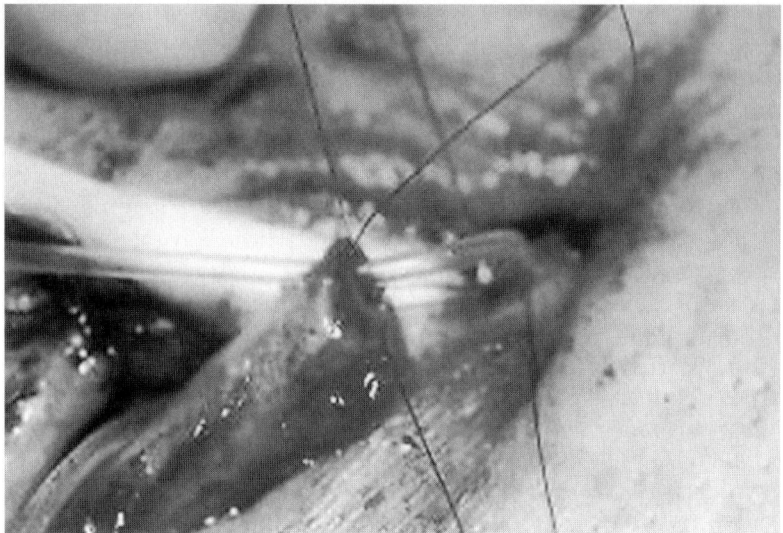

FIGURE 9.1. Repair of a lid margin laceration involving the canaliculus.

or infratrochlear) can offer superior anesthesia without distortion of the traumatized tissues.

If possible, canalicular lacerations should be probed before repair in the operating room to assure disruption of the lacrimal apparatus. Tetanus immune status should be achieved and treated appropriately. Preoperative treatment with intravenous antibiotics for contaminated wounds should be considered. The nose should be prepared for possible intubation by decongesting it with topical phenylephrine or other nasal decongestants (e.g., oxymetazoline). If general anesthesia is not given, the nasal mucosa should be anesthetized (e.g., topical lidocaine or cocaine). The surgeon must thoroughly irrigate the wound. Internal splinting of the canaliculus is mandatory to repair the laceration, and there are several materials that may be used successfully. End-to-end anastomosis of the canaliculi can be achieved using two or three 7-0 or 8-0 absorbable sutures placed equidistant around the wound edges (Figure 9.1).

Many methods and a variety of materials have been described for stenting a lacerated canaliculus (e.g., metal rods, polyethylene tubes, absorbable sutures, etc.). When silicone stents were introduced, they rapidly became the material of choice.

Monocanalicular Intubation

Monocanalicular stenting can be accomplished using the Mini Monoka (FCI Ophthalmics, Marshfield Hills, MA) monocanalicular intubation set. This hollow silicone tubing (40 mm) is attached to a patent silicone plug. Once in place, it offers a pathway for escape of tears while the repaired laceration heals. When a monocanalicular stent is used, the opposing canaliculus does not have to be violated and usually the nose does not need to be entered.

The surgeon passes the Mini Monoka stent through the punctum and distal canaliculus into the laceration and then pushes it into the proximal end of the canaliculus and the nasolacrimal canal. The pericanalicular tissue is then reapproximated using interrupted 7-0 absorbable sutures (e.g., Vicryl or chromic sutures), one inferior and one superior to the canaliculus if there is minimal tension on the wound. In cases in which significant tension exists, 5-0 Vicryl or chromic gut should be used to close the deep subcutaneous tissue first.

Before closing the deep tissue, the medial canthal tendon should be evaluated and, if the tendon is involved in the laceration, 5-0 Vicryl suture on a small half-circle needle (P-2) should be used to reapproximate it to the periosteum above the lacrimal crest. If both ends of the cut tendon are visible, it can be attached to itself. The distal end of the stent with the cap is designed to fit snugly into the punctum and ampulla and no stitch should be required (Figure 9.2). The stent is left in place for several weeks while the canaliculus heals. Although the Mini Monoka is the authors' preferred stent, standard silicone tubing can be used. The distal end of the tubing is tied into a knot to prevent it from slipping into the canaliculus and sutured to the eyelid skin near the lash line.

Bicanalicular stenting can be used to repair monocanalicular lacerations. This is useful when the laceration involves the papilla or ampulla. Because the authors have had such good results with the Mini Monoka monocanalicular stent, they reserve bicanalicular stenting for bicanalicular lacerations.

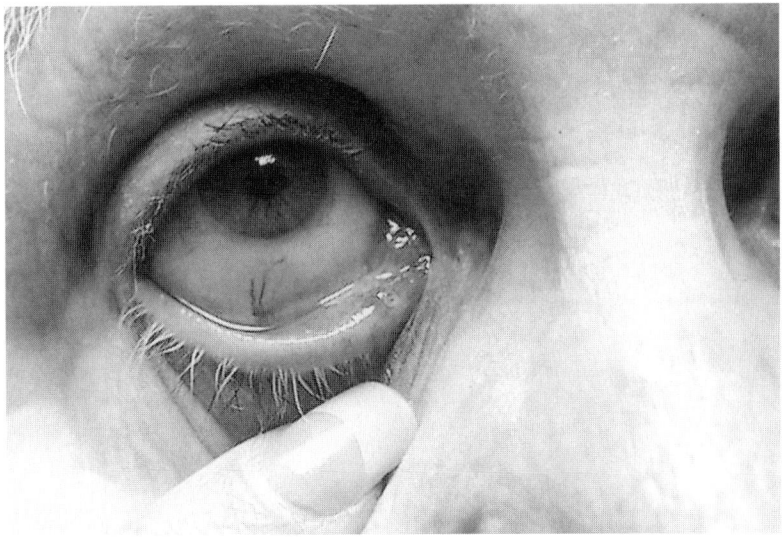

FIGURE 9.2. Well-seated Mini Monoka flange in right lower eyelid punctum.

Bicanalicular Intubation

There are a variety of bicanalicular lacrimal intubation systems [e.g., Crawford, Ritleng FCI Ophthalmics (Marshfield Hills, MA), BD Visitec (Franklin Lakes, NJ)]. Each contains a length of silicone tubing that is fixed to rigid or semirigid probes, one at each end of the tubing. Most have a retrieval instrument (e.g., hook or guide) that is used to remove the tubing from the nose.

Once the distal and proximal ends of the lacerated canaliculus are found, one probe is inserted through the punctum, into the wound, and out the distal end of the lacerated canaliculus. The tissue around the proximal end of the lacerated canaliculus is gently supported while providing countertraction; the same probe is continued through the open end of the proximal canaliculus. The probe is directed in the usual manner through the nasolacrimal sac and canal and into the nose. The appropriate retrieval instrument is used to remove the probe from the nose. The canaliculus is repaired over the tubing as described above (Figures 9.3 and 9.4). The same process is repeated for the opposite canaliculus.

The silicone tubing is tied to itself with multiple knots once the Crawford probes are removed. The silicone tubing can be anchored to the mucocutaneous junction inside the lateral nasal wall with 6-0 Prolene suture. If a combined upper and lower canalicular laceration is present that cannot be reanastomosed or if the medial end of the canaliculus is too damaged to allow identification, a standard dacryocystorhinostomy dissection can then be executed opening the

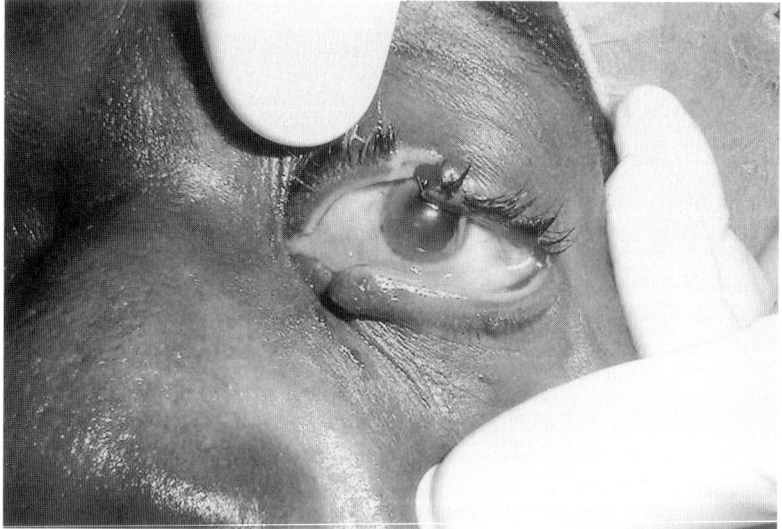

FIGURE 9.3. Upper and lower eyelid lacerations involving the left lower eyelid canaliculus.

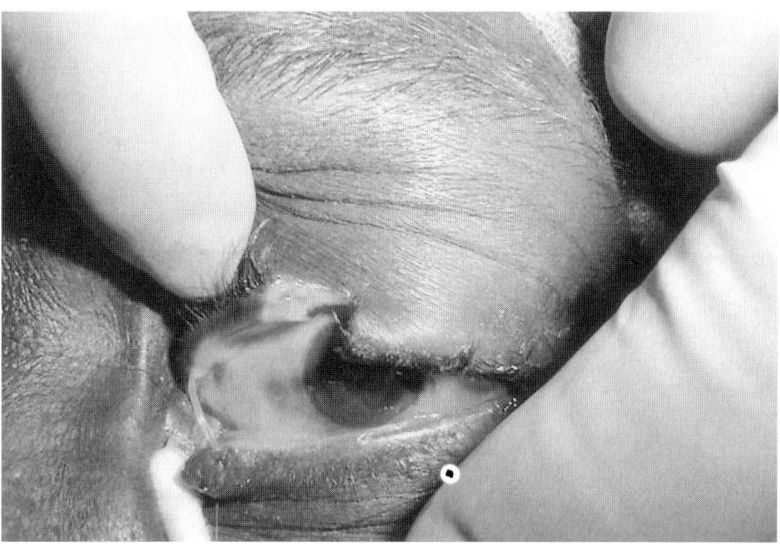

FIGURE 9.4. Same patient in Figure 9.3 after bicanalicular intubation.

lacrimal sac vertically. The lacrimal probes can then be guided into the lacrimal sac through the soft tissue after the common internal punctum has been enlarged. An absorbable 5-0 suture (e.g., Vicryl or chromic) is used to close the sac and the skin is closed in the standard manner. If this is not possible and the extent of the damage is too great or appears irreparable, it is acceptable to repair the laceration and return at a later date for Jones tube placement or a standard dacryocystorhinostomy.

Canaliculotomy

The most common organism responsible for causing canaliculitis is *Actinomyces israelii*. Concretions, which may be up to 5 mm in diameter, develop in the canaliculus (Figure 9.5). Several methods of treatment are available. The least invasive is removal of the stones with a 2-mm curette through a dilated punctum. If that is not sufficient, the surgeon may make a horizontal incision through the posterior lid, curette out the stones, and repair the wound.

Our preferred method is to pass a probe into the canaliculus and make a horizontal incision through the skin to open the canaliculus and expose the probe. The incision should begin about 2 mm medial to the ampulla and be about 8 mm in length. Once the canaliculus is opened, the probe is removed and the stones are extracted with a small curette. The canaliculus may be irrigated with antibiotic solution. A silicone tubing stent such as a Mini Monoka is passed into the canaliculus and the wound is closed with small absorbable sutures. The tube is removed in a few weeks.

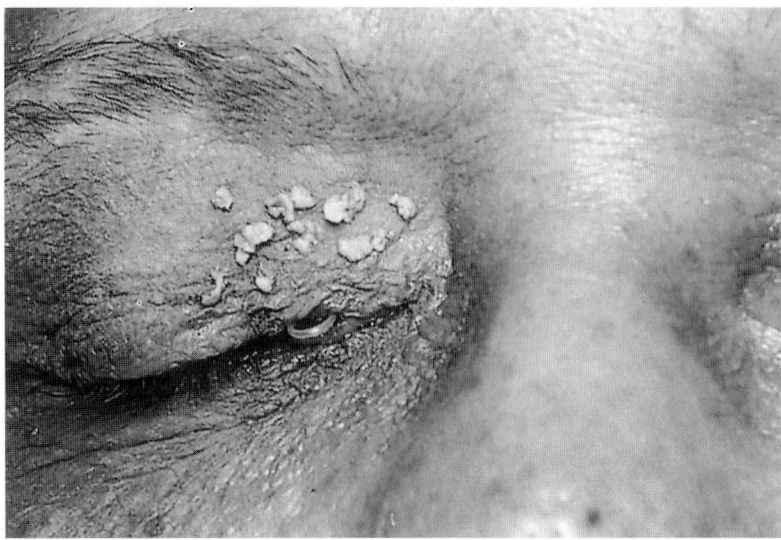

FIGURE 9.5. Canalicular concretions secondary to a canaliculitis.

References

1. Tanenbaum M, McCord CD Jr. The lacrimal drainage system. In: Duane TD, ed. Clinical Ophthalmology. Vol 4. Philadelphia: JB Lippincott; 1992:1–33.
2. Katowitz JA. Lacrimal drainage surgery. In: Duane TD, ed. Clinical Ophthalmology. Vol 5. Philadelphia: JB Lippincott; 1992:1–32.
3. Hirschbein MJ, Stasior GO. Lacrimal system. In: Chen WP, ed. Oculoplastic Surgery: The Essentials. Stuttgart: Thieme; 2001:253–288.
4. Dutton JJ. Orbit and oculoplastics. In: Yanoff M, Duker JS, eds. Ophthalmology. London; 1999:71.1–717.8.
5. Kanski JJ. Disorders of the lacrimal drainage system. In: Kanski JJ, ed. Clinical Ophthalmology. Oxford; 1999:44–54.
6. The Foundation of the American Academy of Ophthalmology. Anatomy and physiology. In: The Foundation of the American Academy of Ophthalmology: Basic and Clinical Science Course 2001–2002 – Orbit, Eyelids, and Lacrimal System. The Foundation of the American Academy of Ophthalmology; 2001:224–230.
7. The Foundation of the American Academy of Ophthalmology. Evaluation and management of the tearing patient. In: The Foundation of the American Academy of Ophthalmology: Basic and Clinical Science Course 2001–2002 – Orbit, Eyelids, and Lacrimal System. The Foundation of the American Academy of Ophthalmology; 2001:231–255.

10

Lacrimal Trauma

Harry Marshak and Steven C. Dresner

Canalicular lacerations are common after blunt trauma to the periorbital region. The tissue surrounding the canaliculi is relatively fragile, as the tarsal plate ends at the punctum, leaving only soft tissue for medial canthal area support. Lacerations from blunt trauma likely result from lateral traction of the eyelid during trauma.[1] The most common mechanism for canalicular laceration is blunt trauma from a fist punch, which accounts for 23% of such injuries.[2] Dog bites account for 19% of canalicular lacerations[3] and are the most common cause of these lacerations in children.[2] Concomitant medial canthal tendon injury has been reported to occur in 36% of insults resulting in canalicular lacerations.[4]

Canalicular lacerations should be repaired within 72 hours to ensure the best possible outcome. Surgery usually involves placement of a stent to assist in apposition of the canalicular edges. If a medial eyelid and canalicular laceration is repaired without placement of a stent, the canaliculus will likely scar closed. Late repair is difficult, and patients often require conjunctivodacryocystorhinostomy (CDCR) to resolve their tearing problem.

Lacerations of the inferior canaliculus occur more frequently than the superior canaliculus. One study used meta-analysis to determine that in patients with canalicular lacerations, 72% were inferior and 16% were superior. Twelve percent of patients had both superior and inferior canalicular lacerarations.[3]

Examination

A thorough ophthalmic examination should be performed in all cases of suspected eyelid and canalicular lacerations (Figure 10.1). Ruptured globe and other sequelae secondary to ocular trauma should be addressed immediately. The eyelids should be examined for lacerations. If an injury lies medial to or involves the punctum, a canalicular laceration must be suspected.

To inspect an eyelid with suspected canalicular laceration, the surgeon should manually inspect tissue with suspected injury. Often,

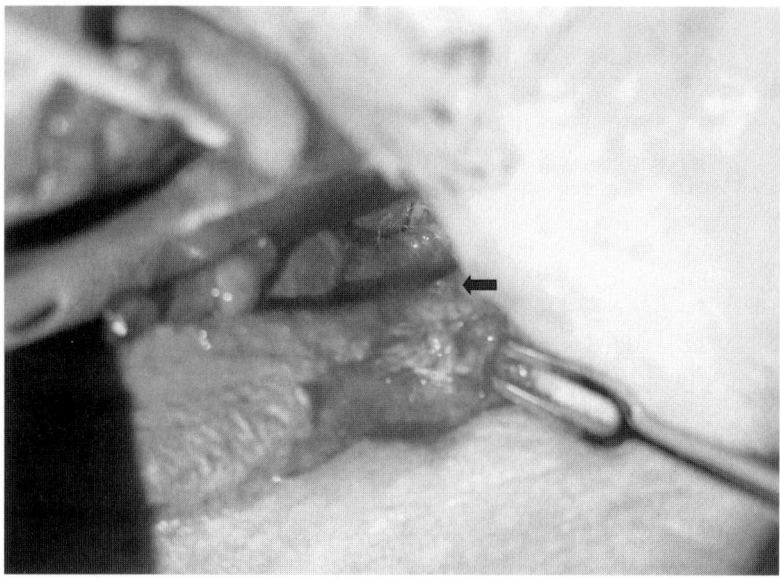

FIGURE 10.1. Canalicular laceration. Medial cut edge is visible (arrow).

an area that appears to have superficial abrasions is determined to have deeper injury. The eyelids should be everted. In unusual circumstances, injury can include the conjunctival surface or a small section of the lid margin, leaving the skin completely intact.

To inspect the canaliculus, the punctum is dilated and a size 0 Bowman probe is passed through the canaliculus until a hard stop is felt at the nose. If complete passage is not accomplished, the suspicion for a canalicular laceration should be high and the eyelid must be meticulously inspected to visualize the probe within the wound. If the probe is not seen, it should be removed. An irrigating cannula should be placed in the proximal canaliculus and gentle irrigation should be performed. Flow of irrigation solution out of the eyelid through the wound confirms the presence of a laceration. The same procedure should be performed for both upper and lower canaliculi.

Dog bites to the face have a propensity to involve the medial canthus and canalicular system. Canine-induced injuries often result in deep facial lacerations without soft-tissue loss.[5] Patients with this type of injury should receive a broad-spectrum antibiotic intravenously and a tetanus toxin injection if indicated. The wound must be irrigated profusely before surgical repair.

Surgical Technique

The traditional method for repair of mono- or bicanalicular lacerations involves repair of the eyelid defect after placement of a bicanalicular stent. This usually entails a procedure in the operating room, using intravenous sedation or general anesthesia. The introduction of mono-canalicular stents has allowed repair of simple monocanalicular lacerations that do not involve the punctum with only local anesthesia, without the need for intranasal manipulation and sedation. Most of these repairs can now be performed in the office, reducing the need for surgery in the operating room.

The most difficult part of canalicular repair is locating the medial end of the severed canaliculus. Under magnification, the edge of a canaliculus appears as a white, glistening ring surrounded by the medial canthal tissue usually posterior to the canthus. As a rule, in more medial lacerations, the distal canaliculus is more difficult to detect. The surgeon should remember that the canaliculus normally progresses posteriorly and further from the skin surface. In other words, the more medial the laceration, the more posterior the cut edges will be. With monocanalicular lacerations, if the cut edge cannot be found, the surgeon may slowly inject viscous lidocaine mixed with methylene blue through the intact canaliculus and observe for reflux from the distal cut end (Figure 10.2).

Choice of Stent

Bicanalicular intubation is the gold standard for mono- or bicanalicular lacerations. This tube creates a "closed loop" system that is unlikely to become dislodged. Placement does, however, require local anesthesia (intranasal packing with topical anesthesia or infiltration with lido-

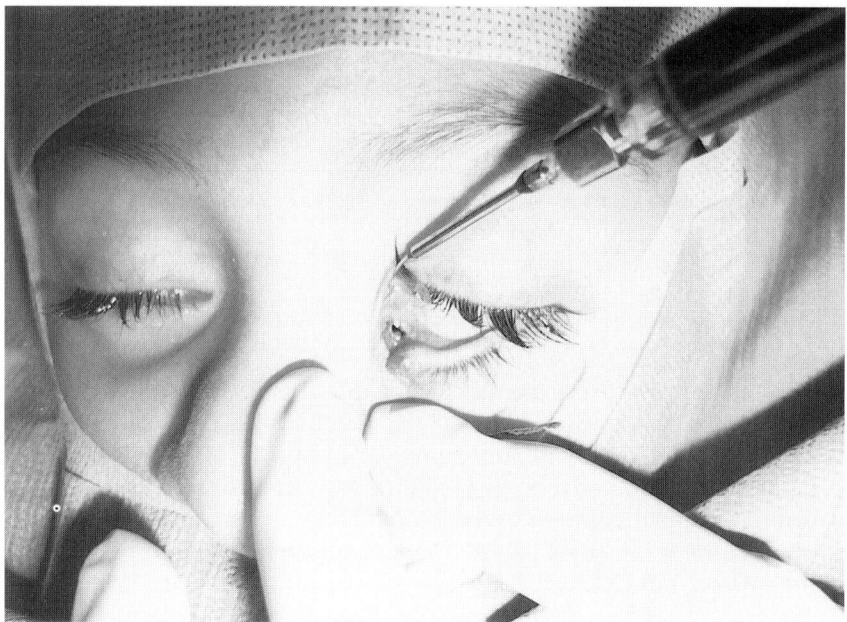

FIGURE 10.2. Technique for finding cut edge of canaliculus. Viscous lidocaine with methylene blue is injected through superior canaliculus. Blue dye shows medial cut edge of inferior canaliculus.

caine with epinephrine) along with intravenous sedation, or general anesthesia.

The main attribute of a monocanalicular stent is it allows for placement under local anesthesia alone or in conjunction with monitored anesthesia care. However, these stents are less secure compared with the bicanalicular type and can be dislodged in children quite easily. Punctal injury precludes the use of a monocanalicular stent.

Bicanalicular Repair

Bicanalicular stent trocars are passed through each punctum and proximal canaliculus (Figure 10.3A–C). Each end is then gently passed into the distal canaliculus and advanced until a hard stop is felt at the nasal bone. The stent is then rotated vertically along the brow and passed into the nasolacrimal duct and nose. An appropriate retrieval device is then used to remove the tubes from under the inferior turbinate.

The authors' preferred stent is a Crawford tube. Once both ends of the stent are brought out through the nose, the tubes should be placed on gentle traction and clamped with a small hemostat at the level of the nostril. This allows the tubes to provide traction on the canthal wound to aid in anatomic reapproximation. If the medial canthal tendon has been avulsed, it is closed by passing a 5-0 polyglactin (Vicryl) suture, preferably on a P-2 needle, through the periosteum of the medial wall and then through the canthal tendon, superior and inferior to the canaliculi. If the punctum is lacerated, it is sutured closed around the stent with 7-0 Vicryl sutures. The pericanalicular orbicularis muscle is reapproximated using a single 7-0 Vicryl mattress suture.[6,7] The medial canthal sutures are then tied. The wound is closed with 6-0 Vicryl deep sutures. The skin is closed with 6-0 gut sutures.

The ends of the tube can be tied in a square knot or can be tied together with an absorbable, long-lasting suture such as polydioxanone. If the tube is not tied, it will likely become dislodged within a few days. The stent is sutured to the lateral wall of the nose at the mucocutaneous junction with a 5-0 Vicryl suture in adults (or 6-0 Vicryl in children). This suture will dissolve by the time the tubes are removed in approximately 6 weeks.

To remove the tube, a drop of topical anesthetic is placed in the eye. The tube is grasped with forceps and elevated approximately 5 mm. Scissors are used to cut the tube, while the surgeon holds the tube with the forceps in the other hand. If the tube is released, both ends can retract into the canaliculi and complicate removal. After a monocanalicular laceration, the tube and knot can be removed from the opposite, uninjured canaliculus, to prevent reinjury. For example, if the superior canaliculus was injured, the surgeon should remove the tube through the inferior canaliculus. The surgeon grasps the tube with forceps and cuts the tube above the forceps. The tube can be gently removed with a single pulling motion.

The tubes can also be removed through the nose. The surgeon can cut the tubes between the puncta and ask the patient to forcefully

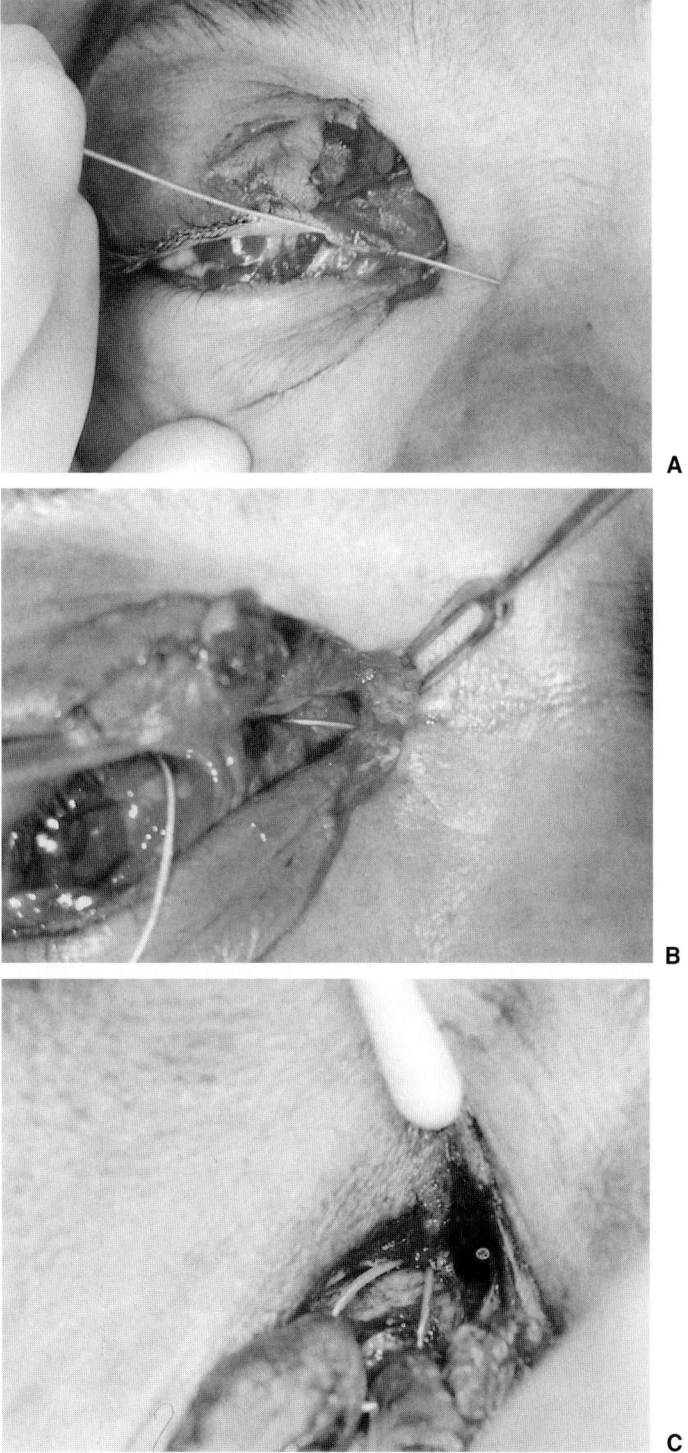

FIGURE 10.3. (A) Probe passed through superior punctum and out through canalicular laceration. **(B)** Stent has been passed across the laceration, through the medial cut edge, and into the nasolacrimal duct into nose. **(C)** Stent passed across superior and inferior canalicular lacerations.

exhale. This method is not as reliable, because the tubes often adhere to the nasal mucosa. Removal through the puncta is especially useful in children, who tend to be more uncooperative during tube removal through the nasal passages. Leaving the cut tube in the nose and assuming it will extricate itself is not recommended. The tubes may remain in place and cause scarring.

Monocanalicular Repair

The monocanalicular stent (Figure 10.4) is a short silicone tube with a phalange at the proximal end. To insert the stent, the surgeon passes the distal end through the punctum and brings it out through the proximal end of the severed canaliculus. The phalange should be fixed securely in the punctum by gently pulling the distal end of the stent (Figure 10.5). The length of the tube may need to be shortened, so that it rests in the lacrimal sac. It does not need to pass into the bony naso-lacrimal duct. When the distal canaliculus is identified, the stent can be threaded into it with forceps.

The monocanalicular stent cannot be used when a laceration to the punctum is present, because the proximal end cannot be fixed. Also, it should not be used with medial canthal avulsion, because the stent cannot provide the adequate inferior and posterior traction to close the wounds, as would a bicanalicular stent tied in the nose.

Pigtail Probe

Canalicular intubation with a "pigtail" probe is a method of last resort when a severed end of a canaliculus cannot be located (Figure 10.6).

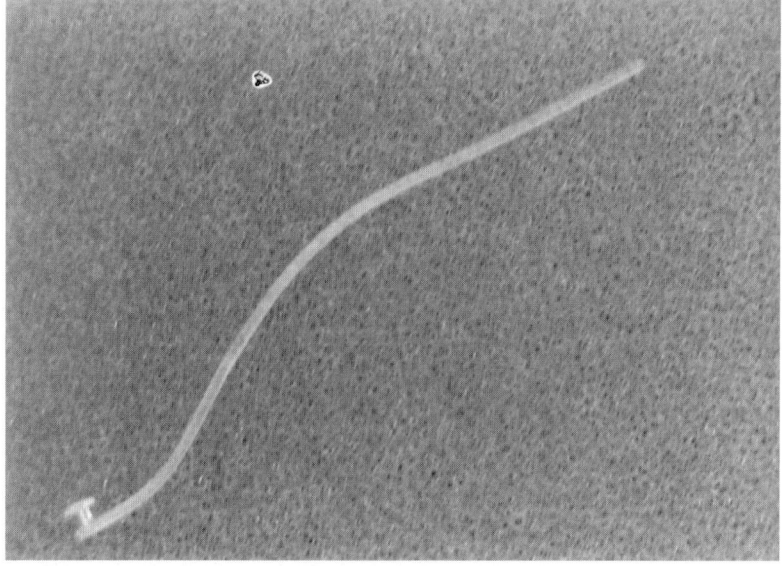

FIGURE 10.4. Monocanalicular stent. Mini Monoka (©FCI Ophthalmics Inc.).

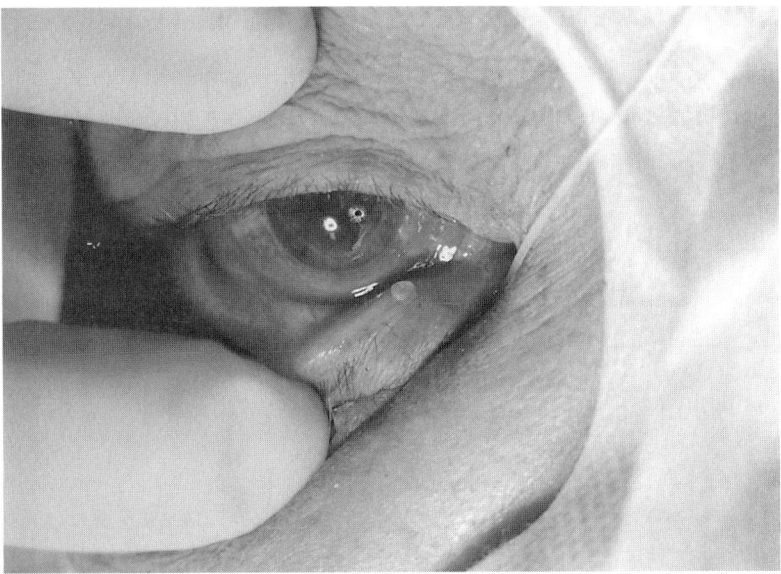

FIGURE 10.5. Monocanalicular stent seated in punctum.

Passing a curved probe around the tight turn of the common canaliculus can inadvertently cause iatrogenic trauma to the patent canaliculus and the lacrimal system.

The pigtail probe, with an eyelet at its tip, is passed through the intact canaliculus with the probe handle maintained in a vertical position. It is gently rotated until the end of the probe is seen exiting the

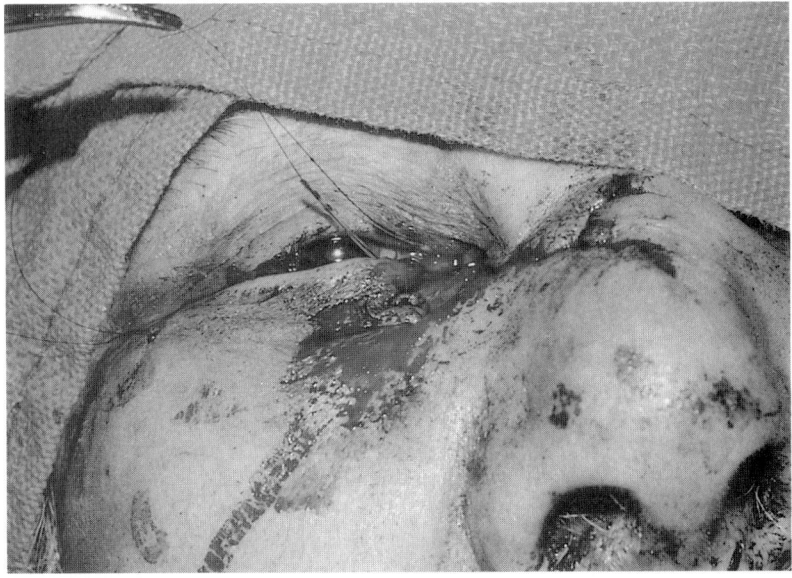

FIGURE 10.6. Both ends of stent after being passed using a pigtail probe.

cut edge of the other canaliculus. A 5-0 nylon suture is passed through the eyelet of the tip of the probe. The probe is rotated backward, out of the canaliculi, bringing the suture with it.

The opposite end of the pigtail probe is passed through the other punctum and into the wound. The nylon is threaded into the probe and the probe is withdrawn. The nylon suture is threaded into a stent tube and a clamp is placed across the tube and suture. The other end of the suture is pulled so that the stent tube passes through both canaliculi. The nylon suture is left in place. The severed canaliculus is sutured over the stent and the laceration is closed. The stent is then trimmed appropriately and the suture is tied to itself, creating a circle within the stent tube. The closed edges of the stent are rotated into the canaliculus.

Stent Removal

Canalicular stents can usually be removed approximately 6 weeks after repair. They are preferably removed from the nose after the loop between the puncta is cut. An endoscope can aid in finding the nasal end of the stent. If this method is not possible, as in a small child, the stent may be removed by cutting the loop between the puncta and pulling the stent out of one of the puncta. Tying the ends of the Crawford tube with suture facilitates removal, because there is only a small knot in the silk suture that must pass through the system, thus avoiding damage to the canaliculus and punctum.

Cutting the stent without removing it, in the assumption that the patient will blow it out of the nose, is not recommended because the stent may remain lodged in the lacrimal duct and lead to granuloma formation.[8]

References

1. Wulc AE, Arterberry JF. The pathogenesis of canalicular laceration. Ophthalmology 1991;98(8):1243–1249.
2. Kennedy RH, May J, Dailey J, Flanagan JC. Canalicular laceration. An 11-year epidemiologic and clinical study. Ophthal Plast Reconstr Surg 1990;6(1):46–53.
3. Reifler DM. Management of canalicular laceration. Surv Ophthalmol 1991;36(2):113–132.
4. Dortzbach RK, Angrist RA. Silicone intubation for lacerated lacrimal canaliculi. Ophthalmic Surg 1985;16(10):639–642.
5. Slonim CB. Dog bite-induced canalicular lacerations: a review of 17 cases. Ophthal Plast Reconstr Surg 1996;12(3):218–222.
6. Kersten RC, Kulwin DR. "One-stitch" canalicular repair. A simplified approach for repair of canalicular laceration. Ophthalmology 1996;103(5):785–789.
7. Baum JL. Canalicular function after "one-stitch" repair. Ophthalmology 1997;104(1):2–3.
8. Dresner SC, Codere F, Brownstein S, Jouve P. Lacrimal drainage system inflammatory masses from retained silicone tubing. Am J Ophthalmol 1984;98(5):609–613.

11

Primary External Dacryocystorhinostomy

Richard H. Hart, Suzanne Powrie, and Geoffrey E. Rose

The watering eye may be the result of excessive tear production, abnormalities of lid position or movement, lacrimal canalicular pump failure, or obstruction of the outflow tract. With external dacryocystorhinostomy (DCR), the lacrimal sac is directly incorporated into the lateral wall of the nose, so that the canaliculi drain directly into the nasal cavity.

The aims of surgery are twofold: to eliminate fluid and mucus retention within the lacrimal sac and prevent sac enlargement (as a mucocele) – the latter leading to intermittent viscous ocular discharge – and to bypass the higher hydraulic resistance of the nasolacrimal duct, thereby increasing tear conductance and aiding the relief of epiphora.

Indications for Surgery

1. Primary acquired nasolacrimal duct obstruction
2. Secondary acquired nasolacrimal duct obstruction attributed, for example, to dacryolithiasis, endonasal surgery, inflammatory nasal or sinus disease, or prior midfacial injury
3. Persistent congenital nasolacrimal duct obstruction, often after unsuccessful probing or intubation of the nasolacrimal duct
4. Functional obstruction of lacrimal outflow with decreased tear conductance as a result of:
   (a) Stenosis, but not occlusion, of the nasolacrimal duct
   (b) Lacrimal canalicular pump failure from age-related laxity of the lower eyelid, or after facial nerve palsy
5. Acute or chronic dacryocystitis; the former group requiring initial treatment with systemic antibiotics

Surgical Principles

External DCR should establish a low-resistance drainage pathway between the conjunctival tear sac and the nasal cavity, by conversion of the lacrimal sac into part of the lateral nasal wall.

Advantages of the external approach to DCR include:

1. Sutured apposition and primary intention healing of mucosal flaps
2. Preparation of a large osteotomy that facilitates future closed placement of glass canalicular bypass tubes, should this be required
3. Direct visualization of abnormalities of the lacrimal sac – including stones, foreign bodies, or tumors
4. Provides ready access for the surgical management of canalicular disease; this includes canaliculo-DCR, retrograde canaliculostomy and intubation, or open placement of a canalicular bypass tube

Anesthesia

External lacrimal surgery may be performed under local or general anesthesia, usually as a day-case admission, and both the patient and surgeon may have a preference for either technique.[1]

Local Anesthesia

The anterior nasal space is sprayed with 4% lignocaine and packed with approximately 2′ (60 cm) of 1/2″ (12.5-mm) ribbon gauze presoaked in 2 mL of a 4% (or 10%) solution of cocaine; this pack provides effective nasal anesthesia and mucosal vasoconstriction. Using angled nasal-packing forceps, successive loops of ribbon gauze are stacked anteriorly to each of the previously placed loops and the packing should be deliberately placed above, and in front of, the anterior end of the middle turbinate.

A mixture of 0.5% bupivacaine with 1:100,000 to 1:200,000 epinephrine is used for local anesthesia: 2–3 mL of this solution is placed in the orbicularis muscle of the medial one-third of the lower eyelid and approximately 2–3 mL infiltrated medially within the orbit, around the anterior ethmoidal branch of the nasociliary nerve. The intraorbital injection is given by passing a 27-gauge needle through the skin at a point 5 mm above the medial canthus, and heading about 20° caudally from the axial plane – thereby reducing the risk of piercing the anterior ethmoidal vessels.

Giving the infiltrative local anesthesia before the surgeon scrubs allows enough time for the epinephrine-mediated vasoconstriction to occur before the start of surgery and topical anesthesia, such as amethocaine 0.5% drops, instilled into both eyes at the time of skin preparation.

Anxiolytic drugs or intravenous sedation – such as a benzodiazepine (oral or intravenous) or low-dose propofol infusion – may be provided as required throughout the procedure.

Advantages of local anesthesia include:

(a) Hemostasis because of the vasoconstriction from injection of local anesthetic solutions containing epinephrine
(b) Avoidance of general anesthetic risk in the elderly, or in patients with multiple medical problems

General Anesthesia

General anesthesia traditionally signaled a need for inpatient care but, with development of short-acting anesthetic drugs, it has become possible to perform day-case surgery under general anesthetic. Rapidly reversible anesthesia and hypotension are beneficial for lacrimal surgery, especially in the day-case setting, and a well-tested technique is described.

After placement of electrocardiogram leads, noninvasive blood pressure monitoring and pulse oximetry, general anesthesia is induced with a bolus dose of propofol and an intravenous infusion of remifentanil. After receiving a small dose of the muscle relaxant rocuronium (e.g., 400 μg per kg), the patient is ventilated with oxygen-enriched air and isoflurane until relaxed; the low-dose of rocuronium is possible because of the respiratory depression caused by the remifentanil and, if the patient has a significant tachycardia, a bolus dose of remifentanil may be given. Endotracheal intubation is undertaken and a pharyngeal pack inserted, which is only done when the patient is sufficiently relaxed to prevent coughing, because an increase in venous pressure at this stage encourages subsequent bleeding during surgery. With a surgeon well-versed in open lacrimal surgery (where bleeding might be minimal), the experienced anesthetist may choose to place a laryngeal mask airway (LMA) because emergence from anesthesia is smoother; LMA should be avoided, however, where there is greater risk of hemorrhage – as with revisional surgery or in hypertensive patients – or where problems might arise in the maintenance of a patent airway.

Some practitioners use total intravenous anesthesia throughout surgery, with continuous infusions of both propofol and remifentanil, and no volatile anesthetic agent, whereas others believe that the following technique allows a more rapid adjustment of blood pressure. A remifentanil infusion, adjusted to maintain relative bradycardia, is used for maintenance of anesthesia and the lungs are ventilated with a mixture of oxygen in air and volatile isoflurane at 0.5 MAC (minimum alveolar concentration).

The patient is placed on the operating table with a head-up tilt to reduce venous congestion at the operative site. Although the intraoperative blood pressure should be related to both the normal status of the patient and the condition at the operative field, bleeding with external lacrimal surgery is typically light with systolic pressures in the region of 80–90 mm Hg. The pulse oximeter trace can, to an experienced anesthetist, give a good indication of tissue blood flow. Local anesthetic infiltration of the operative site before skin incision will reduce the noxious stimulation that normally increases systemic blood pressure. After preparation of the sterile field, vasoconstriction of the nasal mucosa may be encouraged by the placement of three cotton-tip buds, moistened with 0.1% epinephrine solution, anterior to the middle turbinate.

At about 10 minutes before the end of the operation, the remifentanil infusion is stopped and the isoflurane increased to 1.0 MAC. An intravenous dose of ketorolac (10–30 mg) may be given to provide postoperative analgesia and only rarely will a patient require opiates in the postoperative period; in most cases, oral paracetamol provides adequate postoperative analgesia. If required, an antiemetic, such as intravenous ondansetron 4 mg, may be given.

At the end of surgery, the pharyngeal pack is removed and suction is applied with special attention given to the posterior nasopharynx. The patient is recovered in a semirecumbent position and is extubated – or the LMA removed – once he or she is breathing spontaneously.

Advantages of general anesthesia include:

(a) Controlled intraoperative hypotension with good control of operative bleeding
(b) Preferred by many patients, who do not wish to be conscious during surgery, and helpful for the teaching of these procedures

Vasoconstriction and Hemostasis

Successful lacrimal surgery depends on a good, blood-free visualization of tissues to permit accurate bone removal, mucosal apposition, and careful attention to the common canalicular opening to remove obstructive membranes or negotiate a retrograde canaliculostomy.

Several techniques help to encourage vasoconstriction and improve hemostasis:

1. With local anesthesia:
   (a) A nasal pack moistened with a 4% or 10% cocaine solution produces mucosal vasoconstriction; best if pack is left in place until the time of nasal mucosal suturing
   (b) Supplementary intramucosal injection of local anesthetic with 1:200,000 epinephrine may be used, but is rarely necessary during the procedure
2. With general anesthesia:
   (a) Three intranasal cotton-tip buds moistened with 1:1,000 epinephrine and placed at, and above, the anterior end of the middle turbinate produces mucosal vasoconstriction in the operative field
   (b) Infiltration of local anesthetic at the site of the skin incision
   (c) Controlled systemic hypotension, with typical pressures of 90/60 mm Hg
3. General measures:
   (a) Head-elevated (reverse Trendelenburg) posture reduces venous congestion
   (b) Use of a continuous suction device in the nondominant hand helps maintain a blood-free field, viewing of tissues, and the displacement and protection of neighboring structures during surgery
   (c) The careful handling of tissues, gentle diathermy of cut edges, suturing of mucosal flaps, and respect for surgical planes
   (d) The judicious use of bone wax for persistent hemorrhage from the cut edges of bone

Surgical Technique

A standard surgical skin cleansing and sterile draping is performed with access to the eye and nose; for local anesthesia, the whole face can be exposed after complete facial cleansing.

Using a no. 15 blade to cut skin alone, a 1/2″ (12-mm) incision – slightly shorter in children – is placed on the flat area alongside the nasion, beginning just above the level of the medial canthal tendon (MCT); positioning of a straight incision in the thicker paranasal skin helps prevent the late scar contracture and bridging often seen with posteriorly placed incisions. Lifting the lateral skin-edge anteriorly, the skin is separated from the underlying orbicularis muscle using blunt-tipped scissors until the MCT is evident (Figure 11.1A). The union

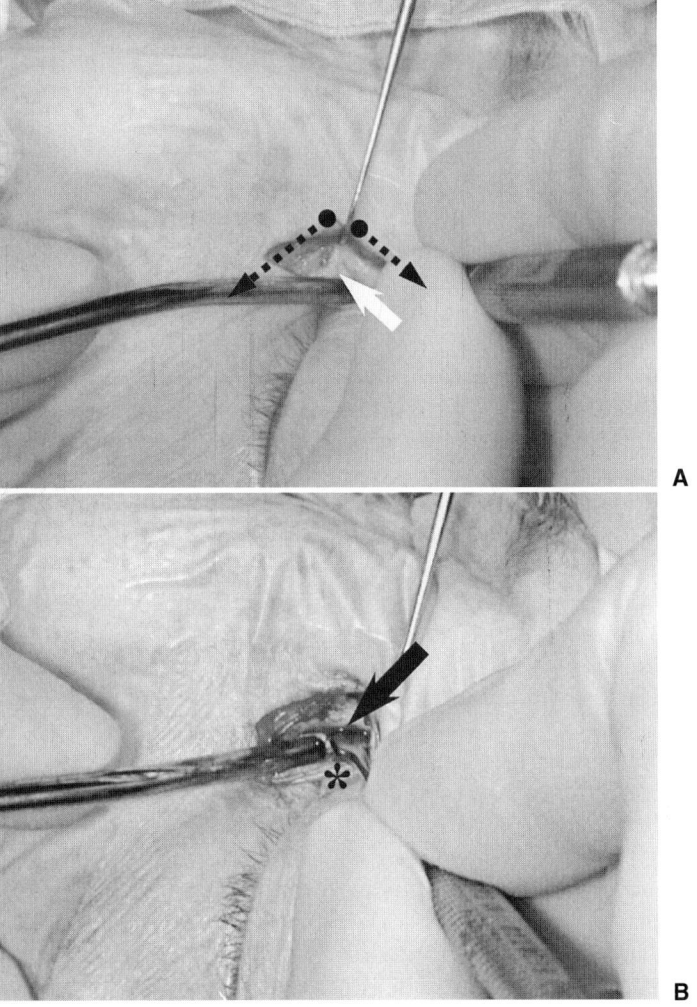

FIGURE 11.1. **(A)** The left MCT is readily evident (white arrow) after undermining the skin and the pretarsal and preseptal orbicularis fibers are separated superolaterally and inferolaterally (broken arrows). **(B)** A rougine is passed behind the anterior lacrimal crest (arrow) to displace the lacrimal sac (*) laterally from its bony fossa.

between preseptal and pretarsal orbicularis fibers is evident at the bony attachment of the anterior limb of the MCT, lateral to the angular vessels, and the two groups of fibers should be separated along this avascular junction using a Rollett's rongine (Figure 11.1A). The surgical assistant should use a squint hook to anteriorly retract the preseptal orbicularis and angular vessels, while the surgeon uses the rougine to incise the periosteum – starting by disinsertion of the anterior limb of the MCT and continuing down the anterior lacrimal crest, using the sharp bone edge as a cutting edge beneath the instrument. The periosteum is raised widely – anteriorly alongside the nose – and posteriorly to elevate the lacrimal sac laterally within the lacrimal sac fossa (Figure 11.1B). Using a right-angled periosteal elevator, the thin bone between the sac and anterior ethmoids is perforated at the suture line between the lacrimal bone and the frontal process of the maxilla. Occasionally, the bone in the fossa is exceptionally strong and it may be necessary to thin the bone with a drill, trephine, or hammer and chisel before perforation; an alternative in this situation is to raise the periosteum to beyond the posterior lacrimal crest and then perforate the very thin lamina papyracea just behind the posterior lacrimal crest.

Once bone has been breached, bone removal should proceed anteriorly across the anterior lacrimal crest and this can be most readily achieved with a Kerrison-style rongeur, crossing the crest close to the skull base – this being the thinnest bone on the crest and also reducing the chance of damage to the nasal mucosa (Figure 11.2A); a periosteal elevator should be swept around the bone edge (every 2 or 3 bites) to separate the nasal mucosa from underlying bone. Nasal mucosa is reached as the anterior lacrimal crest is crossed and, at this point, it is best to slightly withdraw the epinephrine-moistened cotton buds. They may be readvanced to the apex of the nasal space once the bone removal is complete. Once across the anterior crest, bone removal should be directed inferiorly to the level of the inferior orbital rim – creating an "L"-shaped rhinostomy. The remaining bone of the frontal process of the maxilla is removed, either with down-cutting rongeurs or straight (Jensen) bone-nibblers, while the lacrimal sac tissues are protected by displacing them laterally with the sucker held in the nondominant hand. The thin hamular process of the lacrimal bone, between the upper part of the nasolacrimal duct and nasal mucosa, is removed with bone nibblers and the upper part of the rhinostomy is extended to the skull base, although care should be taken here to avoid shearing forces that may fracture the cribriform plate and cause a cerebrospinal fluid leak. At this stage, the rhinostomy should be approximately 1/2"–3/4" (12–18 mm) in diameter and extend from the fundus of the sac at the skull base, approximately 1/4"–1/2" (up to 10 mm) in front of the anterior lacrimal crest, and inferiorly to expose the upper part of the nasolacrimal duct (Figure 11.2B). Anterior ethmoidectomy should be performed, using nontoothed forceps or a fine artery clip to palpate and avulse the fragment of bone and mucosa, because this creates a wide-open space that facilitates easy apposition and suture of the posterior mucosal anastomosis.[2]

A "00" Bowman probe is passed into the lacrimal sac through the lower canaliculus, and the assistant maintains gentle medial pressure to "tent" the medial wall of the sac while the medial face of the sac is opened with a no. 11 blade; this blade should be directed away from the internal opening of the common canaliculus (Figure 11.3A). Once in the sac, the closed blades of a Westcott spring scissor should *easily* pass into the lumen of the sac and duct (Figure 11.3B); difficult passage

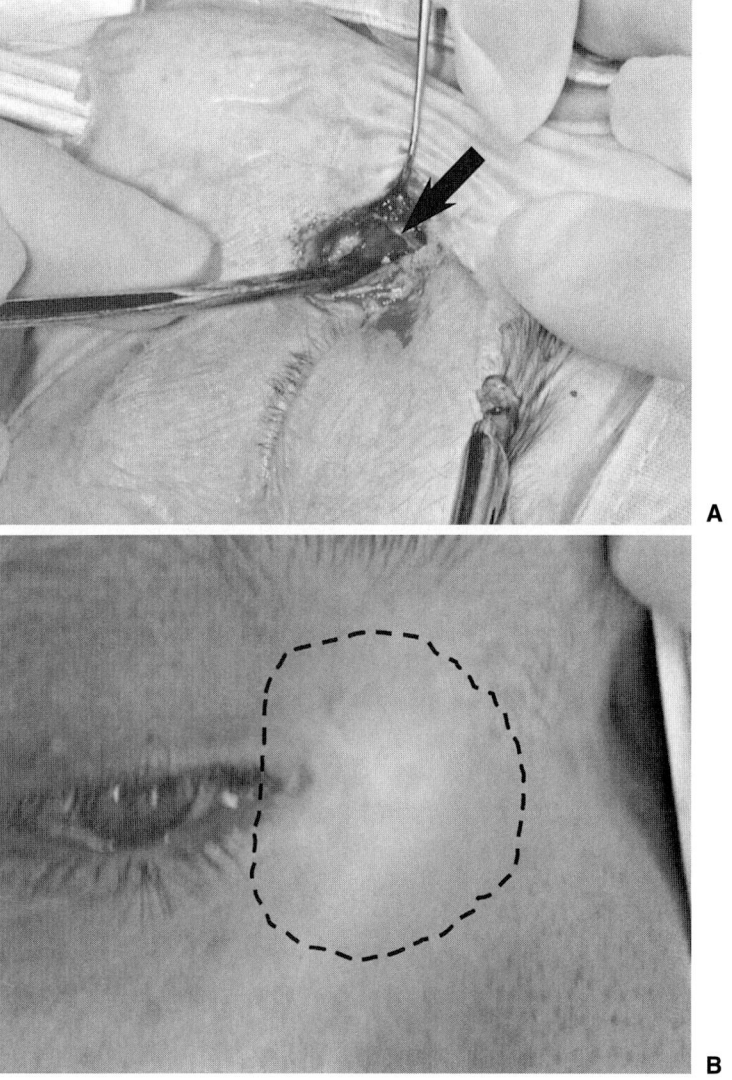

A

B

FIGURE 11.2. **(A)** A large rhinostomy is being created during left DCR, after having creating a defect across the anterior lacrimal crest; the anterior cut edge of bone is evident (arrow). Note the presence of epinephrine-moistened cotton tips in the nasal space. **(B)** The final size of a typical osteotomy is outlined by endonasal transillumination.

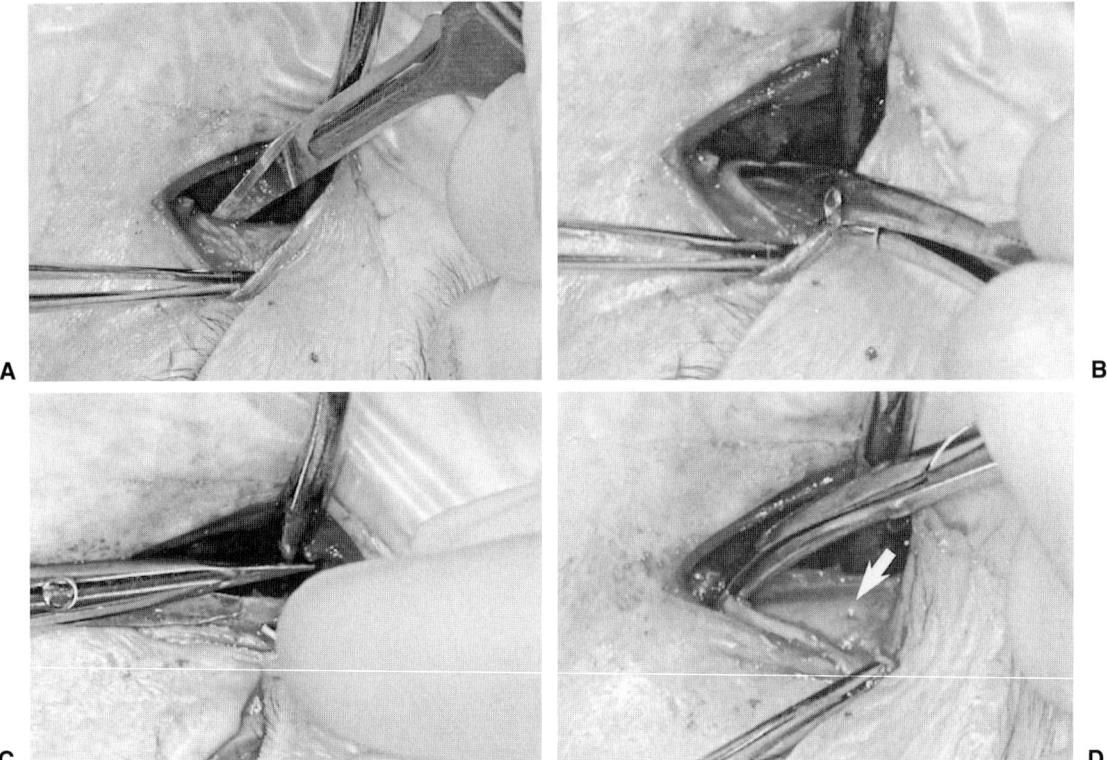

FIGURE 11.3. (A) A no. 11 blade is used to make a small incision, below the level of the common canalicular opening, during left DCR. **(B)** The nasolacrimal duct is "sounded" with the closed spring scissors and the mucosal incision continued inferiorly into the upper end of the duct. **(C)** After likewise "sounding" upward to the fundus of the sac, the mucosa is incised up to the skull base. **(D)** Relieving incisions are performed at the sac–duct junction and at the skull base, which leaves the sac opened widely and the internal opening of the common canaliculus readily evident (arrow).

frequently indicates that lacrimal fascia alone has been opened and the blades have entered the resistant submucosal (extraluminal) plane. The entire sac is opened by extension of the blade incision in both directions (Figure 11.3C) – from the fundus down to the duct, and the sac is further opened with relieving incisions at the skull base above and the nasolacrimal duct below (Figure 11.3D); cautery of the sac–duct junction is advisable before the relieving incisions, because there is a rich vascular plexus at this site.

The internal opening of the common canaliculus should be clearly visible and deliberately inspected (Figure 11.3D): Where membranous obstruction is present, the adherent valve of Rosenmüller should be excised by grasping it with a pair of fine, toothed forceps and excising approximately $1\,mm^2$ using a no. 11 blade. Likewise, biopsy of suspicious lesions within the sac, or removal of any debris (such as stones), is readily accomplished with the sac opened widely.

Using the no. 11 blade with the cotton buds protecting the nasal septum, the nasal mucosa is opened in a superior–inferior direction and the incision placed 3–4 mm anterior to the "arch" formed by the inflexion of the nasal mucosa into anterior insertion of the middle turbinate; this arch is only evident after anterior ethmoidectomy. The anterior flap is created by superior- and inferior-positioned relieving incisions (Figure 11.4A) and the posterior flap is similarly created after

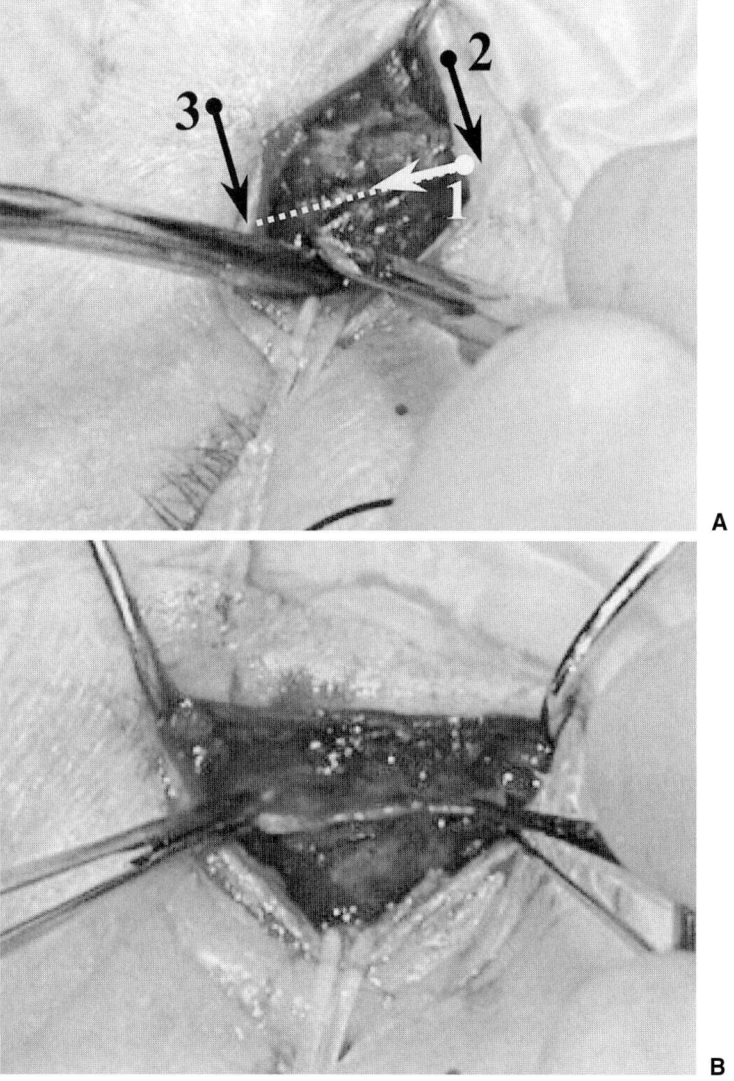

A

B

FIGURE 11.4. **(A)** Fashioning a large anterior flap of nasal mucosa: the first incision – made using a no. 11 blade against intranasal cotton tips – is (anatomically) vertical, and the other two incisions pass anteroposteriorly along the edges of the osteotomy. **(B)** The resulting large nasal mucosal flap should be hung aside by a weighted suture placed across the nasal bridge.

mucosal cautery. A 6-0 soluble suture (e.g., Vicryl W9756; Ethicon) is passed through the orbicularis muscle on the anterior lip of the incision and then through the middle of the free edge of the anterior nasal flap (Figure 11.4B), the suture is clipped and draped across the nasal bridge – this keeps the anterior flaps out of the surgical field during posterior suturing.

The posterior mucosal flaps are apposed – from the skull base (Figure 11.5) to the entrance of the nasolacrimal duct – with a locked continu-

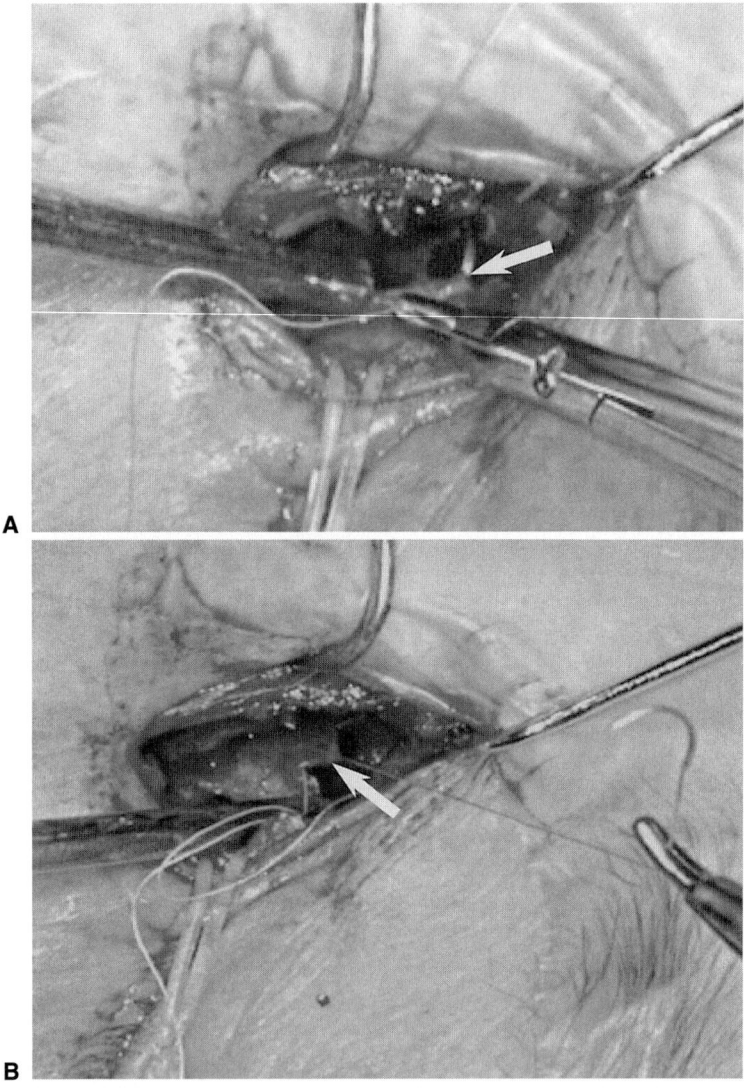

A

B

FIGURE 11.5. (A) Prior anterior ethmoidectomy facilitates suturing of the posterior mucosal flaps using an 8-mm diameter, half-circle needle – here being passed through the upper end of the posterior sac flap (arrow). (B) The posterior nasal flap (arrow) has just been engaged to start the sutured anastomosis that should extend from the skull base to the sac–duct junction.

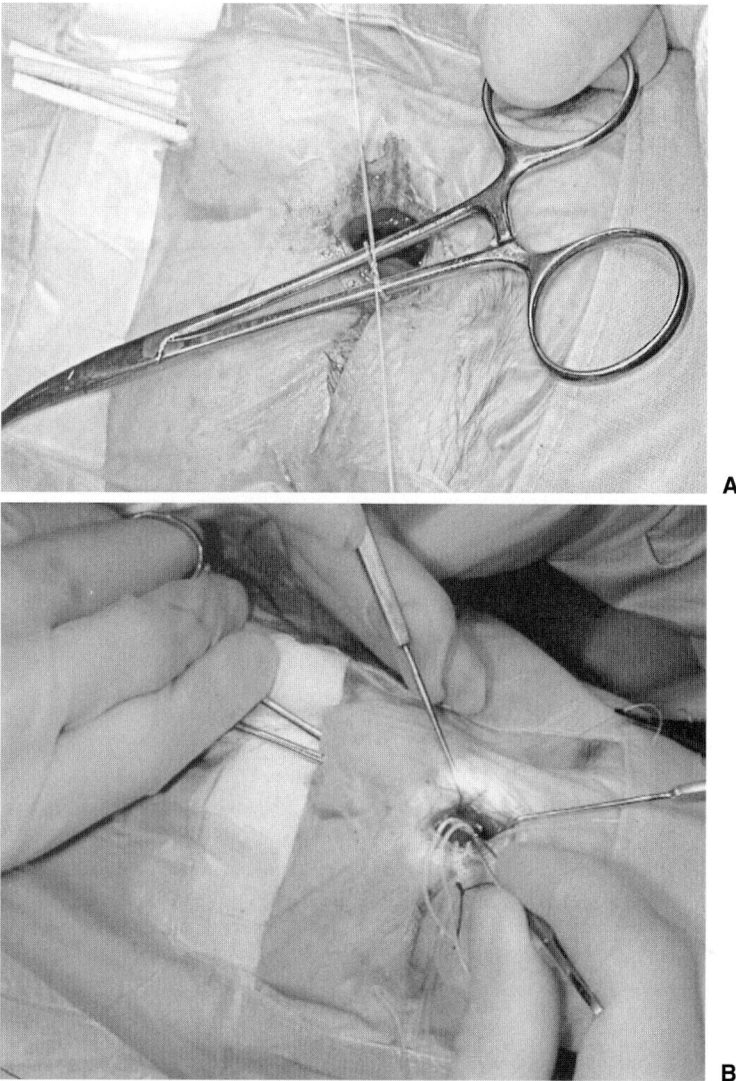

FIGURE 11.6. **(A)** Postoperative ride-up of intubation is almost unknown if the intubation is passed through the section and tied over the shank of an instrument. **(B)** The tied tubes are then retrieved in the jaws of an artery clip passed into the anterior nasal space.

ous 6-0 Vicryl suture and the suture secured by a triple locking throw. Silicone tubes are passed through the upper and lower canaliculi, retrieved through the incision using a curved hemostat, the metal bodkins removed, and the tubes tied over the shank of the closed hemostat resting across the incision (Figure 11.6A). While the assistant holds both tubes elevated, a 2–0 silk ligature is tied just above the silicone knot and the ends are left approximately 15 mm long to facilitate identification within the nose; the tube ends are then passed into the nose and retrieved with a curved hemostat passed from the nasal entrance (Figure 11.6B).

Closure of the anterior mucosal flaps is best accomplished with three 6-0 Vicryl sutures using "suspension" from the orbicularis fibers: The most superior suture is passed successively through the medial orbicularis (avoiding the angular vessels), the edge of the anterior nasal flap, the edge of the anterior sac flap, and finally through the anterior limb of the MCT (Figure 11.7A); the middle suture has already been

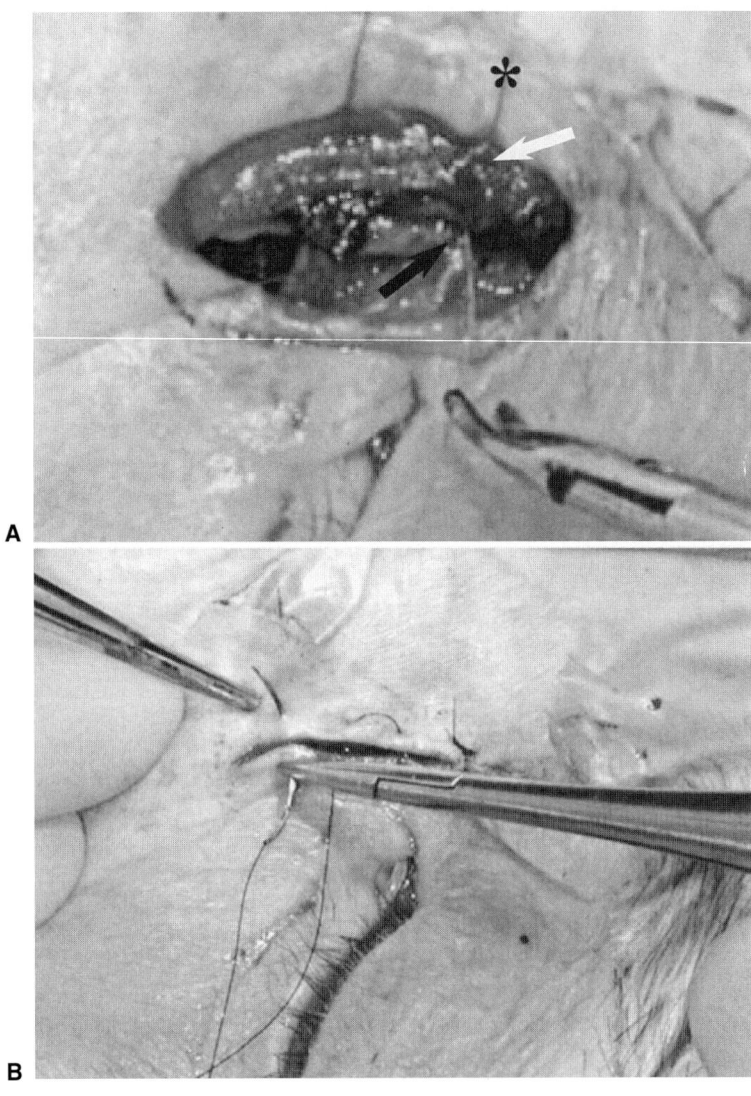

FIGURE 11.7. **(A)** Three sutures are used to suspend the anterior mucosal union from the orbicularis muscle fibers: here the uppermost suture (*) has been passed through the anterior, preseptal orbicularis (white arrow), through the upper end of the anterior nasal and sac mucosa (dark arrow), and finally through the MCT. **(B)** After suture of the deep tissues, the skin is closed with mattress 6-0 nylon.

passed through the anterior structures and only needs to be passed through the anterior sac mucosa; the inferior suture is finally passed through the various layers and the sutures are all tied to close both the mucosa and the orbicularis in one maneuver. The skin is then closed with a running mattress 6-0 nylon suture (Figure 11.7B), antibiotic ointment is instilled in the eye, and a firm, nonadhesive pad is placed on the incision for 12–24 hours. The silicone tubes are left long and taped to the dressing, until trimmed just before hospital discharge – this permits easier nasal packing if necessary in the unlikely event of primary hemorrhage.

If no contraindications exist, cefuroxime (typically 750 mg) is given intravenously during surgery to reduce the risk of postoperative wound infection.

Postoperative Care

The patient should rest for a few hours after surgery, seated half-reclining to reduce nasal venous congestion, and hot drinks and food should be avoided for approximately 12 hours to reduce the chance of epistaxis caused by heat-induced nasal vasodilation.

The dressing may be removed at home on the first postoperative day and a combined topical antibiotic/steroid, such as prednisolone-neomycin, should be used 3–4 times a day. To reduce the low risk of secondary hemorrhage, the patient is asked to avoid nose blowing for a week. The skin sutures are removed at approximately 1 week and the silicone stent at approximately 4–5 weeks, when epithelial healing is complete (Figure 11.8).[3,4]

Complications

1. Intraoperative
   (a) Hemorrhage
       i. For troublesome intraoperative hemorrhage, use cautery to soft tissues and wax on the cut edge of bone
       ii. If persistent, try pressure packing the operative site for 5 minutes with an epinephrine-moistened gauze
       iii. Consider packing the nasal space with an absorbable surgical cellulose sponge
   (b) Canalicular injury
       i. May be avoided by gentle handling of probes and stents during surgery
       ii. When passing a probe or tube, ensure that the eyelid is held taut, to avoid a "concertina" effect in the canaliculus and creation of a false passage
   (c) Cerebrospinal fluid leak
       i. Inadvertent fracture of the cribriform plate may rarely result in cerebrospinal fluid leak

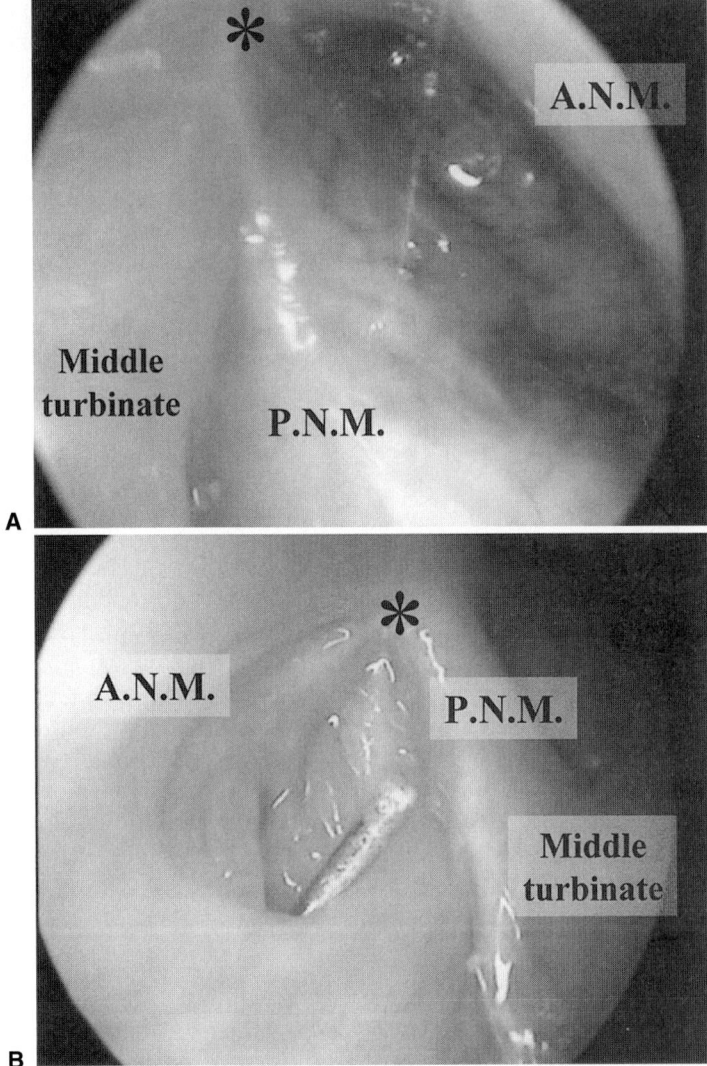

FIGURE 11.8. Healed external DCR, showing **(A)** the left lacrimal sac opened widely to the nasal space and **(B)** a successful right-sided anastomosis, with intracanalicular probe. P.N.M., posterior nasal mucosa; A.N.M., anterior nasal mucosa; asterisk marks the area of secondary intention healing on the skull base.

    ii. Small leaks may be sealed by occlusion with a tiny slip of orbicularis muscle fibers

    iii. Postoperative antibiotics should be administered and vigilant monitoring maintained for symptoms and signs of meningitis; a neurosurgical opinion might be sought in certain circumstances

(d) Inadvertent orbital entry
   i. Orbital fat prolapse may occur during ethmoidectomy or incision of the sac
   ii. Traction on the orbital fat should be avoided to reduce the risk of motility disturbance or, more rarely, orbital hemorrhage

2. Postoperative
   (a) Hemorrhage
      i. Simple measures, such as a head-up posture and nasal ice packs, may be all that is required
      ii. If hemorrhage continues, pack the nose with 1/2″ (12.5 mm) ribbon gauze moistened in 1 : 1,000 epinephrine and leave the pack undisturbed for 5 days. Oral antibiotics should be given for a week after hemorrhage
   (b) Wound infection
      i. Prophylactic systemic antibiotics reduce the risk of wound infection
      ii. A single intraoperative dose of a broad-spectrum antibiotic is as effective as a postoperative course of oral antibiotics
      iii. Consider using postoperative antibiotics in the setting of preoperative infection, simultaneous bilateral surgery, with placement of a nasal tamponade, or with postoperative epistaxis
   (c) Wound necrosis and fistula formation
      i. May occur in the setting of previous radiotherapy or overwhelming skin infections
   (d) Stent prolapse or canalicular "cheese-wiring"
      i. With tying over the handle of forceps, prolapse is almost never encountered
      ii. If prolapse should occur, the silicone tubes can be retrieved with nasal endoscopy in almost all cases
      iii. Medial migration ("cheese-wiring") of stent arises where it is not passing through the fibrous annulus of a lacrimal punctum – as, for example, after punctoplasty or retrograde canaliculostomy
   (e) Hypertrophic scar or bowing of the incision
      i. Generally caused by a posteriorly placed incision, in the concavity of the inner canthus (Figure 11.9)
      ii. May be exacerbated by excessive diathermy or placement of large numbers of subcutaneous sutures
   (f) Failure of drainage
      i. Most often caused by fibrosis at the site of a too-small soft-tissue anastomosis
      ii. If caused by fibrous obstruction at the internal opening of the common canaliculus, this may be treated by transcanalicular trephination and intubation
      iii. A redo-DCR may be required if there has been inadequate bone removal

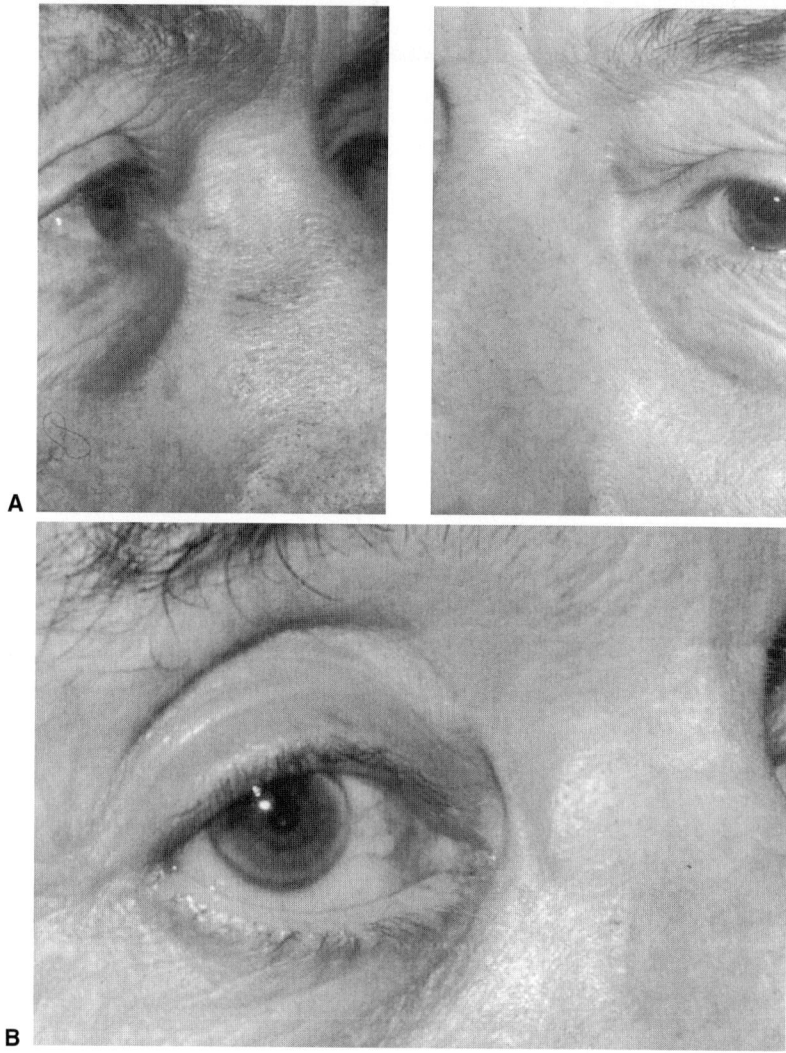

FIGURE 11.9. **(A)** Well-placed incision for external DCR, with an "invisible" scar at 1 year after right-sided surgery. **(B)** Bowing of a DCR scar in the convexity of the inner canthus; this bowing is common with superior and posterior placement of the incision.

iv. Failure because of canalicular obstruction at a more proximal level usually requires placement of a glass canalicular bypass (Lester Jones) tube.

References

1. Hanna IT, Powrie S, Rose GE. Open lacrimal surgery: a comparison of admission outcome and complications after planned day-case or in-patient management. Br J Ophthalmol 1998;82:392–396.
2. McLean CJ, Cree I, Rose GE. Rhinostomies: an open and shut case? Br J Ophthalmol 1999;83:1300–1301.

3. Vardy SJ, Rose GE. Prevention of cellulitis after open lacrimal surgery: a prospective study of three methods. Ophthalmology 2000;107:315–317.
4. Walland MJ, Rose GE. Soft tissue infection after open lacrimal surgery. Ophthalmology 1994;101:608–611.

12

Primary Endonasal Dacryocystorhinostomy

Francois Codere and David W. Rossman

External dacryocystorhinostomy (DCR) has been the procedure of choice for many decades to treat nasolacrimal duct obstruction. The procedure, first described by Toti[1] at the turn of the twentieth century, has been refined over the years and is still currently adopted by most ophthalmologists. It consistently yields excellent results and can be routinely done under local anesthesia on an outpatient basis using minimal instrumentation. The intranasal approach to lacrimal surgery was first described by Caldwell[2] in 1893; however, it quickly fell out of favor because of difficulties viewing the intranasal anatomy through the nose. Attention returned to the intranasal approach after Heermann[3] in 1958 introduced a direct technique for endonasal lacrimal surgery using an operating microscope that produced very good results.[4] Routine utilization of endoscopes by ears, nose, and throat surgeons led to renewed interest in approaching the lacrimal duct from the nose. The first modern endonasal DCR procedures using endoscopes were described by McDonogh and Meiring[5] in 1989. Especially in America, early endonasal DCR techniques frequently included the use of lasers to burn through the mucosa and create the osteotomy.[6] However, the laser-assisted endonasal DCR yielded inferior results compared with the external route. This was likely the result of the generation of excess granulation tissue and char around the ostium in the postoperative period.[7] Careful compliance to endoscopic surgical techniques with minimal tissue damage, the preservation of mucosa, and the creation of mucosal flaps has enabled this technique, in most cases, to become a positive alternative to external DCR with comparable outcomes.[8]

Endonasal DCR has significant advantages over external DCR. It avoids a skin incision and scar, especially important in younger individuals or in patients with a history of keloid formation. Dissection is limited to the inner wall of the lacrimal fossa, leaving intact the medial canthal anatomy and lacrimal pump function and avoiding a surgical site that goes from the skin to the nasal cavity. Postoperative pain is minimal, if at all present, and most patients can resume their normal activities a few days after surgery. The surgery requires less tissue dissection, often resulting in less intraoperative bleeding and a shorter surgical time than external techniques.[9] Endonasal DCR can also be performed early to manage definitively acute dacryocystitis with abscess formation, minimizing the need to decompress the sac from the skin side.[10]

There are also limitations. An anterior diverticulum arising from the lacrimal sac may not be effectively managed via the endonasal approach. Patients with a history of midfacial trauma may have altered anatomy involving the bones surrounding the lacrimal sac, making endonasal DCR hazardous with less predictable outcome. A lacrimal sac neoplasm is best treated with an external DCR. Finally, there is a steep learning curve with using the nasal endoscope that may hamper early success if proper training has not been obtained.[9]

Patient Selection

The most frequent indication for endonasal DCR is chronic epiphora caused by acquired dacryostenosis. Other indications include acute or chronic dacryocystitis with or without the presence of a dacryolith. The technique is useful in children with recurrent dacryostenosis despite probing and lacrimal intubation. In addition, endonasal DCR has produced good results in patients with functional nasolacrimal duct obstruction as determined by dacryocystography and lacrimal scintigraphy.[11]

The investigation of the lacrimal system begins with the examination of the punctum to exclude agenesis, stenosis, ectropion, or any other abnormality. The medial canthal area is palpated to look for any firm mass that might represent a mucocele, dacryolith, or a tumor. If tumor is suspected or there is a history of midfacial trauma, further evaluation with computed tomography scan and/or bone subtraction dacryocystography is necessary. Lacrimal system irrigation will confirm obstruction and allows the assessment of the common canaliculus and internal punctum because exploration of the common canaliculus cannot be performed easily during endonasal DCR.

Careful evaluation of the nasal cavity using an endoscope is crucial to assess the nasal access to the lacrimal sac. A large medial turbinate, nasal polyps, granular inflamed mucosa, tight nostrils, and septal deviations are all potential problems that can make endonasal DCR more difficult or impossible.

Preparation of the Nose

Preoperative vasoconstriction of the nasal cavity using a long-acting nasal decongestant 2 hours and 1 hour before the operation helps visualization and minimizes intraoperative bleeding. Patients with seasonal allergies or with upper respiratory tract infections should wait for remission of their nasal congestion before having surgery. In cases of severe septal deviations, corrective surgery may be necessary before lacrimal surgery, either as a combined procedure or as a separate operation. However, in those patients with septal anomalies or tight nostrils, an external DCR is an excellent option that should be considered in most cases.

Anesthesia

Endonasal DCR can be performed safely under local or general anesthesia. Conditions favoring general anesthetic include acute dacryocystitis, prior surgery in the lacrimal area, difficult nasal anatomy with a tight access, and patient preference. However, in experienced hands and a normal nasal anatomy, local anesthesia can be offered, making the procedure particularly suitable to an ambulatory care unit without a full recovery room.

In both types of anesthesia, the lateral wall of the nose and middle turbinate are infiltrated with a solution of lidocaine 2% with epinephrine 1:100,000 and the nostril is then packed with gauze soaked in either 5% cocaine or a solution of neosynephrine 0.25%–lidocaine 3%. This induces long-lasting vasoconstriction and decongestion of the nasal mucosa allowing optimal visualization and minimizing bleeding. With local anesthesia, an anterior ethmoidal block from the orbital side along the medial orbital wall, 1–1.5 cm behind the medial canthal tendon, provides deep anesthesia of the sac area, the anterior ethmoids, and surrounding bones. The superficial tissues around the medial aspects of the lids should also be infiltrated and the cornea anesthetized with topical eyedrops.

Surgical Equipment

It is mandatory when performing nasal endoscopic procedures to use proper high-quality instruments. A 4-mm, 0-degree endoscope is the instrument most often used, although a 30-degree tip is useful for certain situations in which an oblique view is necessary. A high-powered light source (Xenon) is essential to keep visualization at an optimal level. A high-resolution monitor at least 19 inches wide should be placed at the head of the patient and at eye level of the surgeon. A secondary light source is also necessary to transilluminate the lacrimal sac with a fiberoptic probe.

Surgical Technique

The puncta are dilated and the fiberoptic probe is gently inserted through the upper canaliculus and passed through the internal punctum into the lacrimal sac. The light probe will transilluminate the lacrimal sac through the thin lacrimal bone. The thicker frontal process of the maxilla does not transilluminate as well so that the anterior part of the transillumination corresponds to the lacrimal suture line. The position of the middle turbinate should be appreciated in relation to the position of the sac.

In some cases, the middle turbinate may be displaced medially using a Freer elevator to enhance exposure to the lateral nasal wall over the lacrimal area. A small ridge formed by the projection of the frontal process of the maxilla can usually be seen. A mucosal incision is made with a crescent blade or the sharp edge of the Freer elevator just anterior to that ridge below the insertion of the turbinate (Figure 12.1). The incision is extended inferiorly for 10mm and should go down to the bone and involve the mucoperiosteum. A Freer periosteal elevator is then used to elevate the nasal flap. To avoid damaging the mucosa, the Freer must be kept in continuous firm contact with maxillary bone while dissecting under the mucoperiosteum. Posterior incisions are then made at the superior and inferior margin of the mucosal flap using Yasargill scissors (Figure 12.2). Using the Freer elevator, the mucosal flap is elevated and displaced medially to the middle turbinate to expose the thin lacrimal bone and the area of transillumination. The thicker bone of the frontal process of the maxilla is anterior and does not transilluminate well. The suture line between the lacrimal bone and the frontal process of the maxilla is easily seen. The osteotomy is started by removing the frontal process of the maxilla with a 2-mm Kerrison rongeur (Figure 12.3). The lacrimal bone does not need to be removed at this stage. With the tip of the rongeur, the edge formed by the thick maxillary bone can be felt and the rongeur is inserted just under it, pushing the lacrimal bone toward the sac. Usually 5 to 6 bites are necessary to uncover the anterior part of the lacrimal cylinder. Care is taken to slip the instrument between the bone and the lacrimal mucosa to avoid undue bleeding and early opening of the sac. The posterior aspect of the lacrimal sac and duct is exposed by removing the lacrimal bone (Figure 12.4). Using a Freer elevator, the thin sheets of lacrimal bone are lifted carefully from the lacrimal mucosa and then removed with microethmoid forceps. When the sac is scarred and has a small lumen, a more superior osteotomy is required. This is more

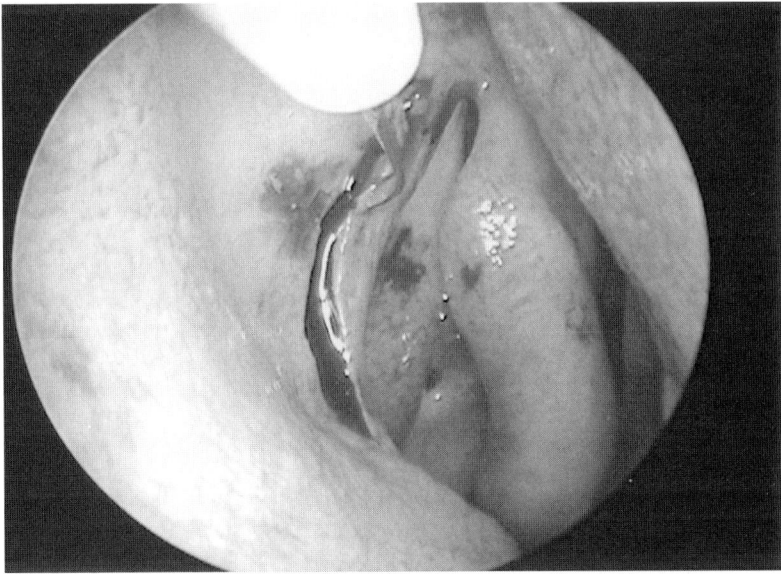

FIGURE 12.1. Incision of the nasal mucosa with a crescent knife.

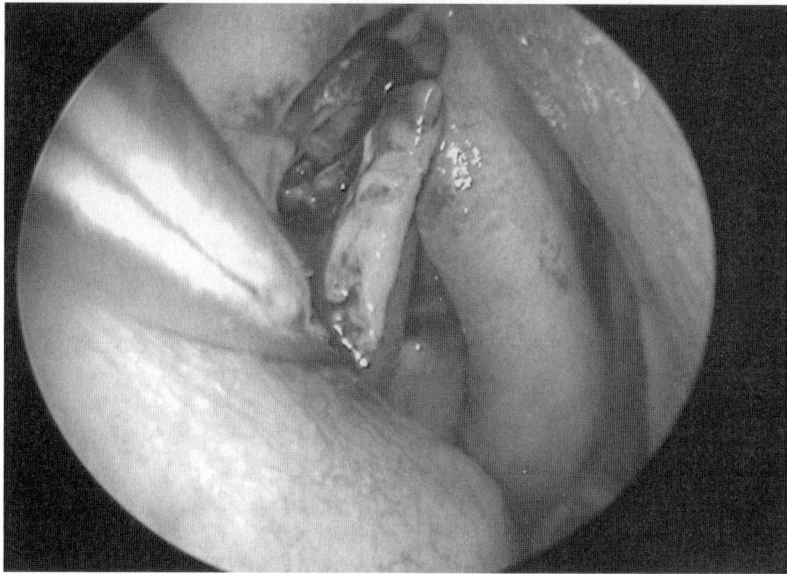

FIGURE 12.2. Inferior incision with scissors. The superior incision has been made.

easily done with a 45-degree tip Kerrison rongeur. Superiorly, the frontal process of the maxilla often has a more posterior projection and removal of the uncinate process may be necessary.

The lacrimal sac is then filled with a viscous solution of methylcellulose. The transillumination probe can be used to tent up the lacrimal sac. A straightened crescent knife is used to create a vertical incision in the anterior portion of the lacrimal cylinder. The incision is directed posteriorly at the superior and inferior end, allowing the large lacrimal

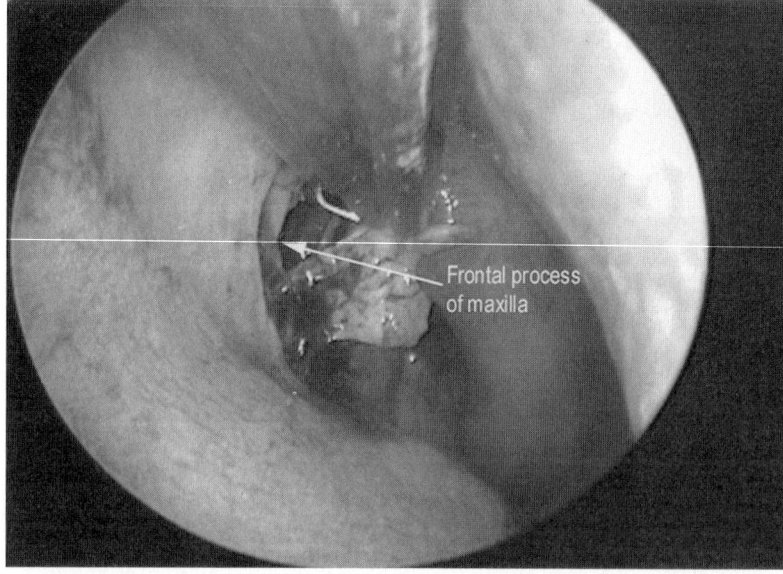

FIGURE 12.3. Osteotomy of the frontal process of the maxilla.

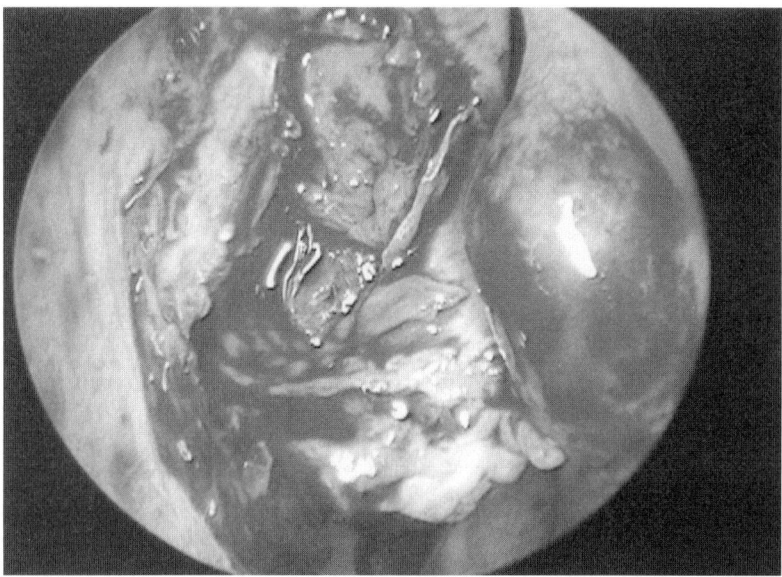

FIGURE 12.4. Lacrimal sac exposed after completion of osteotomy with light probe in the superior portion.

mucosal flap to be hinged posteriorly (Figure 12.5). Massage of the sac at the inner canthus allows for visualization of the fundus of the sac and removal of any dacryolith that may have caused obstruction. The lacrimal mucosa can also be biopsied and sent for histopathologic examination if it is thought to be abnormal.

A Freer elevator is used to mobilize the nasal mucosal flap laterally to come in contact with the posteriorly directed lacrimal sac flap (Figure 12.6). Having the flap edges in close apposition on the lateral nasal wall

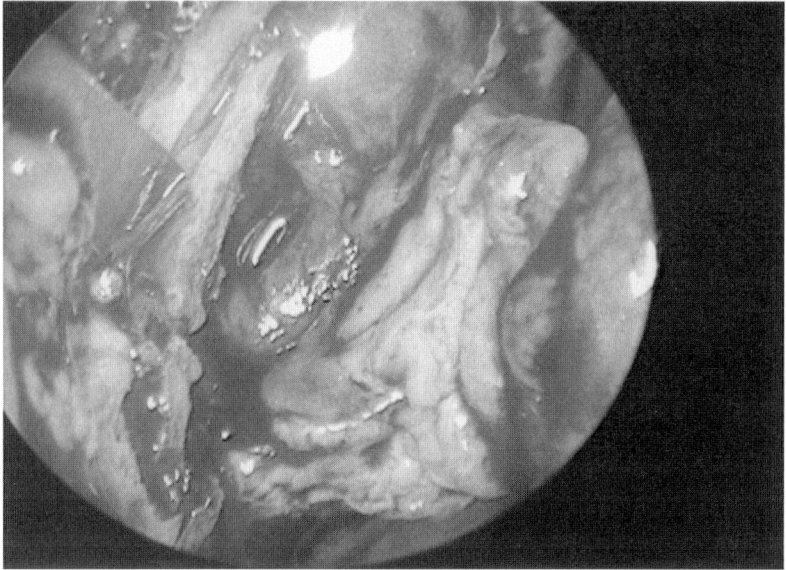

FIGURE 12.5. Incision of sac with light probe showing through in upper portion of the sac.

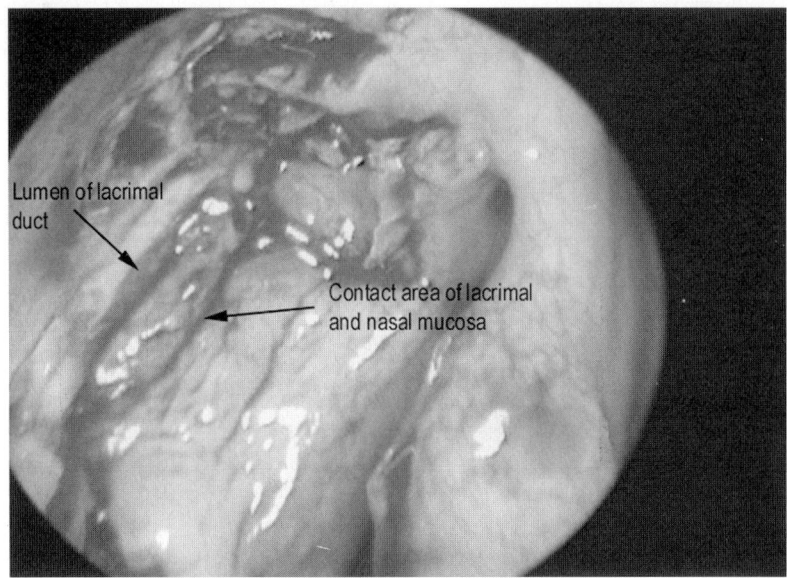

Lumen of lacrimal
duct

Contact area of lacrimal
and nasal mucosa

FIGURE 12.6. Apposition of lacrimal and nasal mucosal flaps.

allows for fusion of the mucosal flaps when healing, creating a mucosal-lined fistula from the sac to the nose.[12] This resembles flap creation in external DCR. At the end of surgery, bicanalicular intubation is done with silicone tubes and the ends are retrieved from the nose with straight microethmoid forceps. Lastly, a small piece of Gelfoam soaked in methylprednisolone 40 mg/cc is slipped over the tubes down on the mucosal flaps to stabilize them and encourage stabilization of the flaps in contact with each other (Figure 12.7).

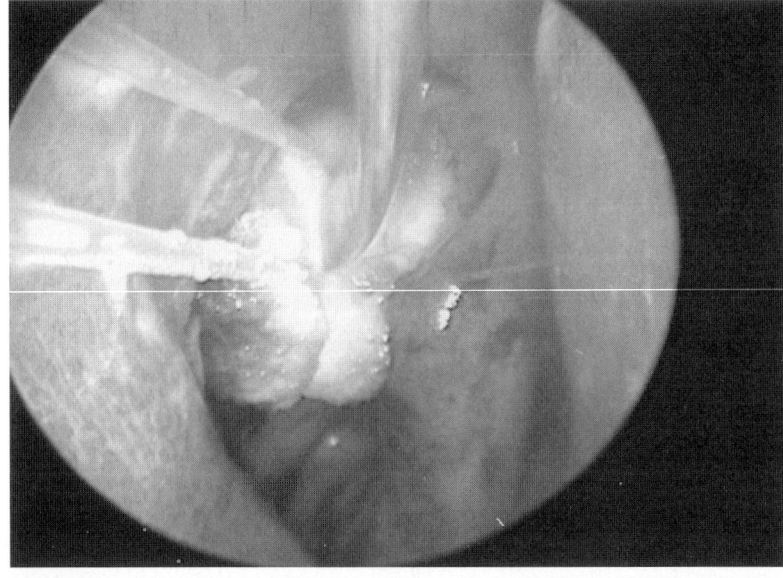

FIGURE 12.7. Gelfoam packing soaked in steroid solution and slipped over lacrimal silicone tubes.

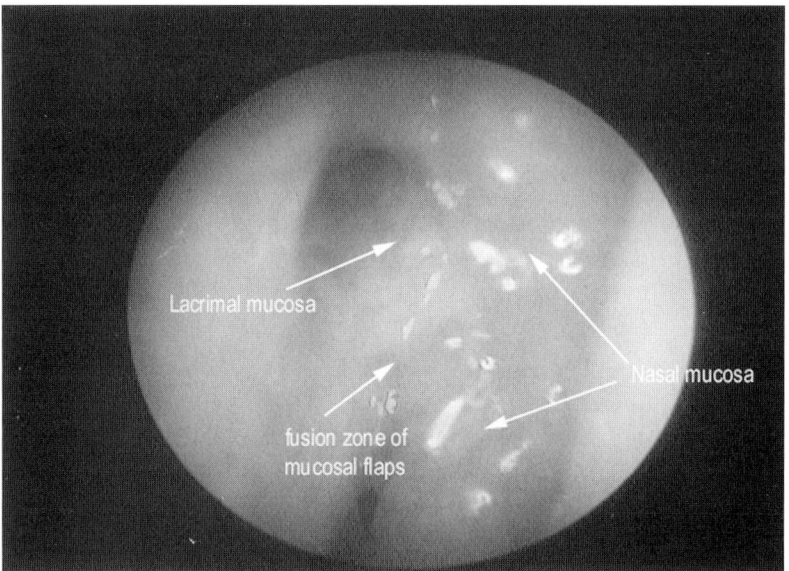

FIGURE 12.8. Endoscopic view 1 month after surgery. The silicone tubes had just been removed. The mucosal flaps were still swollen and hyperemic but the flaps were well fused and the lumen of the DCR clearly visible.

Postoperative Care

Patients are instructed to avoid nose-blowing for 10 days. Prophylactic systemic antibiotics are used only if significant infection is present. Washing of the nostril with saline sprayed in the nose is done for 1 week, 3 or 4 times daily. An antibiotic–steroid combination eyedrop is used for a week in the operated eye. The lacrimal system is irrigated at 1 week and at 1 month. The tube is removed at 1 month. Endoscopy can be performed at 1 week if cleaning of the nostril is believed to be necessary and at 1 month to confirm adequate healing of the surgical site (Figure 12.8). A final follow-up is done at 3 months to confirm the patency of the lacrimal passage and rehabilitation of the nasal anatomy (Figure 12.9).

Complications

Intraoperative or early postoperative bleeding is one of the chief concerns with endonasal DCR surgery. Prevention is the key and involves patients stopping systemic anticoagulants and adequate preoperative preparation to obtain maximum vasoconstriction of the nasal mucosa. Minimal bleeding during the operation is managed with suction. With moderate intraoperative bleeding, the area can be packed with neurosurgical sponges and the suction can be used as well to draw blood into the sponges, further drying the field. If profuse, uncontrollable bleeding occurs, obscuring visualization, the surgeon should consider

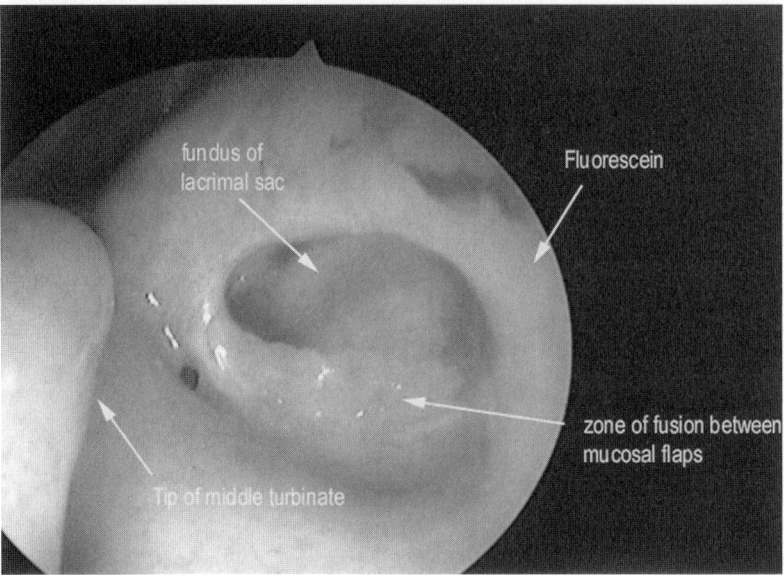

FIGURE 12.9. At 3 months, the dye test was frankly positive at 1 minute and the mucosa was now back to a normal appearance with good continuity of the mucosal flaps.

aborting the operation instead of pursuing the dissection blindly. In the rare instance when significant bleeding occurs in the early postoperative period, the nose is packed overnight and packing removed 24–36 hours later. Patients are given instructions to avoid aspirin-containing compounds and to avoid heavy exercise or Valsalva during the first 10 days after surgery.

Invading adjacent structures is a known complication of endoscopic nasal surgery. Confirming surgical landmarks at every step of the operation will prevent deep invasion of surrounding structures. Temporally, the orbit can be violated, leading to damage of the orbital fat or medial rectus and inferior oblique muscles.[13] A hemorrhage could also result from this complication and any hematoma under tension in the deep medial orbit should be considered for evacuation in extreme cases. Injury to the skull base should not be a risk as long as the proper landmarks are respected. The placement of the light probe in the sac determines the superior landmark, which should be at the level of the internal punctum. However, despite this measure, should a cerebrospinal fluid leak occur, the dissection should be stopped and the patient should be placed on the appropriate antibiotics prophylactically. Bed rest, and in some cases, a lumbar shunt may be necessary to collapse the leak.

Postoperative synechia between different structures in the nose can create problems.[14] The most frequent is a small adhesion between the tip of the middle turbinate and the lateral nasal wall in cases with tight nostrils. Allowing the synechia to mature and then cutting it with scissors a few months later is often all that is necessary. However, excessive dissection and trauma to the nasal mucosa can lead to more extensive synechiae formation. In these difficult cases, more extensive revision with application of antifibroblastic agents such as mitomycin may be the only solution.[9] Granulation tissue may form at the inner ostium of the DCR site in the early postoperative period, resulting in obstruction of the lacrimal drainage system and epiphora. Using the endoscope, the granulation tissue can be removed from the ostium site with straight microethmoid forceps, relieving the blockage. This complication may occur if direct damage to the mucosal lining of the sac is done at the time of the initial surgery.

Conclusion

Endonasal DCR has increasingly been shown to be as successful as external DCR to treat nasolacrimal duct obstruction.[11] Creation of mucosal flaps at the time of surgery is likely responsible for these excellent results. The mucosal healing without granulation promotes the formation of a predictable mucosal-lined fistula into the nose, similar to an external DCR. Endonasal DCR has numerous advantages over external DCR. It is a minimally invasive procedure, which, with experience, can be performed faster than an external DCR.[15] Therefore, in appropriate patients, the endonasal DCR has become the procedure of choice for nasolacrimal duct obstruction.

References

1. Toti A. Nuovo metodo conservatore di cura radicale delle suppurazioni croncihe del sacco lacrimale (dacriocistorinostomia). Clin Mod Firenze 1904;10:385–387.
2. Caldwell GW. Two new operations for the radical cure of obstruction of the nasal duct with preservation of the canaliculi and an incidental description of a new lacrimal probe. NY Med J 1893;57:581.
3. Heermann H. Uber endonasale Chirugie unter Verwendung des binocularen Mikroskopes. Arch Ohren Nasen Kehlkopfheilkd 1958;171:295–297.
4. El Khoury J, Rouvier P. Endonasal dacryocystorhinostomy (95 cases). Acta Otorhinolaryngol Belg 1992;46(4):401–404.
5. McDonogh M, Meiring H. Endoscopic transnasal dacryocystorhinostomy. J Laryngol Otol 1989;103:585–587.
6. Massaro BM, Gonnering RS, Harris GJ. Endolaser laser dacryocystorhinostomy. A new approach to nasolacrimal duct obstruction. Arch Ophthalmol 1990;108:1172–1176.
7. Hartikainen J, Grenman R, Puukka P, Seppa H. Prospective randomized comparison of external dacryocystorhinostomy and endonasal laser dacryocystorhinostomy. Ophthalmology 1998;105:1106–1113.
8. Tsirbas A, Wormald PJ. Endonasal dacryocystorhinostomy with mucosal flaps. Am J Ophthalmol 2003;135:76–83.
9. Woog JJ, Kennedy RH, Custer PL, Kaltreider SA, Meyer DR, Camara JG. Endonasal dacryocystorhinostomy: a report by the American Academy of Ophthalmology. Ophthalmology 2001;108:2369–2377.
10. Lee TS, Woog JJ. Endonasal dacryocystorhinostomy in the primary treatment of acute dacryocystitis with abscess formation. Ophthal Plast Reconstr Surg 2001;17:180–183.

11. Wormald PJ, Tsirbas A. Investigation and endoscopic treatment for functional and anatomical obstruction of the nasolacrimal duct system. Clin Otolaryngol 2004;29:352–356.
12. Goldberg RA. Endonasal dacryocystorhinostomy: is it really less successful? Arch Ophthalmol 2004;122:108–110.
13. Dolman PJ. Comparison of external dacryocystorhinostomy with nonlaser endonasal dacryocystorhinostomy. Ophthalmology 2003;110:78–84.
14. Fayet B, Racy E, Assouline M. Complications of standardized endonasal dacryocystorhinostomy with unciformectomy. Ophthalmology 2004;111: 837–845.
15. Malhotra R, Wright M, Oliver JM. A consideration of the time taken to do dacryocystorhinostomy surgery. Eye 2003;17:691–696.
16. Massegur H, Trias E, Adema JM. Endoscopic dacryocystorhinostomy: modified technique. Otolaryngol Head Neck Surg 2004;130:39–46.

13

Transcanalicular Dacryocystorhinostomy

Hans-Werner Meyer-Rüsenberg and Karl-Heinz Emmerich

Imaging procedures such as dacryocystography, computed tomography, magnetic resonance imaging, high-resolution ultrasound, and scintigraphy are of great importance in diagnosing mechanical dacryostenosis. The aim is locating the mechanical stenosis and allowing for selection of a suitable operative procedure to eliminate the lacrimal obstruction. However, none of the imaging procedures enable direct visualization of pathologic changes such as mucosal or neoplastic changes, dacryoliths, or foreign bodies. The use of rigid endoscopes for preoperative endonasal assessment of the nasal mucosa or for postoperative evaluation has yielded important results for diagnosis and management of diseases of the lacrimal passage for many years.

Dacryoendoscopy

The need to directly visualize pathologic changes in the lacrimal passages led to the development of rigid and flexible endocanicular endoscopes.[1] Because of the narrow lumen of the canaliculus, which is barely more than 1 mm in diameter, the first endoscopes could not provide a satisfactory image quality and thus did not represent a true advancement in diagnostics. Superfine flexible endoscopes (with a diameter of 0.3–0.7 mm) resulting as a modification of gastroduodenal endoscopes were developed for transcanalicular diagnostics.[2,3] With a diameter of 0.3 mm, an image of 1500 pixels could be transmitted with fair quality, but details could not be interpreted and only a rough outline could be attained. By extending the diameter to 0.5 or 0.7 mm, 3000 or 6000 pixels could be transmitted, resulting in a much better image.

Technical Equipment

A modified Juenemann probe was used as the first flexible diagnostic endoscope (Figure 13.1) along with an irrigation channel.[2,4] The exterior diameter was 0.9 mm. The endoscope had a 70° angle view and a 0° direction view. It was illuminated by a Xenon cold light source (Figure 13.2)

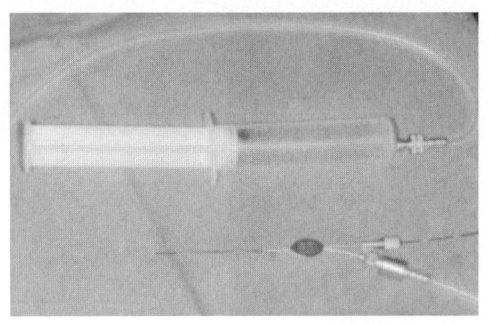

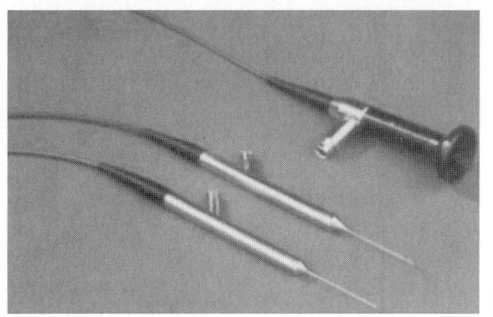

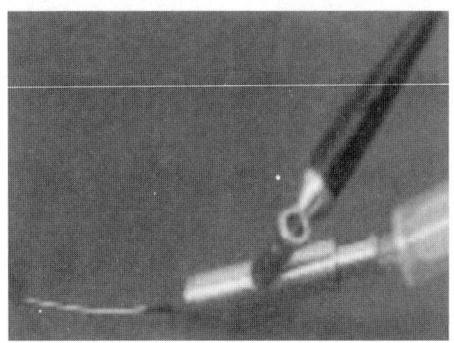

FIGURE 13.1. Development of the dacryoendoscopes. **(A)** Modified Juenemann probe, 3000 pixels. **(B)** Rigid dacryoendoscope (Vitroptic), 6000 pixels. **(C)** Flexible Vitroptic T, 6000 pixels.

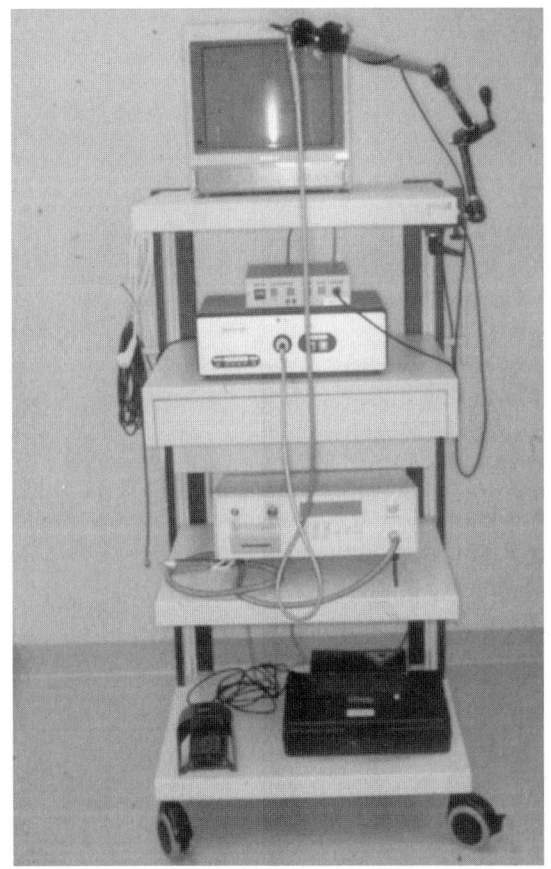

FIGURE 13.2. Endoscopic system (from the top to the bottom): monitor and camera, Xenon light source, erbium:YAG laser, video recorder.

and was connected to a camera by a TV adapter. The camera had a residual light amplification and a high shutter speed of up to 1/2,000,000 of a second. The picture was visible on a high-performance monitor and recorded simultaneously through a video output and documented on a video recorder. It is important to understand that the quality of the actual video picture is much better than the pictures in the text, which were taken from a still video picture. With the exception of the configuration of the endoscopes, e.g., the Vitroptic (Figure 13.1C), the system is unchanged. Future digitalization of the picture may improve its quality.

Performing Dacryoendoscopy

Before performing dacryoendoscopy, the puncta must be dilated (Figure 13.3). Using an astringent solution, the passage is irrigated gently and the endoscope is inserted via the upper or lower canaliculus. The endoscope is advanced forward as far as possible to reach the stenosis or the inferior turbinate. It is then retracted, allowing for a complete evaluation of the lacrimal passage. Retracting and advancing the endoscope with simultaneous irrigation requires a certain amount of practice to obtain quality images. An unobstructed view demonstrates the normal anatomic sequence of transcanalicular endoscopy,

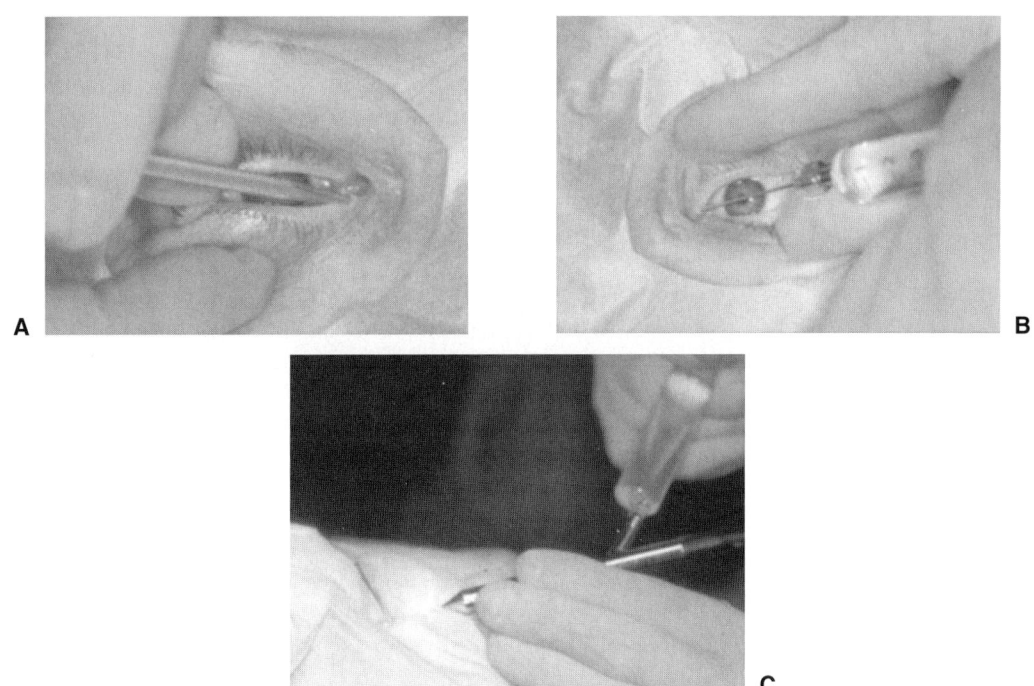

FIGURE 13.3. Steps of dacryoendoscopy. **(A)** Dilating punctum. **(B)** Irrigation. **(C)** Endoscopy and irrigation.

showing canaliculus, lacrimal sac, nasolacrimal duct, and nasal mucosa of the inferior turbinate.

The canalicular mucosa appears white and is quite different from the reddish color of the mucosa of the lacrimal sac. The nasolacrimal duct can be recognized by its narrow shape and its reddish color. The nasal cavity is an intensively red structure, with a smooth surface and large width (Figure 13.4).

Endoscopy permits differentiation of abnormal findings such as membranes, scars, acute or chronic mucosal inflammation, and foreign bodies. Even small blood deposits on the mucosa resulting from manipulation of the lacrimal passage are obvious (Figure 13.5).

From the results of the endoscopy, an appropriate operative procedure can be selected. In Germany, some centers have performed more than 10,000 endoscopic procedures. Injuries caused by the endoscope are comparable to other surgical interventions of the lacrimal passage, such as irrigation or intubation. In general, it is possible to perform a dacryoendoscopy with anesthetizing eye drops, irrigation of the lacrimal passage with 4% cocaine solution, and an anesthetizing nose spray. Most endoscopy procedures are performed under general anesthesia.

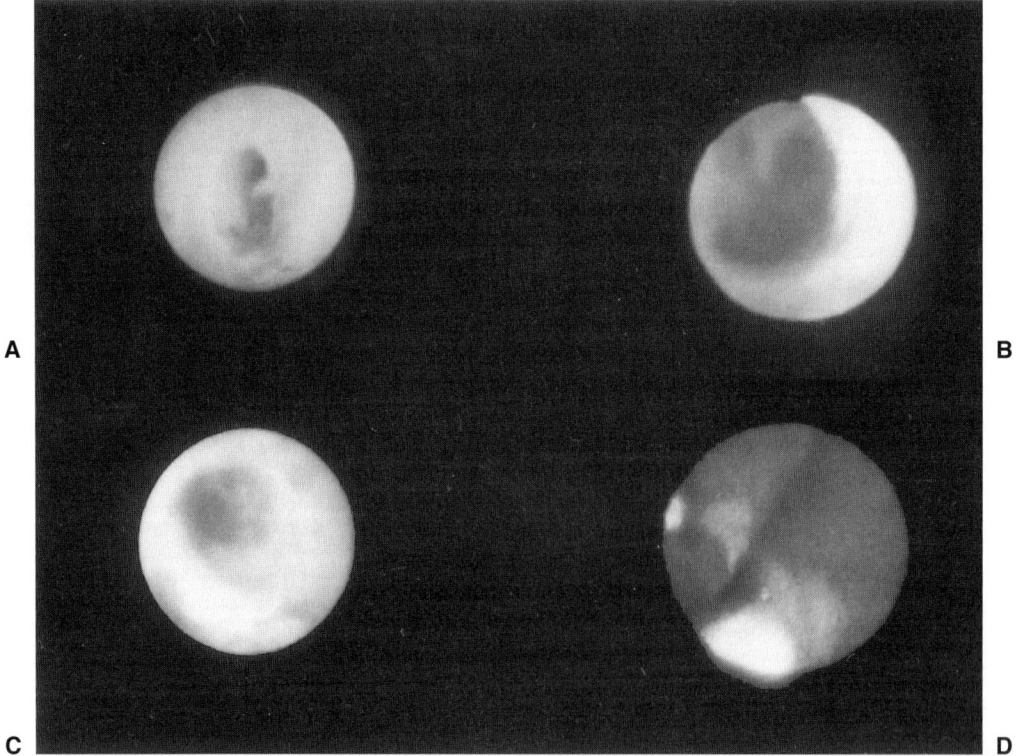

FIGURE 13.4. Endoscopic view of the normal anatomy of the lacrimal passage. **(A)** Canaliculus. **(B)** Rosenmüeller's valve. **(C)** Passage from sac to nasolacrimal duct. **(D)** Nasal cavity and inferior turbinate.

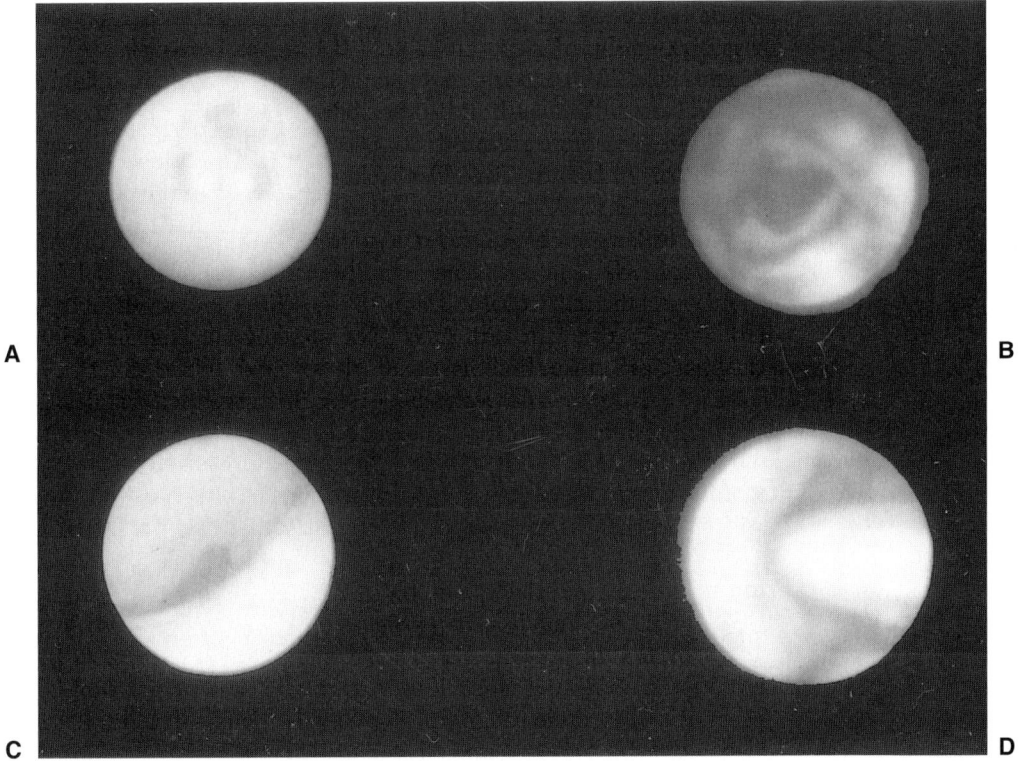

FIGURE 13.5. Endoscopic view to pathologic findings. **(A)** Adhesions of the canaliculus. **(B)** Lacrimal sac stenosis with acute inflammation. **(C)** Mucocele. **(D)** Residual silicone tube after incomplete removal.

Pediatric Endoscopy

In children under the age of 2 years, a purely diagnostic dacryoendoscopy should only be performed in exceptional cases, because the small diameter of the lacrimal passage increases the risk of injury. Diseases of the lacrimal system in newborns and infants are mainly deformational in nature and in these cases, endoscopy does not provide any essential information. Only in cases of failure after prior procedures will endoscopy with simultaneous endoscopic therapy be performed to attempt to avoid a pediatric dacryocystorhinostomy (DCR).

Minimally Invasive Procedures

The desire for lacrimal surgery without scars led to the endonasal DCR technique. Over the years, diverse modifications have been developed. The introduction of microscopes and flexible nasal endoscopes were valuable contributions to this field. The combined approach of anterograde imaging and illumination of the lacrimal system with simultaneous endoscopically controlled nasal surgery provided excellent results.[5] To minimize operative trauma, these endonasal techniques were supplemented by the use of various lasers such as Holmium, potassium titanyl phosphate (KTP), or carbon dioxide.

Laser Dacryoplasty

Holmium:YAG Laser

First attempts of a laser canaliculoplasty were performed using a holmium:YAG laser.[6] Without being linked to an endoscope, a 1-mm cross-sectional connection to the nose was created in the case of canalicular stenosis. The laser had an energy level of 100 mJ, which was delivered by a quartz fiber. After 6 months, the postoperative success rate resulted in an improvement in 57% in 17 examined.

Potassium Titanyl Phosphate Laser

The KTP laser is a very powerful solid-state laser and provides a maximum energy of 10 W, delivered by a 0.3-mm semiflexible fiber that can be connected to an endoscope. The energy released from it is sufficient for creating holes in bones.[7] This laser has been used in a small number of patients and is not frequently used at this time.

Erbium:YAG Laser

A modified, miniaturized erbium:YAG laser[3,4,8] often used for glaucoma surgery has been in use since 1996 (Figure 13.6). A 375-μm sapphire fiber delivers at most 50 mJ with 1–3 Hertz.

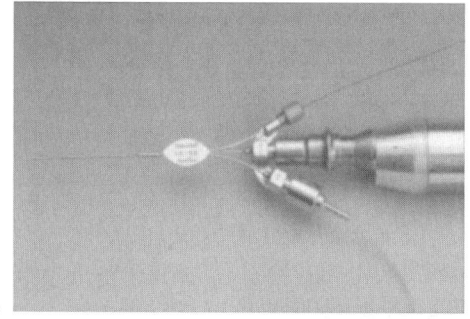
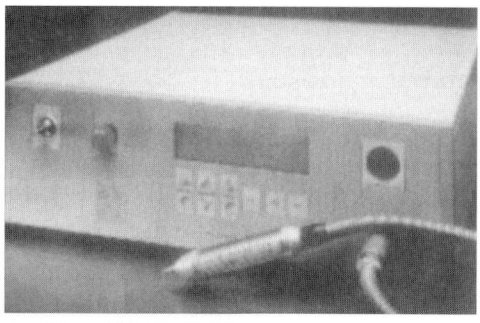
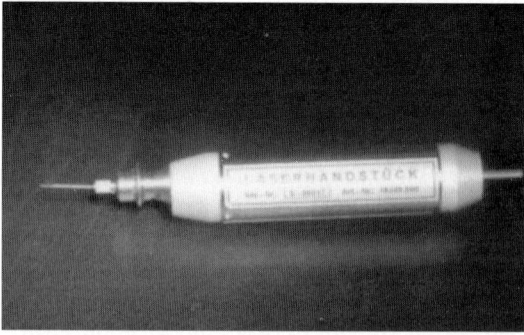

FIGURE 13.6. Erbium:YAG laser components. **(A)** Miniaturized handpiece and early version of a probe. **(B)** Erbium:YAG laser. **(C)** Canaliculus tip.

Miniaturized handpiece	Yes
Wavelength	294 μm
Energy	Maximum 100 mJ
Frequency	1–3 Hertz
Fiber length	11 cm
Zone of necrosis	10–20 μm

The erbium:YAG laser is a photoablative laser, and its maximum absorption occurs in water. Mucosal cells have a water content of 77% so ablation results quickly, but the main effect on a stenotic lacrimal passage is the resulting cavitation blister and not tissue ablation. This blister can extend over several millimeters, allowing for punctal stenoses to be opened with just a few pulses. The energy penetrates the tissue for only a few microns and its low thermal effect creates small necrosis zones of 10–20 μm, making it unsuitable for ablation of bone.

After changing the diagnostic probe from a two to a three working-channel handpiece, therapeutic interventions could be performed. Since 1996, an additional short tip of 4 cm has been developed for treating canalicular stenoses (Figure 13.6C).

Technique of Laser Dacryoplasty

Initially, a diagnostic endoscopy is performed using the same probe, Vitroptic T (Figure 13.6), before the laser application takes place. The procedure is continued until free irrigation without resistance is present and the endoscopic image confirms an opening of the mechanical stenosis. Then, bicanalicular intubation using a silicone tube is performed for preventing postoperative adhesions of the mucosa. The tube stays in place for at least 3 months. Alternatively, in cases of isolated canalicular stenosis, a monocanalicular probe can be used according to the methods of Bernard and Fayet.[9] The postoperative therapy is the same as following bicanalicular intubation in other cases.

Results of Laser Dacryoplasty

The success rate of laser dacryoplasty (LDP), judged as reduction of epiphora, is 60%–70% for all cases (n = 184). The postoperative follow-up was 20.4 months. Considering all canalicular stenoses (n = 44, follow-up more than 12 months), the success rate is 68%, and it increases to 86% for common canaliculus stenosis. These results are better when compared with those after microsurgical procedures performed without endoscopy.[8,10]

Indications for Laser Dacryoplasty

An LDP is indicated in cases of canalicular stenosis, intra- and/or postlacrimal sac lesions, and membranous occlusions after failed DCR. It has been mostly performed on canalicular and lacrimal sac stenoses with chronic infections. Unsuitable scenarios for LDP are acute dacryocystitis, mucoceles, widespread adhesions after viral infections, or stenosis caused by bone displacement after midface fractures.

Microdrill Dacryoplasty

Soon after the development of the LDP, a second technique was introduced for endoscopic transcanalicular manipulation using a microdrill, according to Busse[11] (Figure 13.7). The microdrill, connected to
the Vitroptic T, consists of a stainless steel probe with a diameter of
0.3mm, a drill driven by a shaft, and a battery-operated motor with
50rpm. The drill is controlled by a foot pedal. After inserting the
Vitroptic T into the lacrimal passage and advancing to the location of
the stenosis, the drill is pulled forward under continuous irrigation.
This allows the drill to be visualized throughout the procedure. After
clearing the obstruction, patency is assessed by irrigation and endoscopy. The postoperative regimen (intubation and medical therapy) is
the same as after LDP.

Results

The success rate of microdrill dacryoplasty (n = 168) for reduction of
epiphora with the follow-up of more than 12 months is almost
78%.[10,12]

Indications

The microdrill is suitable for membranes, dacryoliths, or other mechanical obstructions, especially subtotal button-holed-style stenosis at the
end of the lacrimal sac 18–20mm distal to the punctum. The drill per-
forms a kind of mucosal curettage; therefore, canalicular stenosis is not
suitable for treatment with the microdrill system. The microdrill cannot
be used to perform a DCR.

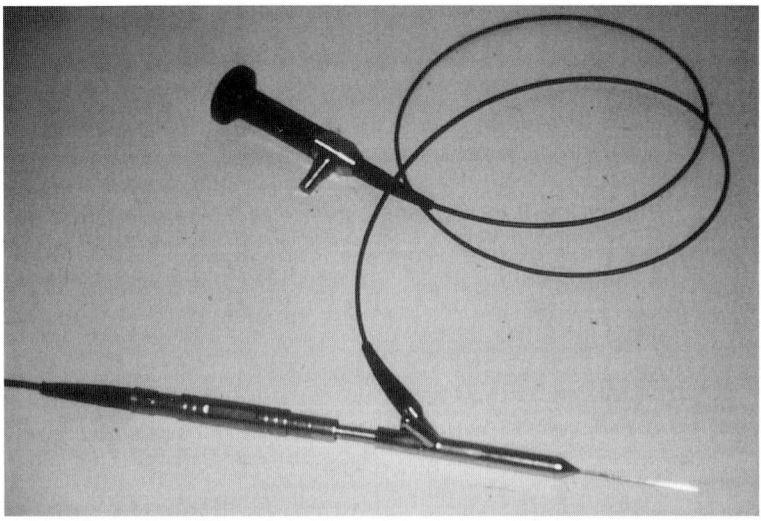

FIGURE 13.7. Microdrill and Vitroptic T.

Conclusion

Transcanalicular dacryoendoscopy combined with simultaneous minimally invasive therapy is a great step forward in diagnostic and operative choices. It has considerably reduced the rate of DCRs that would otherwise have been necessary to perform.

Transcanalicular endoscopy enables new insights into the pathology of the diseases of the lacrimal system. Today, one can directly visualize lesions and decide immediately on appropriate interventions, whereas in the past, only indirect imaging was available.

References

1. Ashenhurst ME, Hurwitz JJ, Katz A. Proceedings of the European Society of Ophthalmic Plastic and Reconstructive Surgery, Vienna, 1990.
2. Steinhauer J, Meyer-Ruesenberg HW, Emmerich KH. Erste Erfahrungen mit der Tränenwegsendoskopie. Sitzungsbericht 158. Versammung des Vereins Rheinisch Westfälischer Augenärzte, 1996, Hagen S., 159–162.
3. Emmerich KH, Luchtenberg M, Meyer-Ruesenberg HW, Steinhauer J. Dacryoendoskopie und Laserdacryoplastik: Technik und Ergebnisse. Klin Monatsbl Augenheilkd 1997;211:375–379.
4. Meyer-Rusenberg HW, Emmerich KH, Lüchtenberg M, Steinhauer J. Endoskopische Laserdacryoplastik – Methodik und Ergebnisse nach 3 Monaten. Ophthalmologe 1999;96:332–334.
5. Michel O, Russmann W. Indikationen und Praxis der simultanen Ophthalmo-Rhinochirurgie. Eur Arch Otorhinolaryngol Suppl 1993;3(1):255–271.
6. Dutton JJ, Holck DE. Holmium laser canaliculoplasty. Ophthalmol Plast Reconstr Surg 1996;12:211–217.
7. Muellner K, Wolf G. Endoskopische Behandlung von Tränenwegsstenosen mit Hilfe eines KTP-Lasers erster Erfahrungsbericht. Klin Monatsbl Augenheilkd 1999;215:28–32.
8. Steinhauer J, Norda A, Emmerich KH, Meyer-Ruesenberg HW. Lasercanaliculoplastik. Ophthalmologe 2000;97:692–695.
9. Fayet B, Assouline M, Bernard JA. Monocanalicular nasolacrimal duct intubation. Ophthalmology 1998;105(10):1795–1796.
10. Emmerich KH, Ungerechts R, Meyer-Ruesenberg HW. Possibilities and limits of minimal invasive lacrimal surgery. Orbit 2000;19(2):67–71.
11. Busse H. Microsurgery in lacrimal disorders. Dev Ophthalmol 1989; 18:50–52.
12. Ungerechts R, Ungerechts G, Meyer-Rüsenberg HW, Emmerich K-H. Promitoa, Meeting of the European Society of Ophthalmic Plastic and Reconstructive Surgery, Gothenburg, Sweden, 11–13 September 2003.

14

Conjunctivodacryocystorhinostomy

Jan Lei Iwata, Robert A. Weiss, and Michael Mercandetti

Conjunctivodacryocystorhinostomy (CDCR) with tube placement is a procedure that Lester Jones, MD pioneered in 1962 as a treatment for irreparable lacrimal canalicular obstruction. Since then, the procedure has undergone various modifications. In 1982, Murube-del-Castillo[1] described a method of total lacrimal bypass that obviated the need for osteal perforation and provided dependable drainage. In 1990, Arden et al.[2] detailed the use of a bipedicle nasal mucosal flap with temporary stenting. In 1991, Gonnering described a CDCR with a partial caruncu-lectomy using a transnasal, endoscopic, CO_2 or potassium titanyl phosphate (KTP) laser-assisted approach with good success in appropriately selected cases.[3,4] Contraindications to this technique included suspicious lacrimal sac malignancy and severe bony deformity of the lacrimal fossa, which would prevent accurate transillumination through the lacrimal bone.

Other modifications to the procedure include: blind canalicular marsupialization in cases of punctal atresia or obliteration[5]; wrapping the tube with mucous membrane,[6] saphenous vein,[7] or buccal mucosal grafts[8,9]; and elimination of a visible cutaneous scar by doing a conjunctival incision for primary CDCR.[10] Modifications of lacrimal bypass tubes included addition of a secondary flange, such as in the Gladstone-Putterman tube, which decreases the extrusion rate,[11] and modifications that allow tube fixation by placement of a stabilizing suture.[12]

The main indication for CDCR surgery is symptomatic epiphora resulting from severe disruption of the canalicular system, including punctal or canalicular agenesis.[13,14] Other causes for obstruction that might require a total lacrimal bypass procedure include herpetic infection, tumors, inflammatory conditions, sarcoidosis,[15] Stevens-Johnson syndrome, systemic chemotherapy, radiation therapy, and lacrimal pump dysfunction in facial nerve palsy.[14] Iatrogenic causes of punctal and canalicular obstruction include chronic use of 0.125%–0.25% echothiophate (phospholine iodide),[16] docetaxel,[17] and permanent punctal (proximal canalicular) occlusion used to manage keratoconjunctivitis sicca.[18,19] Trauma and idiopathic disease remain the most common causes of lacrimal canalicular obstruction, as reported by Sekhar et al.,[20] and Zilelioglu and Gunduz,[21] with 34.8% and 68.5% (13.5% trauma), respectively. Common infectious causes of lacrimal drainage obstruction include: trachoma, *Aspergillus*, *Actinomyces*, *Diphtheria*, and *Streptococcus* organisms.[22] Stagnant lacrimal sac contents can act as culture media for microorganisms such as *Staphylococcus*, *Streptococcus*, gram-negative organisms,[23] and tuberculosis.[24]

Procedure

CDCR is a dacryocystorhinostomy performed in conjunction with placement of a total lacrimal bypass tube such as a Jones, or Gladstone-Putterman, or Cooper tube. Most tubes are made of Pyrex glass (Weiss Scientific Glass Blowing Company, Portland, OR) (Figure 14.1).

After exposing the lacrimal fossa, attention is directed toward placement of the tube. A linear slit is made in the caruncle or subtotal removal of the caruncle is performed so the tube will be well situated in the nasal end of the interpalpebral fissure. A large-gauge needle, von Graefe knife, or 15 blade, is passed into the nose through the caruncular slit and ostomy in an anteromedial and inferior direction (Figure 14.2). The tip of the instrument should be located anterior to the top of the middle turbinate. The intranasal septum must be sufficiently away from the lateral wall of the nose for adequate space of the distal end of the tube. A fine Quickert-Dryden lacrimal intubation probe is placed through the needle lumen into the nose. As the needle is withdrawn from the nose, the distance from the caruncle to the nose should be measured, to determine the length of the tube that is needed. Alternatively, the probe can be passed through the opening made with

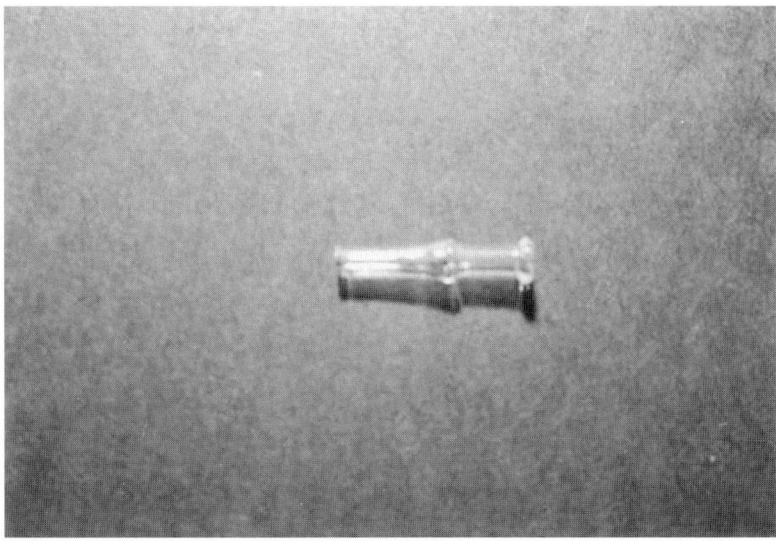

FIGURE 14.1. Gladstone-Putterman tube.

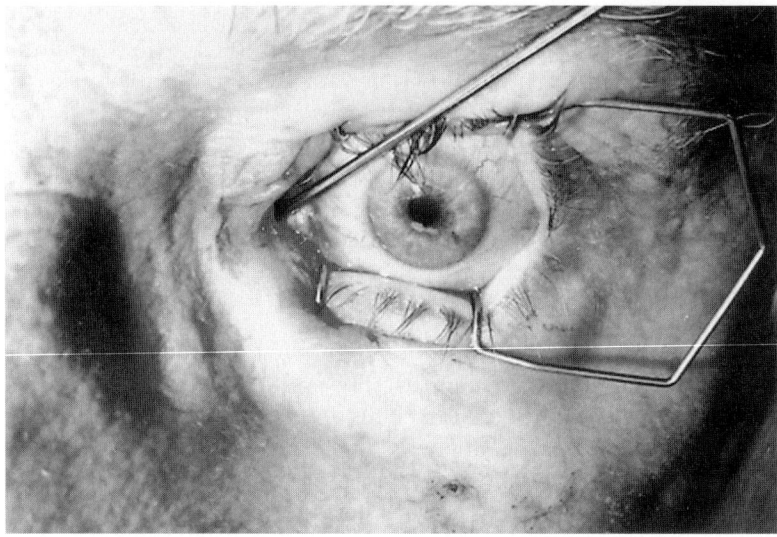

FIGURE 14.2. Creation of a linear slit through caruncle.

the knife or blade. The probe is used as a guide for passing the glass tube directly into the nose (Figure 14.3). A suture is placed around the neck of the collar or through a fixation hole in the collar to anchor the tube to adjacent tissues. Another method for placing the tube is to use a glaucoma trephine over a solid guide.

The authors prefer a 3.5- to 4.0-mm collar size on a straight tube. Tubes come in many collar sizes and can be angulated. When the tube becomes well seated, it is not unusual to need a smaller collar size and different length tube. If it is necessary to change tubes, a gold dilator can be placed to keep the passage open (Figures 14.4 and 14.5).

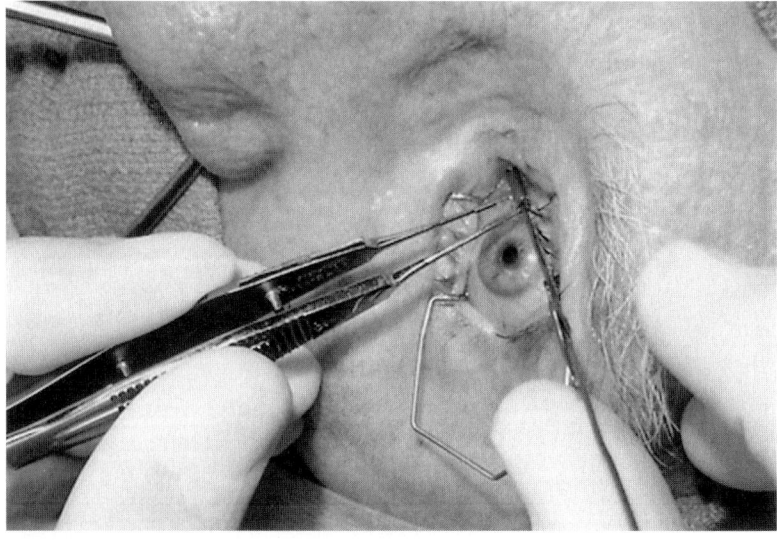

FIGURE 14.3. Passage of total bypass tube over lacrimal probe.

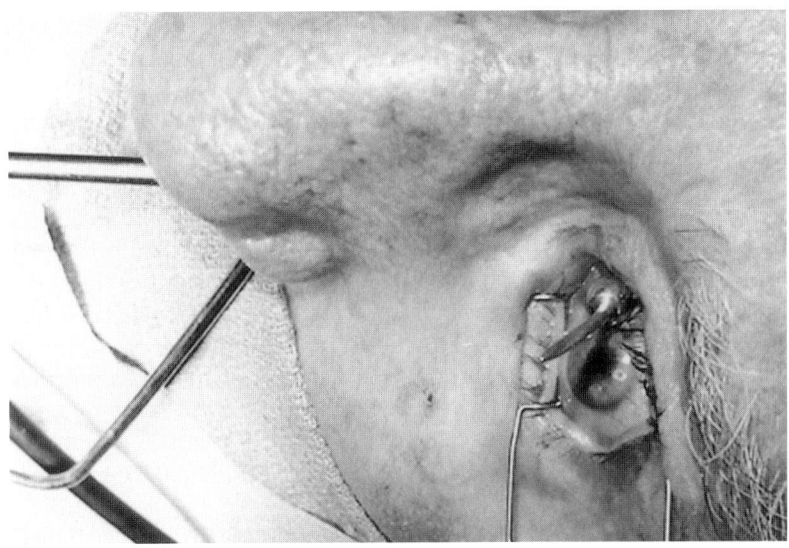

FIGURE 14.4. Gold dilator.

Postoperatively, the patient should be treated with topical antibiotics or antibiotic/steroid eye drops. The patient should be encouraged to irrigate water or saline through the tube daily on a long-term basis to prevent protein buildup[25] and mucous plugging. Having the patient temporarily occlude the contralateral nostril can help the flow through the tube. It is important to inform the patient to close the eyelids when sneezing to avoid reflux or displacement of the tube.

Patients who lose their tubes are at risk of fistula track closure.[8] Steinsapir et al.[26] believe that the tube should remain permanently in

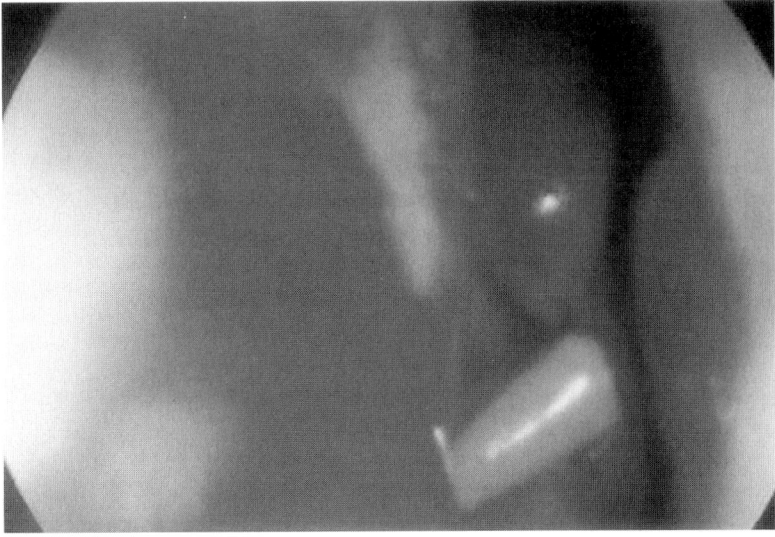

FIGURE 14.5. Endoscopic view of total bypass tube in the left nasal vault.

place, based on their study of 75 patients over a 16-year period. Jones[27] believed that once the fistula tract was epithelialized, the tube could be removed. Lim et al.[28] reported on five eyes in which the tube had been lost; one was a complete success, two were moderate successes, and one was a failure.

In a small series of patients, Leone[8] described similar findings to Campbell et al.,[6] in which 17 patients had a full-thickness buccal-mucosal graft to line the CDCR tract, to prevent closure in the event that the tube came out. Two patients lost their tube from rubbing their eye, one was lost in the nasal cavity, and two elected to have their tubes removed after 6 months. All of these patients remained asymptomatic with primary dye tests demonstrating patency of their reconstructed lacrimal apparatus. Twenty-four percent of grafted patients remained asymptomatic after removal of the Jones tube, between 6 months and 3 years after surgery. Lower success rates (2 of 11 patients) were reported by Can et al.[9]

After CDCR, the conjunctival flora of the eye (in some patients) became similar to nasal flora secondary to retrograde flow of lacrimal and nasal secretions. This may be important in terms of infection risk, especially in patients who are candidates for intraocular surgery. In a study by Can et al.,[9] the number of cases (20 eyes) in which bacteria was isolated from the operated eye and nose (50%) but not from the nonoperated eye included: *Staphylococcus aureus*,[4] *Corynebacterium* sp.,[2] a-hemolytic streptococci,[1] gram-negative bacilli,[1] and pneumococcus.[1]

Overall complication rates postoperatively have ranged from 51%[21] to 63.6%,[9] of which the primary complication was extrusion of the lacrimal bypass tube. Can et al.[9] reported that complications rates were less (21.4%) when CDCR procedures were performed in conjunction with buccal grafts, because there was less irritation resulting in conjunctival overgrowth and granuloma formation, which accounted for 31.8% of complications resulting from standard CDCR. The rate of complication seen in a series of 121 patients who had CDCR performed in the study by Rosen et al.[29] was similar (49%).

Reports of significant and symptomatic medial conjunctival inflammation that developed after CDCR despite aggressive medical treatment were described by Abel and Meyer.[30] Inflammation persisted despite the removal of the Jones tube, and the second patient had what resembled an injected pterygium that formed and was later excised. Histopathologic examination revealed conjunctival tissue with fibrosis, without subepithelial elastotic degenerative changes.[30]

Persistent episcleritis and atypical facial pain, scleral erosion and ulceration, and lower eyelid inflammatory masses have been described by Bartley and Gustafson[31] as complications seen in a limited series of patients who underwent bilateral CDCRs. Other complications include conjunctival overgrowth, internal extrusion, and bypass tube malposition. Some complications such as obstruction, anterior migration, infection, discomfort, including irritation and pain, and diplopia on extreme lateral gaze caused by scarring of the medial bulbar conjunctiva can be prevented or corrected by correct placement of the fistulous tract.[28]

In another report, extrusion was seen in 57.9%, 40 of 69 eyes, of which 57.5% of the extrusions were seen in the first 3 months after the operation.[20] Can et al.[9] found that extrusion and migration accounted for 50% of cases. This complication occurred in most cases within the first 6 months postoperatively. Additional postoperative complications mentioned by Kulwin et al.[32] (1990) included pyogenic granuloma of the caruncle, corneal abrasion, granulation tissue in the nose, wound infection, nasal septal hematoma, and mucous obstruction. They advocated middle turbinectomy and septoplasty to enlarge the middle meatal air space, so that the tube can project 3 mm beyond the lateral nasal wall mucosa, and away from the septum.

Functional outcome is, of course, the key to determining the level of satisfaction with using the Jones tube in the CDCR procedure. A completely successful outcome was defined as a comfortable, epiphora-free eye despite frequent complications. The success rate using this definition ranges from 92.6% (Rosen et al.[29]) to 98% (Sekhar et al.[20]), and 94% (Lim et al.[28]) with complete or significant improvement of epiphora in 49 cases, of which 32 patients (70%) were satisfied with the result; 35% reported tube maintenance to be troublesome. This is somewhat higher than what was reported by Rosen and colleagues[29] who reported an 11.6% dissatisfaction rate of successfully treated patients. Overall, success rates have ranged from 83% from the original Jones tube procedure, up to 90%[21] and 94%–95% with regard to complete relief of epiphora and lacrimal obstruction; the success rate is somewhat higher for endoscopic CDCR in well-chosen patient populations.

The highest rate of dissatisfaction was in patients over 70 years of age (22%), and under 19 years of age. Complaints included tearing in the recumbent position, fogging of eyeglasses, and air blowing in the eye upon sneezing or blowing the nose. Successfully patent mucous membrane-lined fistulous tracts after Jones tube expulsion have been reported.[25,33]

Acknowledgment. The authors appreciate the work of Debra Nation, CST, who assisted in preparation of this chapter.

References

1. Murube-del-Castillo J. Conjunctivodacryocystorhinostomy without osteal perforation. Arch Ophthalmol 1982;100(2):310–311.
2. Arden RL, Mathog RH, Nesi FA. Flap reconstruction techniques in conjunctivorhinostomy. Otolaryngol Head Neck Surg 1990;102(2):150–155.
3. Gonnering RS, Lyon DB, Fisher JC. Endoscopic laser-assisted lacrimal surgery. Am J Ophthalmol 1991;111(2):152–157.
4. Watkins LM, Janfaza P, Rubin PA. The evolution of endonasal dacryocystorhinostomy. Surv Ophthalmol 2003;48(1):73–84.
5. Rumelt S. Blind canalicular marsupialization in complete punctal absence as a part of a systemic approach for classification and treatment of lacrimal system obstructions. Plast Reconstr Surg 2003;112(2):394–403.

6. Campbell CB 3rd, Shannon EM, Flanagan JC. Conjunctivodacryocystorhinostomy with mucous membrane graft. Ophthalmic Surg 1983;14(8):647–652.

7. Soll DB. Vein grafting in nasolacrimal system reconstruction. Ophthalmic Surg 1983;14(8):656–660.

8. Leone CR Jr. Conjunctivodacryocystorhinostomy with buccal mucosal graft. Arch Ophthalmol 1995;113(1):113–115.

9. Can I, Can B, Yarangumeli A, Gurbuz O, Tekelioglu M, Kural G. CDCR with buccal mucosal graft: comparative and histopathological study. Ophthalmic Surg Lasers 1999;30(2):98–104.

10. Liu D. Conjunctival incision for primary conjunctivodacryocystorhinostomy with Jones tube. Am J Ophthalmol 2002;129(2):244–245.

11. Migliori ME, Putterman AM. Recurrent Jones tube extrusion successfully treated with a modified glass tube. Ophthal Plast Reconstr Surg 1989;5(3):189–191.

12. Ma'luf RN, Bashur ZF, Noureddin BN. Modified technique for tube fixation in conjunctivodacryocystorhinostomy. Ophthal Plast Reconstr Surg 2004;20(3):240–241.

13. Duffy MT. Advances in lacrimal surgery. Curr Opin Ophthalmol 2000; 11(5):352–356.

14. Mandeville JT, Woog JJ. Obstruction of the lacrimal drainage system. Curr Opin Ophthalmol 2002;13(5):303–309.

15. Chapman KL, BarleyGB, Garrity JA, Gonnering RS. Lacrimal bypass surgery in patients with sarcoidosis. Am J Ophthalmol 1999;127(4):443–446.

16. Wood JR, Anderson RL, Edwards JJ. Phospholine iodide toxicity and Jones' tubes. Ophthalmology 1980;87(4):346–348.

17. Esmaeli B, Valero V, Ahmadi A, Booser D. Canalicular stenosis secondary to Docetaxel (taxotere): a newly recognized side effect. Ophthalmology 2001;108(5):994–995.

18. Pratt DV, Patrinely JR. Reversal of iatrogenic punctal and canalicular occlusion. Ophthalmology 1996;103(9):1493–1497.

19. White WL, Barley GB, Hawes MJ, Lindberg JV, Leventer DB. Iatrogenic complications related to the use of Herrick lacrimal plugs. Ophthalmology 2000;108(10):1835–1837.

20. Sekhar GC, Dortzbach RK, Gonnering RS, Lemke BN. Problems associated with conjunctivodacryocystorhinostomy. Am J Ophthalmol 1991;112(5):502–506.

21. Zilelioglu G, Gunduz K. Conjunctivodacryocystorhinostomy with Jones tube, a 10-year study. Doc Ophthalmol 1996–97;92(2):97–105.

22. Smolin G, Tabbara K, Whitcher J. Infectious Diseases of the Eye. Baltimore: Williams and Wilkins; 1983:57.

23. Hyde KJ, Berger ST. Epidemic keratoconjunctivitis and lacrimal excretory system obstruction. Ophthalmology 1988;95(10):1447–1449.

24. Al-Malki AF, Issa TM, Riley F, Karcioglu ZA. Nasolacrimal tuberculosis in a patient with conjunctivodacryocystorhinostomy. Ophthal Plast Reconstr Surg 1999;15(3):213–216.

25. McCord CD, Tanenbaum M, Nunery WR. Oculoplastic Surgery. 3rd ed. Lacrimal System Drainage. New York: Raven Press; 1995:363–376.

26. Steinsapir KD, Glatt HJ, Putterman AM. A 16-year study of conjunctival DCR. Am J Ophthalmol 1990;109(4):387–393.

27. Jones LT. Conjunctivodacryocystorhinostomy. Am J Ophthalmol 1965;59:773–783.

28. Lim C, Martin P, Benger R, Lourt G, Ghabrial R. Lacrimal canalicular bypass surgery with the Lester Jones tube. Am J Ophthalmol 2004;137(1): 101–108.
29. Rosen N, Ashkenazi I, Rosner M. Patient dissatisfaction after functionally successful conjunctivodacryocystorhinostomy with Jones tube. Am J Ophthalmol 1994;117(5):636–642.
30. Abel AD, Meyer DR. Refractory medial conjunctival inflammation associated with Jones tubes. Ophthal Plast Reconstr Surg 2003;19(4):309–312.
31. Bartley GB, Gustafson RO. Complications of malpositioned Jones tubes. Am J Ophthalmol 1990;109(1):66–69.
32. Kulwin DR, Tiradellis H, Levartovsky S, Kersten RC, Shumrick KA. The value of intranasal surgery in assuring the success of a conjunctivodacryocystorhinostomy. Ophthal Plast Reconstr Surg 1990;6(1):54–59.
33. Nagashima K. Fistulous tract after conjunctivodacryocystorhinostomy. Ophthalmic Surg 1986;17(12):809.

15

Endoscopic Conjunctivodacryocystorhinostomy

Geoffrey J. Gladstone and Brian G. Brazzo

Preoperative Evaluation

The evaluation of a patient with complaints of epiphora involves investigating causes of excess lacrimation as well as lacrimal outflow obstruction. There are many causes of excess lacrimation. Dry eyes are one of the most common but entropion, trichiasis, and any other cause of ocular irritation are frequently seen. Mild punctal ectropion can cause significant epiphora. Idiopathic hypersecretion, although a diagnosis of exclusion, is an important consideration.

A basic secretor test, a careful slit lamp examination with and without corneal staining, and an evaluation of the conjunctiva for signs of inflammation, symblepharon, or infection are performed. An evaluation of eyelid position should include a search for entropion, ectropion, trichiasis, and eyelid notching. When idiopathic hypersecretion is suspected, a Schirmer 1 test is indicated.

Evaluation of the outflow pathway involves probing and irrigation. Traditional Jones 1 and Jones 2 testing is rarely performed. A 23-gauge lacrimal irrigating needle is used to probe the upper and lower canaliculi. Stenosis or blockage of the canaliculi is noted. Irrigation of the system is attempted through the lacrimal sac. The ease of irrigation into the nasopharynx and the amount of reflux of irrigant back to the eyes are noted. Significant blockage of a canaliculus is an indication for an endoscopic conjunctivodacryocystorhinostomy (CDCR).

A dye retention test is occasionally used. In patients with no or limited outflow obstruction (as demonstrated with probing and irrigation), this test can help make the diagnosis of lacrimal pump failure. It can also be helpful in cases of partial canalicular stenosis. The test is most useful with unilateral epiphora where the side in question can be compared with the normal side. A drop of fluorescein is placed in both eyes. The patient is asked to not wipe his or her eyes. The amount of fluorescein remaining in the tear meniscus is observed after 2 minutes. When a normal outflow tract is present, only a trace amount of fluorescein is present in a normally small tear meniscus. A significant increase in the amount of fluorescein present and in the size of the tear meniscus indicates an outflow obstruction or lacrimal pump failure.

When considering whether to perform endoscopic CDCR, evaluation of the caruncle and medial canthus is important. There must be an appropriate place for the proximal end of the tube to rest. A previously placed medial tarsorrhaphy or other abnormality of the eyelids secondary to trauma or resection of tissue can require correction before the placement of the tube.

Nasal endoscopy can be performed to evaluate the amount of room between the septum and lateral nasal wall and the presence or absence of intranasal tumors. Intranasal tumors can cause an outflow obstruction and need to be evaluated and treated when appropriate. Benign intranasal tumors can impinge on the distal end of the tube after surgery. A deviated nasal septum can make endoscopic surgery difficult or impossible. Visualization of the operative site just anterior to the middle turbinate is decreased and a constant blockage of the endoscope tip by blood can occur. Additionally, the distal end of the tube must rest between the septum and the lateral nasal wall. If insufficient space is available, a septoplasty needs to be performed before endoscopic CDCR.

Gladstone-Putterman Modified Jones Tube

The original Jones tube is susceptible to internal or external migration and to ejection with nose blowing, sneezing, or coughing. To alleviate these problems, an additional flange can be added to the Jones tube. This internal flange is 4mm distal to the external flange. It acts similar to an arrowhead, locking the tube in position (Figure 15.1). This modi-

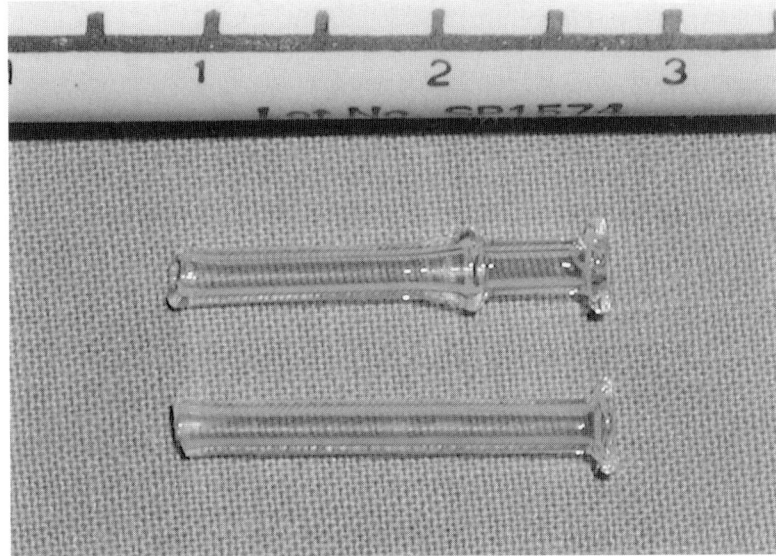

FIGURE 15.1. Comparison of Gladstone-Putterman tube (above) and Jones tube (below).

fied tube, known as the Gladstone-Putterman tube, is inserted in a similar manner as the original Jones tube.

Indications for Endoscopic Conjunctivodacryocystorhinostomy

The most common indication for endoscopic CDCR is canalicular blockage. This blockage may be secondary to trauma, previous surgery, or systemic chemotherapeutic agents such as 5-fluorouracil or Taxotere. A unicanalicular or bicanalicular blockage can cause epiphora, as can a significant common canalicular stenosis.

When canalicular stenosis is present, Silastic intubation can be attempted. If this fails to eliminate the epiphora, then an endoscopic CDCR is indicated. With canalicular blockage, a dacryocystorhinostomy will not be effective because the tears cannot progress to the lacrimal sac. A complete bypass of the lacrimal outflow tract is necessary.

Lacrimal pump failure frequently occurs after Bell's palsy and other causes of facial paralysis, which are common after removal of acoustic neuromas and squamous cell carcinomas. A normal probing and irrigation of the lacrimal system can be performed, but a dye retention test may be quite abnormal with a great deal of dye remaining in the enlarged tear meniscus. Some degree of lagophthalmos, ectropion, and corneal staining may be present. It is important to exclude these as causes of the epiphora before proceeding with endoscopic CDCR. In normal patients, the lower eyelid punctum moves medially with each blink. This is seen most easily if the upper lid is held open and the patient is asked to blink. The absence of this movement can be an indication that an old facial paralysis is not completely resolved and that a lacrimal pump failure may be present.

The final indication for endoscopic CDCR is a patient with idiopathic hypersecretion. This diagnosis of exclusion is made when the outflow tract is normal and there are no identifiable factors causing increased lacrimal gland secretion. Results from the Schirmer 1 test will be much higher than normal. Referral for an external disease consultation should be considered before proceeding with surgery. In these cases, the modified Jones tube provides an additional and larger outflow tract to accommodate the increased tear production.

Advantages of Endoscopic Technique

Endoscopic CDCR offers a number of advantages over external CDCR. These advantages include absence of scarring, absence of ecchymosis and edema, less surgical manipulation of medial canthal tissues, and better visualization of the modified Jones tube and adjacent structures once the tube has been placed. Because no external incision is made, no external scar is present. Because there is minimal external tissue manipulation, it is rare to have ecchymosis or medial canthal edema.

With endoscopic technique, no medial canthal skin incision is used and no dissection of deeper tissue is performed. This lack of tissue manipulation is important in the healing process. A properly placed modified Jones tube is more likely to stay in the proper position. With the external technique, there is a greater chance of the tube shifting its position as the tissues heal. This change can lead to malposition of the proximal end of the tube. Additionally, the angle of the tube can be altered. It is important that the tube maintain an approximately 45° downward angle. If this angle decreases as tissues heal, a decrease in tear drainage can occur.

Once the modified Jones tube is placed, endoscopic intranasal inspection of the distal end of the tube is performed. This process allows an accurate assessment of two potential problems. Tube length is evaluated. A tube that is too short does not protrude far enough from the lateral nasal wall and is at risk for being covered by mucosa. A tube that is too long will touch the nasal septum and can be painful and can lead to external tube extrusion or poor tear drainage. Either of these problems is easily correctable at the time of surgery if recognized.

The relationship of the distal end of the tube to the middle turbinate is evaluated endoscopically. The middle turbinate is often infractured at the onset of surgery to provide easier access to the uncinate process. Postoperatively, the turbinate will often assume its preoperative position. This can bring the turbinate into apposition with the distal end of the modified Jones tube. If the surgeon believes that the shift will result in blockage of the tube, a partial turbinectomy can be performed at that time.

Surgical Technique

Thirty minutes before the procedure, the patient is asked to blow the nose and is then given two sprays of 0.05% oxymetazoline in the nasal cavity ipsilateral to the planned procedure. This process is repeated in 5 minutes. The majority of cases are performed under monitored intravenous sedation and local anesthesia, although some patients require general anesthesia. The nasal cavity is packed with 18 inches of 1/2-inch plain gauze soaked in 4% cocaine solution. The packing is removed after 5 minutes.

Under direct visualization with a 0° rigid endoscope, local injection of 2% lidocaine with 1:100,000 epinephrine mixed 50:50 with bupivacaine 0.75% with 1:200,000 epinephrine is administered to the submucosa of the anterior middle turbinate, uncinate process, and area anterior and superior to the uncinate process. The nasal cavity is repacked, carefully filling the space between the middle turbinate and the lateral nasal wall with 4% cocaine-soaked gauze for another 5 minutes. This regimen of packing is necessary to obtain adequate hemostasis. The face is draped in an appropriate manner, but a sterile field is not required.

Under endoscopic visualization, the middle turbinate and its relationship to the lateral nasal wall are inspected (Figure 15.2). If the

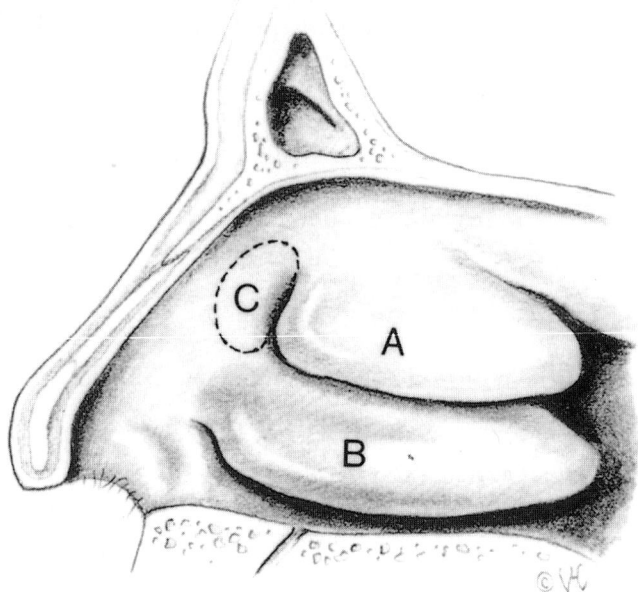

FIGURE 15.2. Normal nasal anatomy. **(A)** Middle turbinate. **(B)** Inferior turbinate. **(C)** Bone and mucosa overlying lacrimal fossa.

turbinate is obstructing the view of the uncinate process, or if the turbinate may obstruct the osteotomy site postoperatively, it may be gently infractured with a blunt periosteal elevator. The same instrument may be used to make an incision at the border of the bony lateral nasal wall and the uncinate process. The uncinate is the first protrusion of the lateral nasal wall encountered under the middle turbinate.

The mucosa overlying the lacrimal fossa is cauterized with monopolar cautery set in the coagulation mode (Figure 15.3). This area extends approximately 10 mm anterior to the uncinate process and from the level of the root of the middle turbinate superiorly and 10 mm inferiorly. The mucosa is scraped from the underlying bone with a periosteal elevator, and removed with Blakesley forceps. Thorough removal of the mucosa is important to prevent bleeding during the next step of the procedure. A medium-size Kerrison bone rongeur creates an osteotomy to correspond to the area from which the mucosa was removed. The rongeur is placed onto the bony edge that was exposed after removal of the uncinate process. Further bone removal proceeds superiorly and anteriorly. Usually four or five bites are needed to obtain an adequate osteotomy. At this point, the lacrimal sac can be identified.

A track for the glass tube is now created. No excision of caruncle is performed because this promotes inward migration of the modified Jones tube. A 12-gauge shielded intravenous catheter (Angiocath, BD, Franklin Lakes, NJ) is bent approximately 30° at its midpoint. A smaller 14-gauge catheter can also be used, but the passage of the Jones tube will be more difficult. Bending the catheter is intended to keep the distal end of the tube relatively anterior in the nose. The Angiocath enters the middle of the caruncle (Figure 15.4). The shaft of the Angio-

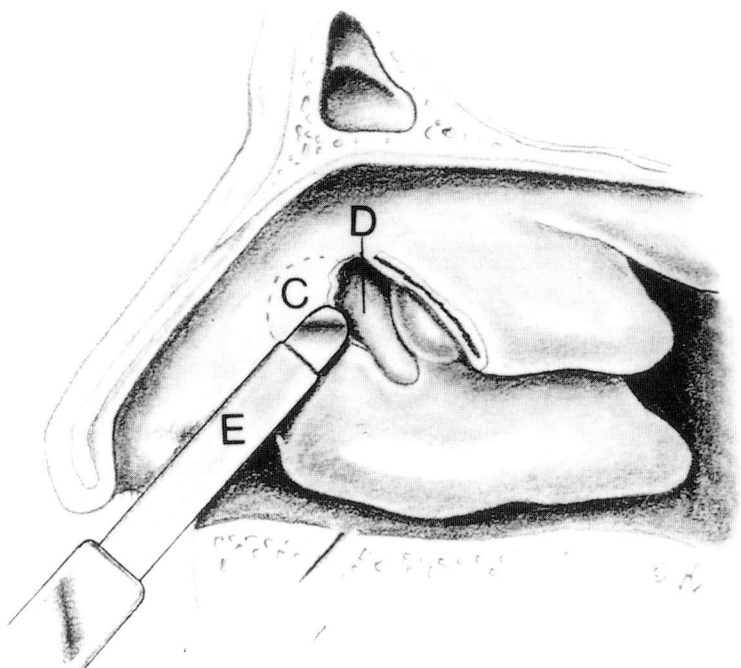

FIGURE 15.3. Guarded monopolar cautery **(E)** applied to nasal mucosa **(C)** and lacrimal fossa bone **(D)**.

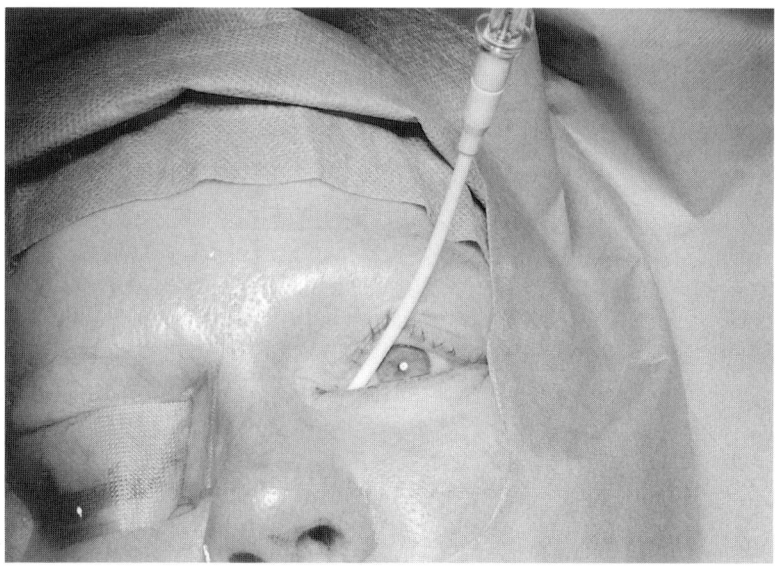

FIGURE 15.4. A 12-gauge shielded intravenous catheter (Angiocath) is bent approximately 30° at its midpoint and advanced through the middle of the caruncle at a 45° angle. The catheter can be visualized entering the nasal cavity with an endoscope.

cath is kept close to the eye as the catheter is advanced in a medial and inferior direction. A downward angle of 45° is attempted. The needle is visualized with the endoscope as it enters the nasal cavity. It can be redirected if necessary so it exits through the osteotomy. The metal needle is removed, leaving only the plastic sheath in position.

A 9-inch-long piece of 20-gauge wire is passed through the plastic sheath and the sheath is removed, leaving only the wire in position (Figure 15.5). The wire acts as a guide for the glass tube placement. A 4 × 19 mm tube is placed over the wire and pushed into proper position (Figure 15.6). When the extra flange encounters the medial canthal tissue, increased resistance will be felt. Both of the surgeon's thumbnails are placed on the proximal end of the tube and used to push it firmly into position. The internal flange will lock the tube in position.

The length and position of the tube are checked with the endoscope. The tube ideally sits halfway between the lateral nasal wall and the nasal septum. If the position is not appropriate, the proximal end of the tube is grasped and the tube removed, leaving the guide wire in place. A longer or shorter tube is inserted. Once an acceptable tube is placed, the guide wire is removed. A 6-0 double-armed silk or polyglactin suture is wrapped twice around the proximal end of the tube. Both needles are brought from the medial side of the tube through the skin. The needles are passed through a small piece of sterile rubber

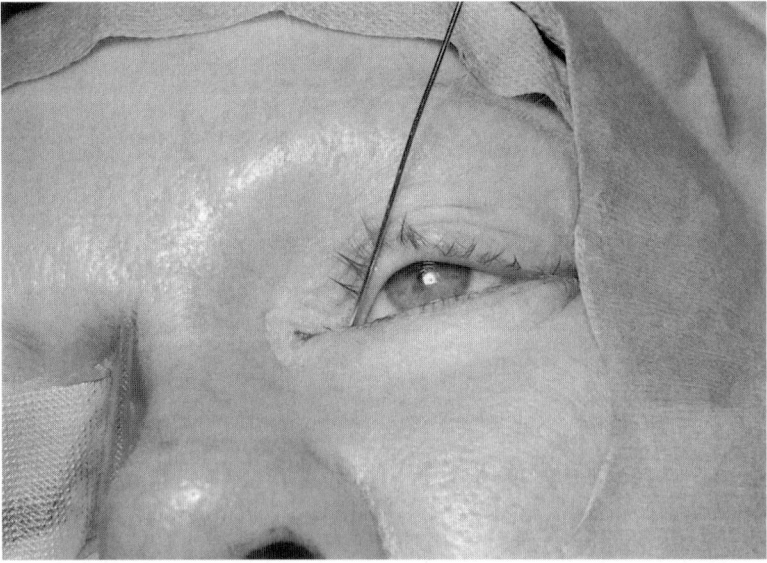

FIGURE 15.5. A 9-inch-long piece of 20-gauge wire is passed through the plastic sheath and the sheath is removed, leaving only the wire in position. The wire acts as a guide for the glass tube placement.

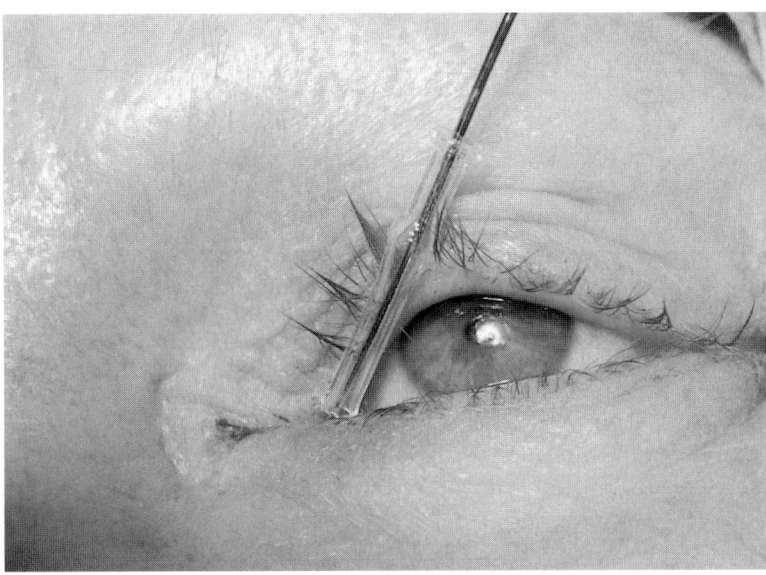

FIGURE 15.6. A Gladstone-Putterman 4 × 19 mm tube is placed over the wire before it is pushed into proper position.

band and are tied with mild tightness. This rubber band bolster and suture are removed after 1 week.

Special Surgical Considerations

After placement of the modified Jones tube, the distal end of the tube must be inspected endoscopically and its relationship to the middle turbinate appraised. If the distal end of the modified Jones tube becomes occluded by the middle turbinate, the change could result in external tube displacement or poor drainage of tears. To reduce the chance of this complication, a partial middle turbinectomy is performed. An additional injection of the local anesthetic mixture is given directly into the turbinate. A small curved hemostat is applied to the turbinate at the inferior border of the area to be removed. The curve of the hemostat is reversed and the instrument applied to the superior border. Care is exercised to avoid crushing the Jones tube. Ideally, the tips of the crushed areas will meet. Right and left angled endoscopic turbinate scissors are used to incise the tissue along the crushed areas. Blakesley forceps are used to gently twist the piece of turbinate and remove it.

An important part of the preoperative evaluation is the intranasal endoscopic examination. If a significant septal deviation is present, it will make endoscopic surgery difficult and allow insufficient room for the modified Jones tube. In these situations, a septoplasty should be performed before the endoscopic CDCR. This procedure can be performed at the time of the endoscopic CDCR but the septum medializes better if the tissue is allowed to contract for a month before proceeding with the endoscopic CDCR. Techniques for performing a septoplasty are beyond the scope of this chapter.

Postoperative Care

For at least several months after surgery, it is important that the patient put a finger over the tube in the medial canthal area during sneezing, nose-blowing, or coughing. This precaution will help prevent external displacement of the tube. Once the medial canthal tissue has contracted around the tube and the extra flange, there is less chance of external displacement. At a minimum, patients should be reminded to tightly close their eyes whenever they perform the above maneuvers. Nose-blowing is discouraged for the first postoperative week because this may cause intranasal bleeding. After 1 week, a nasal saline rinse is used as much as desired to help cleanse the nasal cavity.

Postoperative Evaluation and Management of Complications

One of the most important aspects of postoperative evaluation is the patient's subjective evaluation of how much his or her epiphora has improved. This subjective evaluation is what patients consider when determining their satisfaction with the procedure.

An objective evaluation of tube function has been devised. The drainage is classified as Class I through IV. Several drops of water are place in the medial canthal area with the head tipped backward. In Class I drainage, the water drains spontaneously. In Class II drainage, the water drains with exaggerated nasal respiration. Class III drainage is present when the water will not drain with respiration but the tube can be irrigated. Class IV drainage is present when no irrigation is possible through the tube.

When Class I or II drainage is present, the patient has a significant improvement in his or her epiphora and is typically satisfied. Class III and IV drainage problems need to be investigated and corrected, otherwise epiphora will continue. Poor drainage can be attributed to many factors including displacement of the tube in an anterior or posterior direction, displacement in an internal or external direction, and blockage of the tube either externally or internally.

A tube whose proximal end is anteriorly displaced is not in position to allow entry of tears into the tube. This tube must be removed and replaced in a more posterior position. It is necessary to utilize the 12-gauge Angiocath and enter the caruncular tissue more posterior than the original placement. Removing the modified Jones tube can be difficult because the medial canthal tissues contract and hold the tube in position. Tying a 2-0 silk suture around the neck of the tube allows the tube to be pulled out of position without the risk of breaking it. Occasionally, it is necessary to use Westcott scissors to cut down to the area of the extra flange to free the tube.

A posteriorly placed tube can irritate the eye or can become blocked at its proximal end by conjunctiva. Removal of the tube and placement more anteriorly will typically be curative.

An internally migrated tube is seen more frequently when a portion of the caruncle is removed. It can occasionally occur without caruncular removal. Usually, the tube can be palpated with forceps through the overlying tissue. Westcott scissors are used to cut down to the proximal end of the tube and a 2-0 silk suture is tied around the proximal flange. This suture is used to pull the tube free. If extensive tissue manipulation is necessary to remove the tube, the canthal tissues should be allowed to heal before implanting another tube. Otherwise, another internal migration is likely.

An external displacement of the tube places the proximal end of the tube in a position where tears cannot enter. The tube may also irritate the eye. Simple manual pressure on the proximal end of the tube may force it back into position, allowing the distal flange to lock in position in the medial canthal tissue. If simple manual pressure is not adequate, endoscopic examination of the distal end of the tube is indicated. A tube that is too long can abut the nasal septum. This tube must be removed and one several millimeters shorter placed. A tube that is too short may not be seen intranasally and should be replaced by a tube of appropriate length. The physician should also consider idiopathic hypersecretion as a diagnosis of exclusion.

A normally placed tube may have its proximal end occluded by redundant conjunctiva. An injection of the tissue with a depo steroid may be curative. If not, excision of the excess tissue can be easily performed.

Blockage of the distal end of the tube can be caused by the lateral nasal wall, the nasal septum, or the middle turbinate. The treatment of these problems has been previously covered.

Occasionally, a perfectly placed and functioning tube may cause irritation of the medial canthal tissues. Topical steroid drops may resolve this condition. If not, an injection of a depo steroid can be used.

16

Pediatric Balloon Catheter Dacryocystoplasty

Bruce B. Becker

Balloon catheter dacryocystoplasty (DCP) is a very effective treatment for congenital nasolacrimal duct obstruction in children who have failed probing or silicone intubation, or as a primary procedure in children older than 12 months of age.

Resolution of congenital nasolacrimal duct obstruction occurs either spontaneously or with the aid of massage and antibiotic drops in 80%–95% of patients.[1–5] Probing is very effective in patients with persistent congenital nasolacrimal duct obstruction, if it is performed before the patient is 13 months of age, with a success rate of 97%.[6] However, the success rate of probing decreases after 12 months of age. Katowitz and Welch[6] found the success rate to be 76.4% when probing is performed on patients from age 13 to 18 months, and 33.3% in patients over 24 months of age. Other studies have confirmed that the success of probing decreases with age, but the rate of decrease has varied significantly among different reports.[7–10] The different success rates for probing reported in the literature can be attributed to criteria for success, ranging from confirmation by telephone interviews to confirmation by examinations with or without fluorescein dye disappearance testing, time of follow-up, and variation of referral patterns.[6]

In addition to the decreasing success rate in older children, probing is much less effective in children with stenoses, obstructions, or diffuse narrowing of the nasolacrimal duct proximal to the level of the valve of Hasner.[11–13] Older children and children who have failed probing often have more proximal stenoses or obstructions of the nasolacrimal duct that can be the result of chronic infection and fibrosis or that may be congenital.[11,14] Paul and Shepherd[3] believe that children with congenital nasolacrimal duct obstruction proximal to the level of the valve of Hasner fail conservative treatment and therefore represent a higher proportion of older children.

Silicone intubation of the lacrimal drainage system has been used for children who fail probing or are older. Silicone intubation has a good success rate, but has significant drawbacks: the tube must be retrieved in the nose – this can be difficult in some patients; the tube must be removed 3–6 months after surgery, requiring a second

procedure; the child may remove the tube prematurely; and elonga-
tion of the puncta ("cheese wiring") can occur because of medial
tension.[15,16]

Unlike probing or silicone intubation, balloon catheter dilatation of
the nasolacrimal duct (DCP) achieves true dilatation. Furthermore,
balloon catheter DCP is technically much easier to perform than silicone intubation, and obviates the need to remove the tube or concerns
about the child removing the tube. A very high success rate can be
achieved. One study of balloon catheter DCP of 61 lacrimal systems in
51 patients with congenital nasolacrimal duct obstruction (age range
from 13 to 73 months, mean 26 months) showed a patency rate of 95%.[17]
Of the patients treated in this series, 44.3% had no previous procedures, 34.4% had one or more failed probings, and 21.3% had failed
silicone intubation. Other studies have also found balloon catheter
DCP to be effective in children with nasolacrimal duct obstruction who
have failed probing, have obstructions proximal to the valve of Hasner,
or who are 13–24 months of age or older at the time of the primary
intervention.[18–21]

The indications for balloon catheter DCP in congenital nasolacrimal
duct obstruction are:

1. Failed probing at any age
2. Failed silicone intubation at any age
3. As a primary procedure in children older than 12 months of age
4. As a primary procedure in children with trisomy 21 at any age.[22]
   Children with trisomy 21 have a very poor response to probing or
   silicone intubation.[22]

Silicone intubation should be reserved for patients with canalicular
stenosis, or used in combination with balloon catheter DCP for patients
who have failed a primary balloon catheter dilatation.

Some physicians believe that probing should be performed after 1
year of age, or in older children if intraoperative findings indicate that
a membrane at the level of the valve of Hasner is the only site of
obstruction.[12,13] Balloon catheter DCP has a higher success rate than
either probing or silicone intubation, and is least likely to lead to recurrence necessitating a second procedure and anesthesia. Balloon catheter DCP is therefore recommended for all children who meet any of
the above four criteria, although each physician must decide on a case-
by-case basis when probing should no longer be performed.

Before and after balloon catheter DCP, a medical regimen helps to
ensure the greatest possible success rate. *It is essential that infection be
eliminated or markedly suppressed before surgery.* Because antibiotic drops
are unreliable and often inadequate, *administration of systemic antibiotics
for 7–10 days before surgery is imperative:* amoxicillin and clavulanate
potassium (Augmentin; total of 40 mg/kg/day in two divided doses) or
cefaclor (total of 40 mg/kg/day in three divided doses). If the infection
has not resolved or has not been markedly suppressed before balloon
catheter DCP, surgery should be rescheduled. Preoperative cultures are
not routinely performed, but cultures can be helpful if there is marked
discharge. The most common organism cultured from patients with

congenital nasolacrimal duct obstruction and dacryocystitis is *Strepto-coccus pneumoniae*, although other organisms may be causative.[17,23]

In the operating room just before surgery, intravenous cefazolin (25 mg/kg) is administered. To allow time for vasoconstriction, the nose is packed with one $1/2 \times 3$ inch neurosurgical cottonoid soaked in 0.25% phenylephrine solution (available as a nasal spray) immediately after the administration of general anesthesia. The cottonoid is grasped along its long axis with a bayonet forceps, and is placed in the nasal cavity along the floor of the nose. In this position, it will contact the inferior turbinate and cause vasoconstriction. The surgical field is then prepped and draped.

The puncta are gently dilated. The cottonoid nasal pack is removed. The 0 or 00 Bowman probe is used to perform probing in the usual manner: placing the probe through the punctum and canaliculus into the lacrimal sac, orienting it vertically, pushing the probe down the nasolacrimal duct into the nasal cavity. It is essential to confirm that the probe has entered the nasal cavity because patients who are older or who have failed probing may have multiple stenoses or obstructions. The surgeon must be sure that the probe has penetrated all obstructions and entered the nose. Touching the probe in the nose with a metal instrument (e.g., another probe or closed mosquito hemostat) and feeling "metal on metal" helps confirm that the probe extends into the nasal cavity. The probe is then removed.

If the inferior turbinate appears tightly apposed to the lateral nasal wall, infracture of the inferior turbinate can be performed before balloon catheter inflation. Infracture of the inferior turbinate did not influence the success rate in Becker's series of 61 lacrimal systems, and is probably not essential.[17] Endoscopic visualization shows that there is usually a gap between the opening of the nasolacrimal duct and the inferior turbinate, even if the anterior inferior turbinate abuts the lateral nasal wall. If infracture is performed, a number 4 Penfield dissector or Freer elevator (both available in all operating rooms) is placed along the floor of the nose 25 mm into the nasal cavity. The curved end of the instrument is then slid along the nasal floor onto the lateral wall with the concavity of the instrument directed toward the lateral nasal wall. The instrument will thus lie between the lateral nasal wall and the inferior turbinate. At this point, the elevator is pushed medially to infracture the inferior turbinate medially (Figures 16.1 and 16.2).

After the probing segment of the procedure is completed, the balloon catheter can be placed. The technique of placing the balloon catheter is precisely the same as that used for probing. The lacrimal balloon catheter is in effect a balloon on a probe – handling and feeling like a Bowman probe and thus enabling any physician experienced with probing to accomplish balloon catheter DCP.

A 2-mm balloon catheter is used for patients 30 months of age or younger, and a 3-mm balloon catheter is used for patients older than 30 months of age. The deflated balloon catheter is pushed through the canaliculus, lacrimal sac, and down the nasolacrimal duct into the nose. The balloon catheter must be pushed all the way to the nasal floor, and confirmation of proper placement by touching the deflated

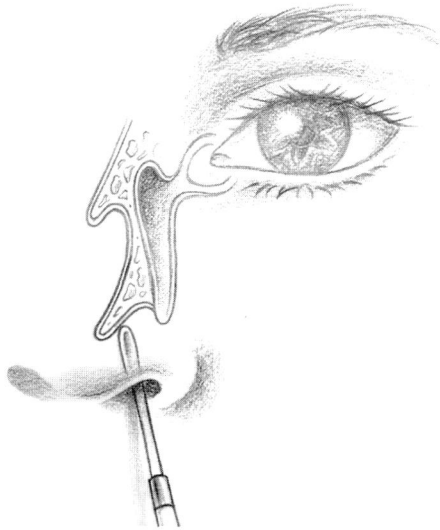

FIGURE 16.1. Infracture of the inferior turbinate (coronal view). The Freer elevator is in the inferior meatus, and is pushing the inferior turbinate medially.

balloon with another instrument is necessary. As mentioned earlier, multiple obstructions may be present, or the balloon may catch on an unusually thick valve of Hasner and stretch the mucosa of the valve without actually entering the nasal cavity. The balloon may be visualized in the nose with a sinuscope, but the use of an endoscope is optional.

Once the lacrimal balloon catheter is positioned in the lacrimal system, it can be connected to the inflation device. Any cardiac balloon angioplasty inflation device can be used, and is obtained from the hospital cardiac catheterization laboratory. Alternatively, the inflation device can be obtained from the same company that makes the lacri-

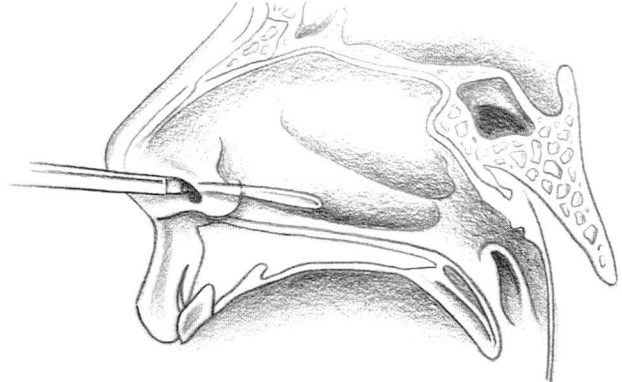

FIGURE 16.2. Infracture of the inferior turbinate (sagittal view).

mal balloon catheter (Atrion, Quest Medical, Allen, TX). Inflation is performed twice for 20 seconds each at a pressure of 8 atmospheres (Figure 16.3). This dilates the distal nasolacrimal duct.

The balloon catheter is then deflated and pulled more proximally so that it lies within the lacrimal sac and proximal nasolacrimal duct. The proximal nasolacrimal duct including the sac–duct junction will thus be dilated. This is essential because an obstruction at the sac–duct junction is present in some older patients or in those who have failed probing.[15] The proximal catheter shaft has a mark 10mm proximal to the beginning of the working (full diameter) portion of the balloon, and a second mark 15mm proximal to the beginning of the working portion of the balloon. The punctum is aligned at a point 5mm distal to the 10-mm mark (i.e., the punctum is 5mm from the balloon). This ensures that the proximal balloon is in the lacrimal sac. An accordion-like contraction of the canaliculus caused by the balloon catheter causes the punctum to be very close to the lacrimal sac. If the balloon catheter is in the common canaliculus, it will slither into the lacrimal sac at the onset of dilation. Inflation is performed to 8 atmospheres of pressure and is again performed twice for 20 seconds (Figure 16.4). After the proximal dilation, the balloon catheter is deflated, all residual fluid is aspirated with a syringe, and the catheter is withdrawn from the lacrimal system. The balloon will not completely deflate passively, and so it is necessary to aspirate the fluid out with a syringe.

Fluorescein-stained fluid is then irrigated through the lacrimal system and recovered in the nose with a soft suction catheter. The fluid should irrigate easily and profusely through the lacrimal system. If not, dilation should be performed again.

Fourth-generation fluoroquinolone drops and 1% prednisolone drops are administered four times a day for 10 days after surgery. The systemic antibiotics are continued for 5 postoperative days.

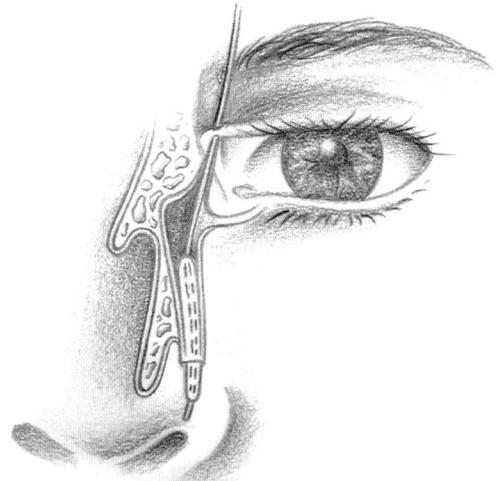

FIGURE 16.3. The lacrimal balloon catheter has been pushed to the nasal floor and inflated.

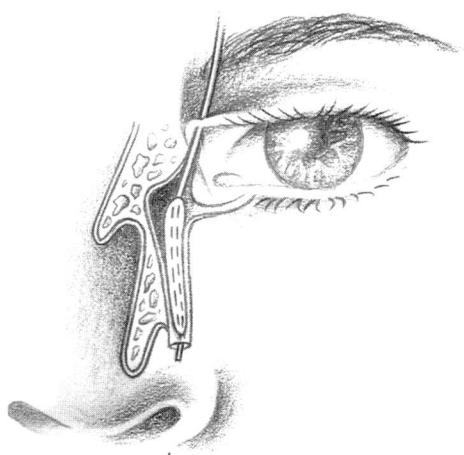

FIGURE 16.4. The lacrimal balloon catheter has been pulled proximally. The balloon lies in the lacrimal sac and extends into the nasolacrimal duct.

Although many physicians are not comfortable with the use of systemic corticosteroids, and good results can be achieved without their use, the author recommends administration of 4 mg of dexamethasone intravenously at the beginning of surgery, prednisolone (15 mg/5 cc) 15 mg a day for 2 days after surgery, then 7.5 mg a day for 2 days. Corticosteroids reduce edema, fibroblast activity, and possibly fibrosis after surgery, but a controlled study has not been performed to determine the efficacy of this and other elements of the medical regimen described here.

Patients are examined at 1 day, 2 weeks, and 6 weeks after balloon catheter DCP to confirm continuing patency of the lacrimal drainage system.

References

1. Nelson LB, Calhoun JH, Menduke H. Medical management of congenital nasolacrimal duct obstruction. Ophthalmology 1985;92:1187–1190.
2. Price HW. Dacryostenosis. J Pediatr 1947;30:302–305.
3. Paul TO, Shepherd R. Congenital nasolacrimal duct obstruction: natural history and the timing of optimal intervention. J Pediatr Ophthalmol Strabismus 1994;312:362–367.
4. Crigler LW. The treatment of congenital dacryocystitis. JAMA 1923;81: 21–24.
5. Peterson RA, Robb RM. The natural course of congenital obstruction of the nasolacrimal duct. J Pediatr Ophthalmol Strabismus 1978;15:246–250.
6. Katowitz JA, Welsh MG. Timing of initial probing and irrigation in congenital nasolacrimal duct obstruction. Ophthalmology 1987;94:698–705.
7. Koxe MP. Treatment of occluded nasolacrimal ducts in infants. Arch Ophthalmol 1950;43:750–754.
8. Robb RM. Probing and irrigation for congenital nasolacrimal duct obstruction. Arch Ophthalmol 1986;104:378–379.

9. Honavar SG, Prakash VE, Rao GN. Outcome of probing for congenital nasolacrimal duct obstruction in older children. Am J Ophthalmol 2000;130:42–48.

10. Mannor GE, Rose GE, Frimpong-Ansah K, Ezra E. Factors affecting the success of nasolacrimal duct probing for congenital nasolacrimal duct obstruction. Am J Ophthalmol 1999;127:616–617.

11. Hurwitz JJ, Welham RAN. The role of dacryocystography in the management of congenital nasolacrimal duct obstruction. Can J Ophthalmol 1975;10:346–350.

12. Kushner BJ. Congenital nasolacrimal duct obstruction. Arch Ophthalmol 1982;100:597–600.

13. Kashkouli MB, Beigi B, Parvaresh NM, Kassaee A, Tabatabaee Z. Late and very late initial probing for congenital nasolacrimal duct obstruction: what is the cause of failure? Br J Ophthalmol 2003;87:1151–1153.

14. Christensen FH, Putterman AM. Management of failed probing in the pediatric patient using dacryocystogram. In: Bosniak SL, Smith BC, eds. Advances in Ophthalmic Plastic and Reconstructive Surgery. Vol 3. New York: Pergamon; 1984:111–132.

15. Patel BCK, Anderson RL. Silicone intubation in adults and children. In: Mauriello JA, ed. Unfavorable Results of Eyelid and Lacrimal Surgery: Prevention and Management. Boston: Butterworth and Heinemann; 2000:491–505.

16. Ratliff CD, Meyer DR. Silicone intubation without intranasal fixation for treatment of congenital nasolacrimal duct obstruction. Am J Ophthalmol 1994;118:781–785.

17. Becker BB, Berry FD, Koller HJ. Balloon catheter dilatation for treatment of congenital nasolacrimal duct obstruction. Am J Ophthalmol 1996;121: 304–309.

18. Leuder GT. Balloon catheter dilation for treatment of older children with nasolacrimal duct obstruction. Arch Opthalmol 2002;120:1685–1688.

19. Tao S, Meyer DR, Simon JW, Zobal-Ratner J. Success of balloon catheter dilatation as a primary or secondary procedure for congenital nasolacrimal duct obstruction. Ophthalmology 2003;109:2108–2111.

20. Lueder GT. Balloon catheter dilation for treatment of persistent lacrimal duct obstruction. Am J Ophthalmol 2002;133:337–340.

21. Hutcheson KA, Drack AV, Lambert SR. Balloon dilatation for treatment of resistant nasolacrimal duct obstruction. J AAPOS 1997;4:241–244.

22. Lueder GT. Treatment of nasolacrimal duct obstruction in children with trisomy 21. J AAPOS 2000;4:230–232.

23. Kuchar A, Lukas J, Steinkogler FJ. Bacteriology and antibiotic therapy in congenital nasolacrimal duct obstruction. Acta Ophthalmol Scand 2000; 78:694–698.

17

Balloon-Assisted Dacryoplasty in Adults

John Pak and Mark T. Duffy

In recent years, there has been an emerging interest in the development and application of alternative therapeutic approaches for the treatment of complete and incomplete nasolacrimal duct (NLD) obstructions (NLDOs). For complete NLDOs, it is generally accepted that an incisional dacryocystorhinostomy (DCR), because of its high rate of success (more than 90%), is the treatment of choice.[1] Despite such efficacy, controversies around anesthetic choices and rare, cosmetically significant scarring have aroused interest in alternative treatment modalities. Increasing attention has recently focused on balloon dacryocystoplasty, a technique based on dilation of a completely or incompletely stenotic aperture along the NLD using a balloon catheter device similar to those used in vascular dilation.

Balloon dacryocystoplasty initially emerged as a fluoroscopic-assisted retrograde technique aimed at dilating the stenotic NLD. This involved the use of a guide wire that cannulated the NLD and, subsequently, placed a balloon catheter through the area of stenosis. Over the past decade, the technique has undergone significant innovations. Most notable is the transition from a retrograde to antero-grade approach using specially designed lacrimal system balloon catheters. Balloon dacryoplasty has also been used in association with temporary silicone tube stenting of the NLD to increase the success rate.[2] Lastly, a recent report also describes significant efficacy in combination with endoscopy.[3] Despite these advances, varying degrees of success have been reported using this technique for complete or incomplete NLDO. In this chapter, the authors examine the efficacy of balloon dacryocystoplasty for complete and incomplete NLDOs.

Procedure

Balloon dacryocystoplasty is performed by the authors using a technique previously published by others.[2] Oxymetazoline 0.05% nasal spray is insufflated or sprayed into the chosen nasal cavity and the corresponding inferior turbinate region is packed with gauze soaked in 0.05% oxymetazoline or 4% cocaine. Topical tetracaine or proparacaine is instilled on the conjunctival surface. An injection of 2% lidocaine with 1:100,000 units of epinephrine is given in the infratrochlear region for a regional nerve block. This will anesthetize the lateral nasal wall, part of the nasal septum, and regionally around the medial canthus. Additional anesthetic can be injected locally in the medial upper and lower lids, and for supraorbital and infraorbital nerve blocks.

The nasal packing is removed. The puncta are dilated. The surgeon probes the upper and lower canaliculi and NLD using Bowman probes in the standard manner. After withdrawal of the probe, intubation of the canaliculus and passage through the NLD is undertaken using a deflated 3-mm LacriCATH™ balloon catheter (Quest Medical, Inc., Allen, TX) from which the protective plastic sleeve has been removed (Figure 17.1). Either the superior or inferior punctum can be used. In general, the upper passage is recommended for several reasons[3]: it provides a more direct route into the NLD, and in the event a false passage is created, the more important inferior canaliculus will remain intact. The deflated catheter is placed within the NLD until the 15-mm marking is adjacent to the punctum. The tip of the catheter can be identified under the inferior turbinate by touching it with a probe or, if endoscopy is performed, the distal balloon can be directly visualized (Figure 17.2A–C).

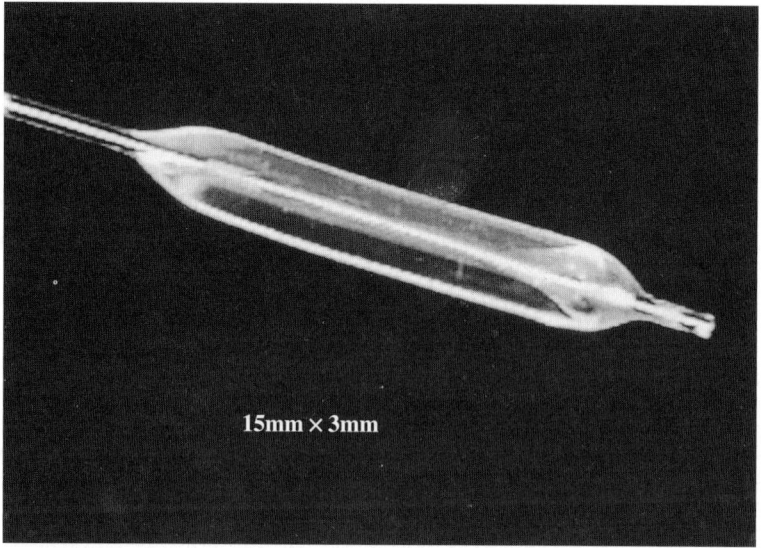

15mm × 3mm

FIGURE 17.1. Balloon catheter 15 × 3mm. (Image courtesy of Michael Mercandetti, MD.)

FIGURE 17.2. (A) Endoscopic view of lacrimal probe exiting inferior opening of lacrimal duct (valve of Hasner) lateral to inferior turbinate, which is displaced medially to the right. (B) Entry of balloon catheter into inferior meatus (same patient as A). (C) Infracture (medial displacement) of inferior turbinate in another patient with visualization of lacrimal probe. (Image courtesy of Michael Mercandetti, MD.)

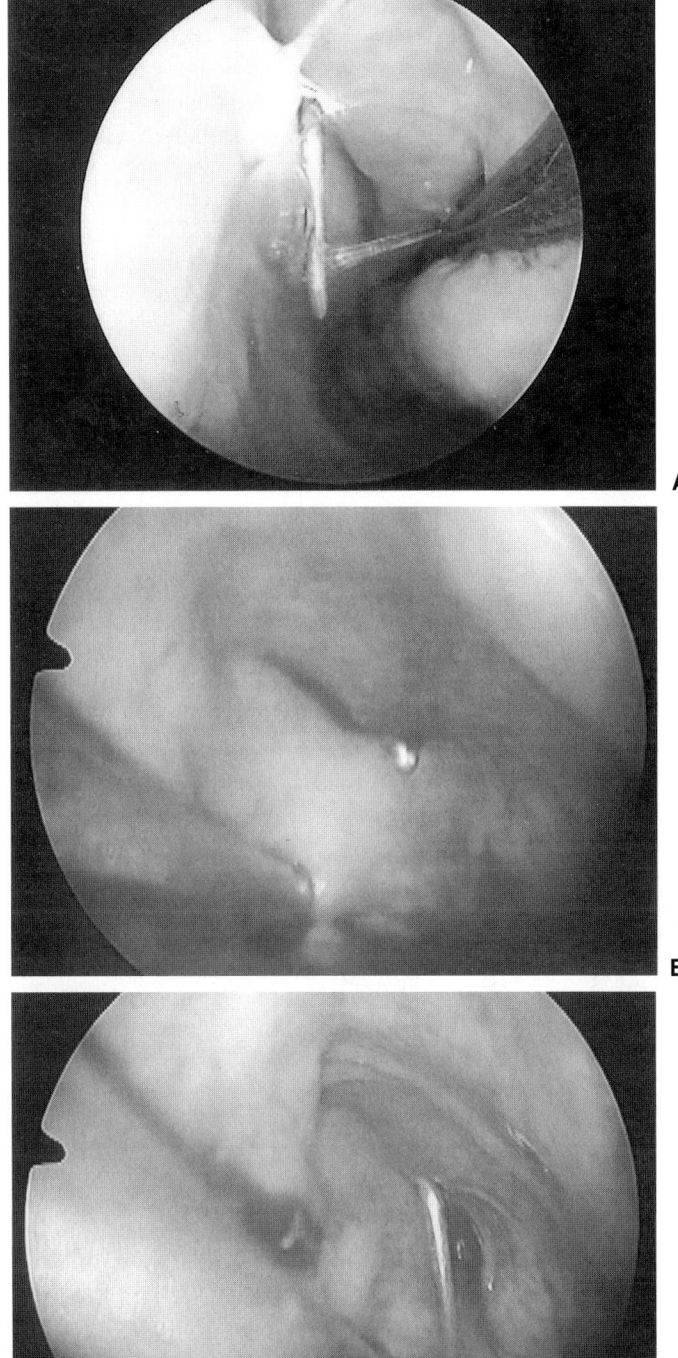

After the catheter is properly positioned, a standard balloon inflation device (Figure 17.3) is attached to the catheter. The balloon is inflated to 8 atmospheres of pressure for 90 seconds (Figure 17.4A and B) and deflated. The catheter is reinflated in the same manner for 90 seconds (Figure 17.5) and deflated. The catheter is reinflated a third time to 8 atmospheres for 60 seconds and deflated. Afterward, the balloon is pulled from the punctal side in order to align the 10-mm marking with the punctum (Figure 17.6). The sequence of inflation and deflation as described above is undertaken. This sequence of positions assures that the valve of Hasner, distal NLD, and proximal NLD are actually dilated by the balloon.

The catheter is removed and irrigation is performed with balanced salt solution. Subsequently, a Monoka silicone lacrimal tube is placed in the standard manner and removed 6–8 weeks postoperatively. Crawford or Guibor tubes can also be placed. However, these are bicanalicular and need to be secured by suture to the lateral nasal wall. This necessitates significant manipulation for removal and usually means repeat general anesthesia in children.

Balloon canaliculoplasty can be performed with a 2-mm balloon after lysis of strictures or scar tissue with a needle or lacrimal probe. Inflation parameters are the same as for NLDO. Bicanalicular intubation is preferred (e.g., Crawford, Guibor) because it allows passage of steroid drops and tears containing growth factors into the canaliculus and NLD, which may maintain patency of the system.

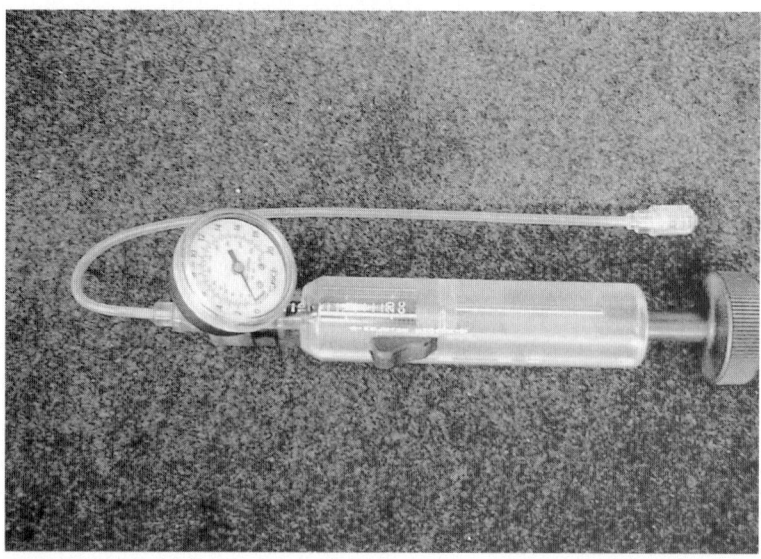

FIGURE 17.3. Inflation device. (Image courtesy of Michael Mercandetti, MD.)

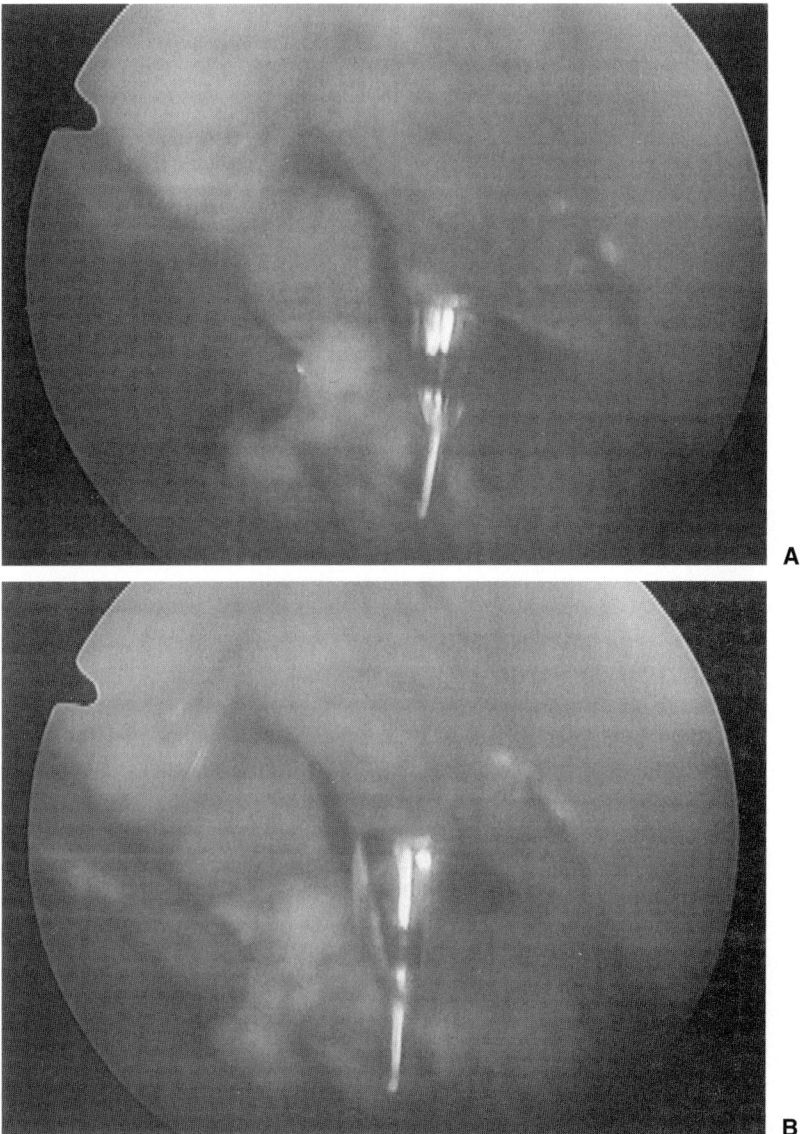

FIGURE 17.4. **(A)** Inflation of balloon catheter. **(B)** Further inflation of balloon catheter. (Image courtesy of Michael Mercandetti, MD.)

Postoperatively, topical prednisolone acetate 1%, one drop four times a day for 2 weeks, is placed on the conjunctival surface. This can be repeated again at the time of lacrimal stent extubation.

Finally, failed or insufficiently patent ostia after DCR can be dilated with either a 5-mm anterograde balloon or endonasally with a right-angle 9-mm LacriCATH™ balloon. This is also followed with bicanalicular intubation and steroid drops.

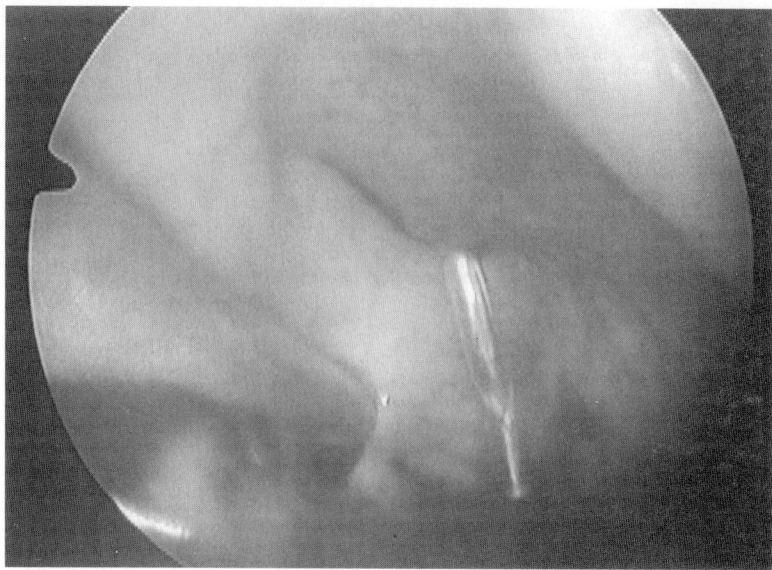

FIGURE 17.5. Balloon catheter deflated. (Image courtesy of Michael Mercandetti, MD.)

Discussion

Balloon Dacryocystoplasty and Complete Nasolacrimal Duct Obstruction

The standard treatment of complete NLDO has been incisional DCR, a procedure that has demonstrated a high success rate (more than 90%).

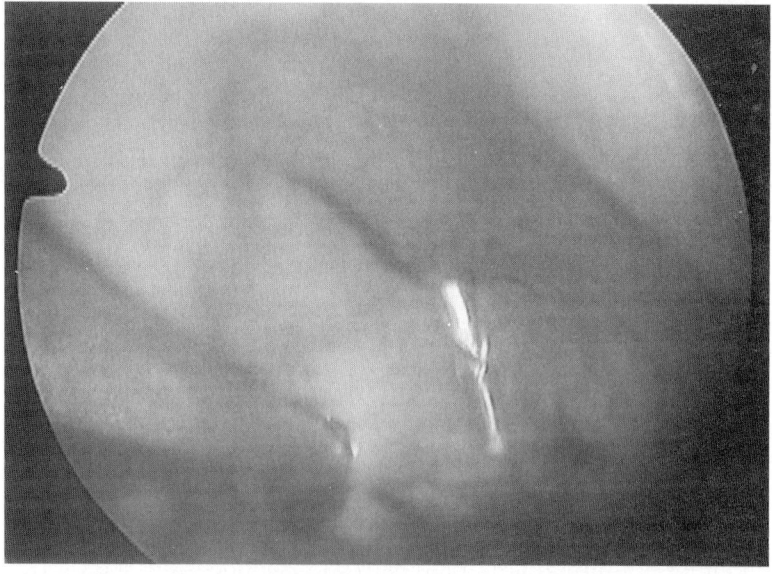

FIGURE 17.6. Balloon catheter further deflated, twisted, and withdrawn. (Image courtesy of Michael Mercandetti, MD.)

Despite the high rate of success, alternative therapies have been sought to obviate the need for general anesthesia and the creation of an external facial scar. Several reports have examined the efficacy of balloon catheter dacryoplasty for cases of complete NLDO.[4,5] Song et al.[5] reported on the efficacy of a retrograde, fluoroscopically guided balloon dacryocystoplasty without subsequent placement of silicone tubing in patients with complete NLDO. In the study, complete NLDO was defined by the absence of contrast medium into the inferior meatus by dacryocystography and by negative Jones I and II tests. The results of the study were disappointing with an initial failure rate of 44%. Additionally, of those NLDs that were initially patent, 45% became obstructed at the 2-month postoperative date.

These findings were supported by other studies that demonstrated similar failure rates. Janssen et al.,[4] also using a retrograde approach without silicone intubation, found a failure rate of 41% (11 of 27 patients). The relatively poor rate of NLD patency in these two studies may be attributed to several key features such as the lack of silicone intubation, a retrograde approach, or use of balloon catheters not specifically designed for NLD catheterization.

In contrast to these disappointing results, some reports have demonstrated moderate success using anterograde balloon dacryocystoplasty with silicone intubation for the treatment of complete NLDO. Using anterograde balloon dacryoplasty with placement of silicone tubes on patients with complete NLDO, defined by canalicular irrigation and transcanalicular endoscopy, Kuchar and Steinkogler[6] found 53.5% (15 of 28 patients) had open NLD, 35.7% (10 of 28 patients) had partially open NLD, and 10.7% (3 of 28 patients) had closed NLD, based on saline irrigation, after 1 year. The difference in patency rates may reflect the changes in technique. Although these findings were favorable, the long-term effects of balloon dacryocystoplasty for the treatment of complete NLDO are unknown.

Balloon Dacryocystoplasty and Incomplete Nasolacrimal Duct Obstruction

The treatment modality most appropriate for the treatment of incomplete NLDO has been a matter of considerable debate. Several studies have examined the efficacy of balloon dacryocystoplasty under these clinical circumstances. In an initial study, 11 of 15 patients (73%) demonstrated patent NLDs (based on unimpeded NLD irrigation) after treatment with balloon dacryocystoplasty and silicone intubation.[2] Similar findings were observed when examining the medium to long-term outcomes (mean follow-up, 36 months) of balloon dacryocystoplasty in incomplete NLDO.

Technical innovations to the procedure have been used in an attempt to augment the success rate of the procedure. One such change has been the use of video-assisted endoscopy. The use of video-assisted endoscopy may be an attractive ancillary component to balloon dacryocystoplasty because it can determine whether the balloon catheter cannulated the valve of Hasner. This is important because one source of failure may be attributed to the inadvertent placement of the balloon catheter in the submucosal space of the nasal cavity. Furthermore, visualizing the nasal cavity and inferior meatus region could help identify abnormal structures or objects that may occlude the outlet of the inferior meatus. Identifying any structural abnormality would aid in the treatment by allowing the use of an appropriate surgical approach. In a recent study, after a follow-up period of approximately 7.5 months, 56% of patients demonstrated complete resolution of their symptoms and 34% of patients demonstrated partial improvement of symptoms.[6] Based on these findings, video-assisted endoscopy seems to be an important ancillary procedure for balloon dacryocystoplasty in adults as well as children with failed probing or previous failed balloon dilation.

Indications

Balloon dacryocystoplasty provides another approach in the treatment of complete and incomplete NLDO. Because of its less rigorous technical requirements compared with DCR, its ability to be done without general anesthesia, and the avoidance of external facial incisions, this technique may be an appropriate first-line treatment modality in certain selected cases.

Currently, there are no long-term studies evaluating the success rate of balloon dacryocystoplasty for cases of complete and incomplete NLDO. However, we support the use of this technique for those individuals demonstrating incomplete NLDO based on epiphora symptoms and imaging studies (e.g., computed tomography-dacryocystography). We continue to advocate surgical DCR as the treatment of choice for complete NLDO, but balloon dacryocystoplasty can be performed on patients who are unable to tolerate general anesthesia or used as a temporizing measure before performing a DCR.

References

1. Yeats RP. Acquired nasolacrimal duct obstruction. Ophthalmol Clin North Am 2000;13(4):719–729.
2. Perry JD, Maus M, Nowinski TS, Penne RB. Balloon catheter dilation for treatment of adults with partial nasolacrimal duct obstruction: a preliminary report. Am J Ophthalmol 1998;126:811–816.
3. Couch SM, White WL. Endoscopically assisted balloon dacryoplasty treatment of incomplete nasolacrimal duct obstruction. Ophthalmology 2004; 111(3):585–589.
4. Janssen AG, Mansour K, Bos JJ. Obstructed nasolacrimal duct system in epiphora: long-term results of dacryoplasty by means of balloon dilation. Radiology 1997;205:791–796.
5. Song HY, Ahn HS, Park CK, Kwon SH, Kim CS, Choi KC. Complete obstruction of the nasolacrimal system. Part I. Treatment with balloon dilation. Radiology 1993;186:367–371.
6. Kuchar A, Steinkogler FJ. Antegrade balloon dilatation of nasolacrimal duct obstruction in adults. Br J Ophthalmol 2001;85:200–204.

18

Balloon-Assisted Lacrimal Surgery

William L. White, Jerry K. Popham, and Robert G. Fante

Instrumentation and Principles

The use of radiologic technology for interventional application in the lacrimal system was first described by Hanafee and Dayton[1] from the University of California, Los Angeles in 1978. They dilated native nasolacrimal ducts (NLDs) with sialography cannulas under fluoroscopy. The use of radiologic instrumentation in the lacrimal system was carried one step further in 1989 when Becker and Berry[2] reported the use of balloon catheters to perform secondary dacryocystorhinostomies (DCRs). They used existing coronary artery angioplasty balloons in their series. This led to the development of what is presently the only commercially available balloon product made specifically for application in the lacrimal system, the LacriCATH lacrimal duct catheters, manufactured by Quest Medical, Inc. (Allen, TX).

The balloon catheter device is used in both nonincisional, endoscopic, balloon-assisted (EBA) DCR and nonincisional balloon dilation of the NLD, also known as balloon dacryoplasty (DCP). Both procedures are currently performed in both adult and pediatric populations. Generally, balloon DCR surgery is more often used in patients with complete NLD obstruction (NLDO) and balloon DCP is more often used in patients with partial or incomplete NLDO.

Balloon catheter dilation of the lacrimal tract as performed in most centers outside of the United States (US) still utilizes clinically available balloon catheters originally manufactured for vascular work and applies a combination of lacrimal and vascular thought to clinical applications.[3–7] In such procedures, a guide wire is passed through the punctum, canaliculus, and NLD. The guide wire is subsequently retrieved in the nose. The balloon catheter is then passed transnasally over the guide wire. Quest Medical has recently introduced the transnasal 9-mm balloon catheter to the US marketplace. This catheter is endoscopically positioned in the ostium after passing the device through the nose, not the canaliculus. It does not require a guide wire for passage.

Most non-US investigations also differ from US investigations in that procedures in the US are generally performed by ophthalmologists in the operating room, or less frequently in an office setting. Outside of the US, most procedures are performed by radiologists in a radiology suite. Long backlogs of surgical patients awaiting traditional DCR outside the US apparently led to the development of specific techniques and interventions that can be performed by non-ophthalmologists.[8] Results of such studies in the literature are difficult to interpret and compare. Most studies of balloon DCP outside the US include patients with incomplete and complete NLDOs.

Quest Medical presently has three different transcanalicular lacrimal dilation catheters with distinct indications for each. Quest Medical has also recently introduced a transnasal balloon device. Two numbers describe the transcanalicular catheters. The first is the outside diameter of the inflated balloon. The second number is the length of the inflated balloon. Both numbers are measured in millimeters. The smallest catheter is a $2 \times 13\,mm$ device and is designed for dilation of the native NLD in congenital NLDO. It is recommended for use in children up to the age of 30 months and is 0.8mm in diameter before inflation. The next larger diameter catheter is a $3 \times 15\,mm$ catheter, which is made to treat incomplete pediatric or adult NLDO through dilation of the native tract in patients who are 30 months of age or older. It is 0.9mm in diameter before inflation. The third and largest diameter transcanalicular catheter available is the $5 \times 8\,mm$ device designed primarily for use in EBA DCR in adults with complete NLDO. It is 1.0mm in diameter before inflation and can be used for primary or secondary DCR. It is not intended for dilation of the native NLD.

It is important to avoid inflation of any balloon before passage through the canaliculus. Inflation or "testing" of the balloon before transcanalicular passage makes the catheter much more difficult, if not impossible, to pass and may increase the risk of canalicular trauma. The catheters slide through the punctum and canaliculus better when they are lubricated with a small amount of an ophthalmic ointment. It is generally advisable to have at least one more catheter available for use in a given case than thought to be necessary in the event that a balloon ruptures during inflation or is contaminated before use. This recommendation also applies to the inflation manometer devices, although they very rarely malfunction.

Each catheter has a luer-lock adapter for attachment to the inflation manometer. It is important to eliminate all of the air present in the inflation manometer before use by filling the device with normal saline or any physiologic solution. The inflation devices typically display the pressure reading within the system in digital or analog format. Clockwise rotation of a knob at the distal end of the inflation device elevates the pressure within the device. Most inflation devices also utilize a release switch for more rapid deflation of the balloon. A small amount of air will enter the manometer after the first inflation, but is typically insignificant in volume and inconsequential in achieving adequate inflation pressures.

Each transcanalicular balloon has two sets of rings outlined to provide approximate information about the depth of balloon placement during a dilation procedure. The catheters have black rings 10 and 15 mm proximal to the beginning of the balloon.

Balloon lacrimal surgery is best accomplished with a videoendoscope to ensure the correct intranasal location of the catheter. Proper placement of the catheter cannot be confirmed without intranasal visualization. Simply passing the catheter without confirming correct intranasal passage can create false channels and compromise upper system lacrimal anatomy for any subsequent procedures. In general, a 3.5-mm-diameter, 0-degree scope is most useful. Occasionally, a 30-degree scope or a smaller 2.7-mm-diameter pediatric scope can be beneficial.

Unless contraindicated, general anesthesia delivered with a laryngeal mask airway (LMA) offers the ideal method of airway management when performing all types of balloon-assisted lacrimal surgery. Because manipulation and instrumentation of the airway is minimized with the LMA as compared with endotracheal intubation, the need for larger doses of sedative/hypnotic agents and muscle relaxants is eliminated, thus reducing the occurrence of side effects. Postoperative recovery is hastened and the incidence of nausea, vomiting, and sore throat is reduced without sacrificing sufficient control and protection of the airway. Balloon-assisted lacrimal surgery can, however, be performed under local anesthesia or with local anesthesia and supplemental intravenous sedation when desired by the surgeon and a cooperative patient. Light mask anesthesia is not recommended in pediatric patients, because the irrigant solution administered after dilation can be sufficient in volume to induce bronchospasm. LMA-delivered anesthesia offers excellent airway control, as seen with endotracheal intubation, and rapid postoperative recovery as seen in local anesthesia cases with supplemental intravenous sedation. LMA anesthesia, therefore, is recommended in balloon lacrimal surgery.

Acquired Adult Dacryostenosis – Complete Obstruction

Acquired, complete obstruction of the NLD with epiphora or dacryocystitis in adults is an indication for DCR. Traditionally, DCR is accomplished through an external incision along the bridge of the nose near the lacrimal sac. A variety of endoscopic techniques have been developed to avoid incisions, scarring, and to minimize operative morbidity. The authors' EBA DCR experience has been limited to the use of the Quest Medical LacriCATH 5×8 mm balloon to create or enlarge a true DCR ostium between the lacrimal sac and the nasal antrum.

The dye disappearance test combined with probing and irrigation of the lacrimal drainage apparatus is used to diagnose the presence of complete NLDO. The Jones' dye tests may also be useful in selected patients. Contraindications to balloon-assisted DCR are generally the same as those for balloon DCP.

EBA DCR may be performed under general or local anesthesia. The authors use general anesthesia for the majority of DCR surgery. Patients are treated preoperatively with 1 g of intravenous cefazolin and 10 mg of dexamethasone. Patients are also treated in the preoperative area with three sprays of intranasal oxymetazoline. Although topical cocaine is an excellent decongestant and anesthetic, its potential interaction with epinephrine used in local anesthetic solution makes it a suboptimal choice in this setting.

After general anesthesia has been induced, the nasal mucosa is infiltrated with lidocaine with epinephrine 1:100,000 at the anticipated ostium site, just beneath the insertion of the anterior tip of the middle turbinate on the lateral nasal wall. This injection is usually given using a nasal speculum and direct visualization, but may also be directed using the nasal endoscope. Infiltration of lidocaine with epinephrine 1:100,000 reduces the need for larger doses of inhalational anesthetics and vasoconstricts the nasal mucosa, thereby reducing bleeding. A temporary, mild increase in blood pressure may be noted after the injection. The nasal antrum in the area of the middle turbinate is packed with $1/2 \times 3$ inch cottonoids soaked in oxymetazoline. The patient is then prepped and draped in the usual sterile manner.

After punctal dilation, the upper and lower canaliculi and common canalicular dilation is performed using increasingly larger lacrimal probes. Preservation of normal punctal and canalicular anatomy through atraumatic dilation is critical to successful outcomes in this operation. With the puncta and canaliculi thoroughly dilated, a no. 3 or no. 4 specially hardened stainless steel lacrimal probe (Storz Instrument Co., St. Louis, MO) is passed through the superior punctum and canaliculus to a hard stop in the lacrimal sac. The probe is directed inferiorly and posteriorly to a weak and thin point in the bony wall between the lacrimal sac and the nasal antrum. Before pushing the probe through the wall of the lacrimal sac fossa, the packing in the nasal antrum is removed.

The nasal endoscope is then passed and directed toward the anterior tip of the middle turbinate. While viewing the intranasal area around the anterior tip of the middle turbinate, the lacrimal probe already in the lacrimal sac is slowly advanced. A bulge in the nasal mucosa may be seen as the probe begins to advance. Alternatively, no change in the nasal mucosa may be seen if the probe is entering the nasal antrum beneath the anterior tip on the middle turbinate. In this scenario, an attempt is made to change the position of the tip of the lacrimal probe in order to allow creation of the ostium just anterior and superior to the anterior tip of the middle turbinate.

It is preferable to position the ostium; this may allow the surgeon to avoid any manipulation of the turbinate. At times, the ostium cannot be placed anywhere but beneath the anterior tip of the middle turbinate. In this circumstance, the middle turbinate must be infractured or conservatively resected. A biting instrument, such as size 0 Thru Bite Blakesley forceps, is particularly helpful in this regard because it tends not to strip mucosa, but to cut it sharply and precisely. In any circumstance, the mucosal lining of the turbinate and the nasal antrum in general must be preserved with as little manipulation and trauma as possible. Any irritation of the mucosa may lead to unnecessary bleeding or formation of adhesions, which can cause obstruction of the ostium.

After the initial ostium opening is created through passage of the no. 3 or 4 lacrimal probe and the position of the ostium is optimized, the probe is repeatedly advanced out of and retracted back into the lacrimal sac in different locations to widen the ostium mechanically. The area of the intended ostium is in effect "honeycombed" with small holes in preparation for the placement of the balloon catheter device. The perforations in the bone are made contiguous with the no. 3 or 4 lacrimal probe. A lubricated 5×8 mm balloon catheter is inserted through the superior punctum and canaliculus, through the common canaliculus and lacrimal sac, and positioned in the ostium previously created with the probe. The endoscope is used to confirm correct positioning of the tip of the balloon catheter at least 2 mm past the nasal mucosa in the nasal antrum.

Once correct position is established, the balloon is attached to the inflation device and is inflated to 8 atmospheres for the first 90-second cycle. At times, the balloon device may push further into the nasal antrum during inflation. The balloon catheter tip is observed during inflation using the videoendoscope. The balloon is then deflated by releasing the pressure with the manometer. The balloon is again positioned in the ostium using the endoscope. It is reinflated to 8 atmospheres of pressure for one additional 60-second cycle. During the second inflation, mucosal or bone fragments are carefully removed from around the perimeter of the ostium and balloon using fine ear forceps. It is important to remove any such fragments to minimize the risk of closure of the ostium during the healing process. Some surgeons may want to enlarge the ostium transnasally with a nerve hook or rongeurs.

After the second inflation, the balloon is completely deflated and removed. Endoscopic observation of the balloon tip in the nose confirms complete deflation of the balloon before withdrawal of the balloon catheter through the upper canaliculus and punctum. Mild resistance may be encountered during withdrawal of the balloon device. For this reason, some surgeons elect to cut the shaft of the metal portion of the balloon catheter and remove the balloon end of the device through the nostril. This maneuver may reduce trauma to the canaliculus.

After removal of the inflation device, the lacrimal stent is prepared for use by lubricating it with an ophthalmic antibiotic ointment. The STENTube is a lacrimal stent manufactured by Quest Medical for this specific application. It is unique because of its variance in diameter. The central 22 mm of the STENTube, designed for placement in the interpalpebral fissure and in the canaliculi, is 0.86 mm in diameter. The remaining portion of the tube is 1.3 mm in diameter, allowing greater mechanical dilation and stenting of the surgical ostium. It is important to ensure that the thin portion of the STENTube is correctly positioned in the canaliculi and interpalpebral fissure. The olive tips of the stylets on the STENTube are designed to be engaged with a standard lacrimal hook to facilitate easy removal through the nostril. It is often easier, however, to grasp the tip of the stylet with a straight hemostat under endoscopic guidance. This maneuver minimizes the risk of abrasion or laceration of the nasal mucosa. Once positioning is correct, the tubing is placed on gentle inferior traction. The two ends of the tube are tied together with a 5-0 polypropylene suture. Excess suture and tubing are cut away, allowing the knot to retract back into the patient's nose. The tubing remains in position for 3–4 months.

Systemic and topical antibiotics are administered for 10–14 days postoperatively. Antibiotic selection may be directed toward specific organisms discovered during preoperative culture and sensitivity testing. Because many patients have already started antibiotics at the time of initial presentation, empiric antibiotic selection is most often necessary. Cephalexin 250–500 mg is often used four times daily. Gentamicin is frequently selected for use as a topical ocular antibiotic and is administered every 2 hours while awake for the first 2 days and continued four times daily for an additional 8 days. Patients who develop any sign of infection while the tubing is in place after initial treatment with postoperative antibiotics are candidates for further topical or systemic antibiotics.

Systemic, topical, and intranasal steroids are administered to reduce inflammation and scarring. Oral prednisone is begun on the day of the surgery at 50 mg per day and is decreased by 10 mg per day every other day. This regimen keeps the patient on the tapering dose for 10 days. Topical prednisolone acetate 1% is used on the same schedule as the topical antibiotics. Intranasal saline spray is used to limit crusting around the ostium and on the lacrimal stent. It is started on the day of surgery and is used at least once daily preceding the nasal steroid spray. The nasal steroid spray most often used is budesonide 32 μg (Rhinocort Aqua, Astra Pharmaceuticals, Westborough, MA). The nasal saline and steroid sprays are continued postoperatively until gone, which is usually in about 2 months. Requirements for pain medication after this procedure are typically minor with acetaminophen usually being adequate in those patients requiring an analgesic.

Lacrimal stent removal is accomplished in the office 4–6 months postoperatively. The nasal mucosa is decongested using oxymetazoline. Some patients may require topical anesthesia of the nasal mucosa using Pontocaine spray. The thicker portion of a STENTube, unlike traditional lacrimal stents, cannot be removed through the canaliculus. The thin portion of the Stentube, therefore, is cut in the interpalpebral fissure and the tubing is removed transnasally. This is most easily and atraumatically accomplished with the guidance of a nasal endoscope. After tube removal, the lacrimal drainage system is irrigated to remove any mucous or debris from the system and to confirm patency of the system. Patients are once again started on the same postoperative regimen of oral and topical antibiotics and steroids and on the nasal saline and steroid sprays. Patients are scheduled for reevaluation 4–6 weeks later and 1 year after the reevaluation. If reobstruction is to occur, it typically occurs within 4–6 weeks of tube removal. Complications of balloon-assisted DCR are generally the same as those seen with traditional incisional DCR and include failed surgery, epistaxis, and canalicular stenosis.

Recurrent Dacryostenosis

The 5-mm-diameter balloon catheter can be used to perform secondary balloon-assisted DCR when traditional incisional DCR, transnasal endoscopic DCR, or primary balloon-assisted DCR fails to provide adequate lacrimal drainage. Nasal endoscopy is performed preoperatively to rule out intranasal pathology, such as severe nasal septal deviation, as a reason for procedural failure. It is also imperative to probe and irrigate such patients to ensure that the obstruction is in the area of the nasal ostium and not the canaliculi, because complete canalicular obstruction cannot typically be overcome by balloon dilation.

Secondary balloon DCRs can be performed under general anesthesia or local anesthesia with IV sedation. Regardless of the technique chosen, the medial canthal area is injected with a local anesthetic mixture containing epinephrine. The nasal mucosa in the area of the ostium is then injected with the same anesthetic mixture. The middle meatus is packed with cottonoids soaked in oxymetazoline or a vasoconstrictant-anesthetic mixture. After the patient is prepped and draped, the puncta are dilated atraumatically.

The superior canaliculus is subsequently probed to a size 3 or 4. A stainless steel size 3 or 4 lacrimal probe is then passed through the previous ostium or scar into the nose. The ostium is then enlarged in the same manner as a primary balloon-assisted DCR with special attention being given to ensure that the middle turbinate or nasal septum does not impact or occlude the ostium. The videoendoscope is critical for this part of the procedure. The 5×8 mm catheter is then passed through the superior canaliculus through the ostium and inflated to 8 atmospheres for 90 seconds, released, and then reinflated for 60 seconds. The catheter is then withdrawn 1 cm or to the distal ring on the catheter and two more inflation cycles are completed. The catheter is withdrawn to the proximal ring and two more inflation cycles are repeated. Rarely are inflations at more than two or three positions necessary. The newly created lacrimal tract is subsequently irrigated.

Some surgeons may elect to apply mitomycin C, 0.4 mg/cc on a 1/2 × 1/2 inch cottonoid for 5 minutes transnasally to the ostium, and then copiously irrigate the ostium transnasally. The optimal concentration, time of application, and specific therapeutic efficacy of such intervention is not currently known.[9] Most surgeons will not likely want to use mitomycin C in pediatric patients or in those in whom adequate informed consent has not been obtained. Silicone tubes are then passed and secured in the nose. Some surgeons may elect to use a traditional lacrimal stent and leave it in place longer rather than using the Stentube. The same medication regimen used in primary balloon-assisted

DCR is initiated. Complications of secondary balloon DCR are the same as those seen with primary balloon-assisted DCR. Results of clinical trials using the 5-mm balloon for repeat DCRs are quite limited.

References

1. Hanafee WN, Dayton GO. Dilatation of the nasolacrimal duct under radiographic control. Radiology 1978;127:813–815.
2. Becker BB, Berry FD. Balloon catheter dilatation in lacrimal surgery. Ophthalmic Surg 1989;20:193–198.
3. Robinson R, Turner N, Brettle P, Chell PB, Chavda SV, Murray PI. The treatment of epiphora with balloon dacryoplasty. Eye 1993;7:687–690.
4. Ilgit ET, Yuksel D, Unal M, Akpek S, Isik S, Hasanreisoglu B. Transluminal balloon dilatation of the lacrimal drainage system for the treatment of epiphora. Am J Radiol 1995;165:1517–1524.
5. Liermann D, Berkefeld J, Fries U, Schalnus RW, Gumpel H. Balloon dacryoplasty: an alternative treatment for obstructed tear ducts. Ophthalmologica 1996;210:319–324.
6. Berkefeld J, Kirchner J, Muller HM, Fries U, Kollath J. Balloon dacryoplasty: indications and contraindications. Radiology 1997;205:785–790.
7. Janssen AG, Mansour K, Box JJ. Obstructed nasolacrimal duct system in epiphora: long-term results of dacryoplasty by means of balloon dilation. Radiology 1997;205:791–796.
8. Kumar NE. Technical note: non-surgical treatment of epiphora by balloon dacryoplasty – the technique. Br J Radiol 1995;68:1116–1118.
9. Kao SC, Liao CL, Tseng JHS, Chen MS, Hou PK. Dacryocystorhinostomy with intraoperative mitomycin C. Ophthalmology 1997;104:86–91.

19

Nine-Millimeter Endoscopic Balloon Dacryocystorhinostomy: A New, Less-Invasive Procedure for Tearing in Adults

David I. Silbert

Toti introduced incisional dacryocystorhinostomy (DCR) in 1904, and modifications resulted in successful outcomes by the 1920s. Aside from variations in the size and location of the incision, silicon tube intubation, and antibiotics, the basics of the procedure have changed little.

Most lacrimal surgeons are familiar with the external approach and its advantages, including a high success rate and excellent visualization of the common canaliculus. In addition, many surgeons believe the external approach affords a better view of the lacrimal sac, which is important in suspected cases of neoplasia, and allows for easier access to tissue for biopsy.

Disadvantages to the external approach are numerous. Recovery can be quite prolonged because of swelling and healing of the external incision. The incision sight often interferes with the nose pads of spectacles, and hypertrophic scarring can occur. Blood loss from inadvertent damage to the angular vessels or infraorbital artery, or from excessive manipulation of the nasal mucosa, which is poorly visualized, can complicate and prolong the procedure. Nasal packing is sometimes required because of excessive bleeding and may be uncomfortable. Bleeding may recur when the packing is removed.

Advantages of the endoscopic balloon (eb)-DCR include the absence of a skin incision and no need for power instrumentation in most cases. When performed properly, there is minimal bleeding and cautery is rarely necessary. Once the surgeon becomes facile with the endoscope, the procedure time decreases significantly compared with the external approach and no flaps or incisions need to be closed. Recovery times are reduced, with less postoperative sequelae. In the author's hands, the success rate is comparable to the external approach.

Indications for eb-DCR include complete or functional (partial) nasolacrimal duct obstruction. In cases of partial obstruction, the patient often provides consent for a 3-mm balloon dacryoplasty (DCP) with the understanding that the surgeon may convert to an eb-DCR. Frequently, in adults, it is impossible to intraoperatively pass probes down the nasolacrimal system, necessitating conversion from DCP to eb-DCR. From the patient's standpoint, the main difference between DCP and eb-DCR is the presence of stenting tubes in the latter procedure.

Suspicion of a lacrimal sac tumor is a contraindication to eb-DCR. However, imaging studies in select cases can help rule out neoplasia. Relative contraindications to the endoscopic approach include severe nasal septal deviation and canalicular obstruction. It was once thought that dacryocystitis was a contraindication to the endoscopic approach; however, this is not the case. Approaching an infected sac and draining it endonasally without creating a skin incision is particularly effective and markedly minimizes the risk of a cellulitis by contamination of the incision site through the external approach.

Anesthesia is either monitored anesthesia care with sedation or general endotracheal or laryngeal mask anesthesia. General anesthesia with a laryngeal mask is a good choice in selected cases. Less patient bucking is encountered when coming out of anesthesia, which decreases postoperative bleeding. A throat pack can be used, but is rarely necessary, in the author's experience.

Local anesthetic is used with both monitored anesthesia care and general anesthesia. Lidocaine 2% with epinephrine mixed 10:1 with bicarbonate is injected submucosally using a 25-gauge spinal needle. This is usually done by using a headlight and nasal speculum immediately after the patient is brought into the operating room and sedated or placed under general anesthesia. Approximately 3 cc of anesthetic is injected into the anterior middle turbinate, and just anterior and inferior to the insertion of the turbinate. Alternatively, the anesthetic can be injected under endoscopic control.

After the endonasal injections are given, the nose is packed with 1/2-inch cottonoids soaked in 4% cocaine mixed 1:1 with oxymetazoline hydrochloride 0.05% nasal spray. The cottonoids are placed beneath the middle turbinate and in the area anterior to the insertion of the turbinate. This is usually done by using bayonet forceps, a nasal speculum, and a headlight.

After the packing of the nose, the patient is prepped and draped and the endoscope is set up. Generally, a right-handed surgeon stands to the patient's right hand side using the left hand to hold the endoscope and the right hand to hold other instrumentation. The monitor is placed 2 feet in front of the head of the bed, leaving room for a Mayo stand with the instrumentation. A 4-mm, straight (0-degree) endoscope is used for the procedure. The patient is placed on a surgical bed with the right arm tucked tightly against the patient to provide ample space for the surgeon.

Equipment on the Mayo stand should include the following:

Punctal dilators
Reinforced Bowman's probe (Quest Medical Inc., Allen, TX)
Dandy nerve hook

Blakesley and Truecut forceps, straight, up-biting, back-biting
Freer elevator
Turbinate scissors
Nasal speculum
4-mm, straight (0-degree) sinuscope
LacriCATH® 9-mm balloon catheter (Quest Medical)
LacriCATH® 5-mm balloon catheter (Quest Medical)
Inflation device (Quest Medical)
STENTubes (Quest Medical)
Frazier suction
Irrigating cannulas
Retinal-style light pipe

   Optional equipment:

Essential shaver
Suction Bovie cautery

Procedure

The punctum is first dilated with a punctal dilator. It needs to be dilated enough to allow passage of the number 3 or 4 reinforced Bowman's probe. A retinal-type light pipe may be used to demonstrate the area of the proposed ostium endonasally. The light pipe is introduced through the superior (or inferior) punctum and directed into the sac. The packing is removed from the nose, and the endoscope is introduced. The endoscope is held with the left hand and the light pipe is manipulated, moving it superiorly, inferiorly, anteriorly, and posteriorly. Performing this maneuver with the light pipe allows visualization of the lacrimal sac location by transillumination. This permits the surgeon to anticipate the location of the ostium. Generally, the ostium will be just inferior to the anterior insertion of the middle turbinate and the uncinate process, although there is considerable variability. The light pipe maneuver also helps determine whether any debulking of the turbinate is necessary.

   The middle turbinate is infractured with a Freer elevator. Care should be taken to avoid overmanipulation, because the middle turbinate originates from the cribriform plate. Disruption of the cribriform plate could result in cerebrospinal fluid leaks and meningitis. If the turbinate interferes with the planned site of the ostium, the anterior portion of the turbinate can be debulked by anterior turbinectomy with turbinate scissors. It is preferable not to debulk the turbinate unless absolutely necessary because excess manipulation can result in bleeding and scarring.

   The reinforced Bowman's probe is introduced through the superior punctum and passed into the sac. It is directed toward the inferior and posterior aspect of the lacrimal fossa where the thinnest bone is present. It is firmly advanced and "popped" through the thin posterior lacrimal bone. At this point, the endoscope is inserted and the location of the probe noted (Figure 19.1). If it is advanced too far, it can penetrate the turbinate. If this occurs, it is repositioned until it rests beneath or ante-

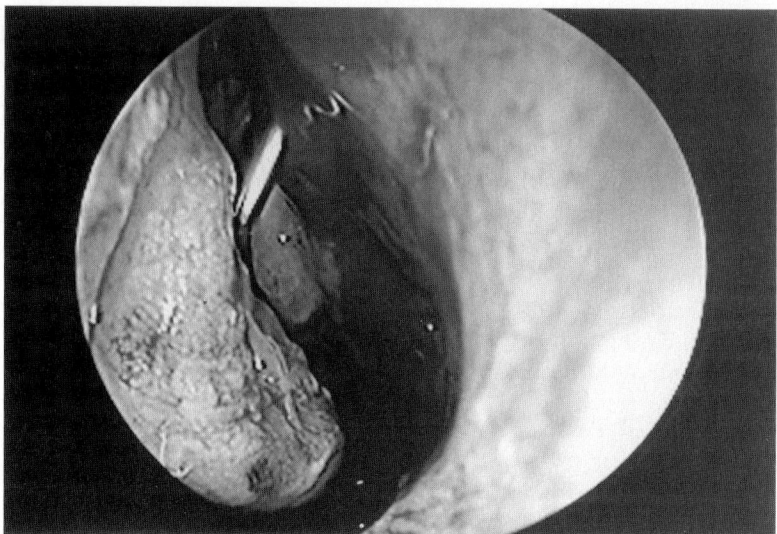

FIGURE 19.1. The reinforced Bowman's probe is introduced through the superior punctum and passed into the sac. It is firmly advanced through the thin posterior lacrimal bone.

rior to the turbinate. The probe is then pulled back under endoscopic control and passed through the thin lacrimal bone as inferiorly as possible. The probe is then pivoted, pushing the external portion of the probe inferiorly, which moves the endonasal portion superiorly, thus "filleting open" the lacrimal sac. Small, up-biting Blakesly forceps are introduced into the nose under endoscopic control. They are placed into the ostium created by the reinforced Bowman's probe. The assistant removes the probe, and the Blakesly forceps are opened and then pulled back into the nose in the open position, thus enlarging the ostium (Figure 19.2).

The surgeon inflates the device halfway with fluorescein-stained saline and removes all air. The 9-mm endonasal balloon is attached to the inflation device. The Bowman's probe is again passed through the ostium and visualized in the nose endoscopically. The probe will be used as a guide when introducing the 9-mm balloon. The balloon probe is then placed into the nose with the balloon portion facing cephalad. It is passed halfway into the ostium and the Bowman's probe is removed (Figure 19.3). The balloon is inflated to 8 atmospheres of pressure and left in place for 1 minute and then pulled into the nose while still inflated. This serves to dramatically enlarge the ostium (Figure 19.4). The probe is then deflated and removed from the nose. If it is impossible to pull the probe out of the ostium inflated, it has likely been inserted too far. It should be deflated, pulled slightly back into the nose, and reinflated.

In many cases, the ostium is now of adequate size. Any fragments of bone and mucosa can be pushed into the nose with the Bowman's probe and removed with Blakesly forceps. At the surgeon's discretion, the ostium may be further enlarged using Blakesly forceps, truecut forceps, or back-biting forceps.

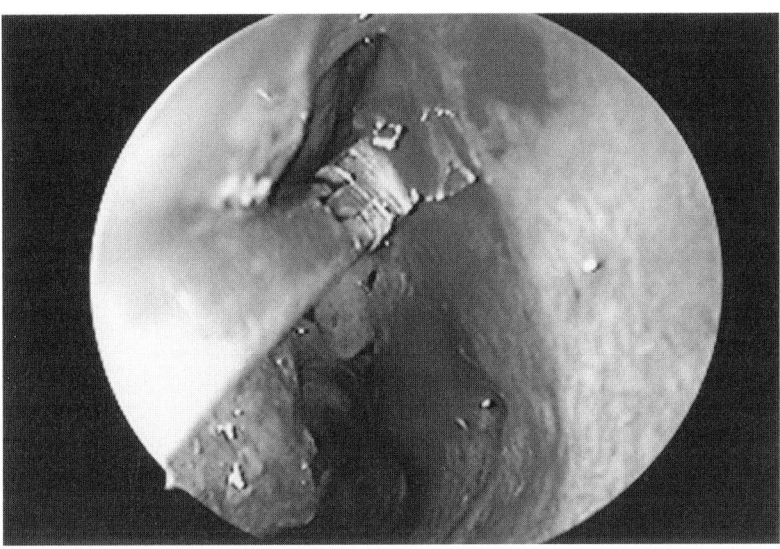

FIGURE 19.2. The ostium is enlarged with Blakesly forceps.

Bleeding is generally minimal during the procedure but if hemorrhaging interferes with visualization, Frazier-tipped suctioning or suction cautery can be used. The surgeon may need to repack the nose with the cocaine and oxymetazoline hydrochloride 0.05% soaked cottonoids until bleeding stops.

If the endoscope fogs during the procedure, special solution ("FRED") can be used to prevent fogging.

Once the ostium is found to be of adequate size, the canaliculus is irrigated with an antibiotic–steroid mixture and intubated with

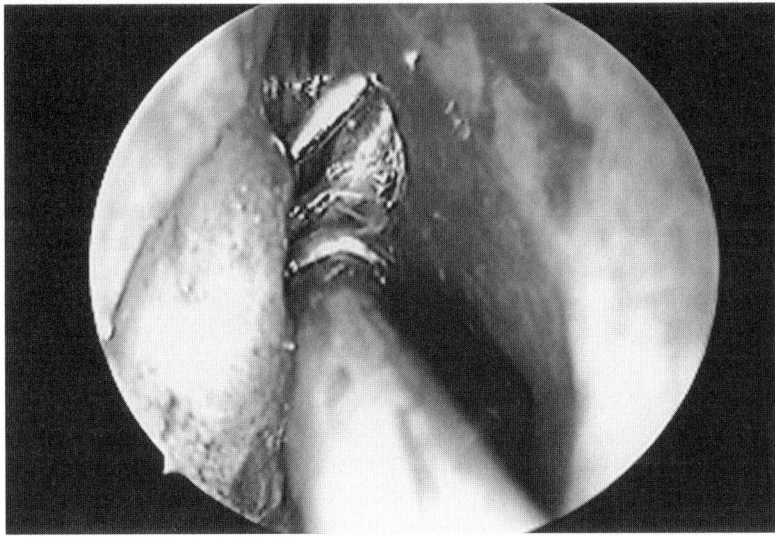

FIGURE 19.3. The balloon probe is then placed into the nose with the balloon portion facing cephalad. It is passed halfway into the ostium and the Bowman's probe is removed.

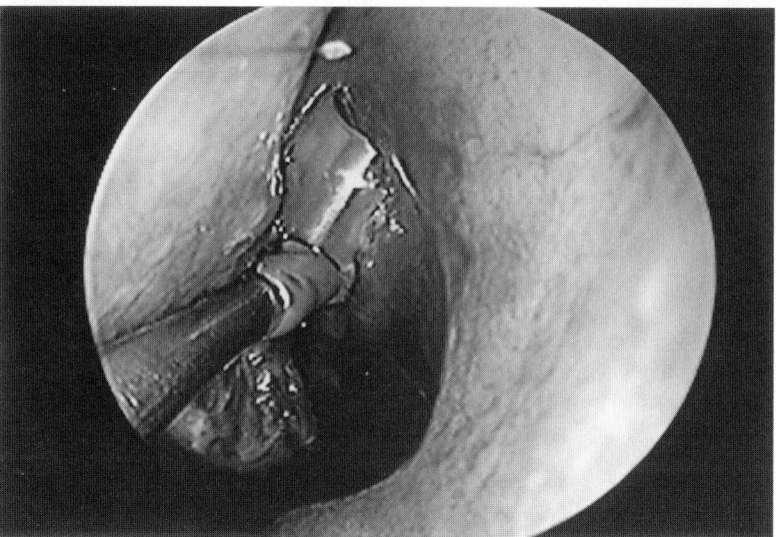

FIGURE 19.4. The balloon is inflated to 8 atmospheres of pressure, left in place for 1 minute, and then pulled into the nose while still inflated. This serves to dramatically enlarge the ostium.

stenting tubes. The stent tubes are typically 0.86mm wide at the canalicular portion, and widen to 1.3mm where they pass through the ostium. The olive-tipped probes are passed through the canaliculus and the ostium, and recovered in the nose with a Crawford hook under endoscopic control. It is important to make sure that the thinner portion of the tubes rests in the canaliculi. The tubes are tied to themselves using two silk ties, cut, and allowed to retract into the nose (Figure 19.5).

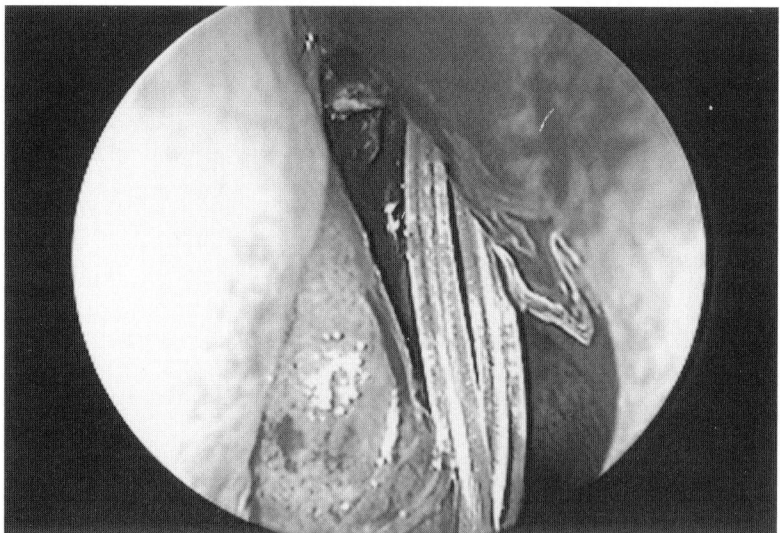

FIGURE 19.5. The olive-tipped probes are passed through the canaliculus and the ostium, and recovered in the nose. It is important to make sure that the thinner portion of the tubes rests in the canaliculi. The tubes are tied to themselves, cut, and allowed to retract into the nose.

It is useful to use a muscle hook to hold the tubes at the punctum while tying the silk sutures, because the tubes are stretched when tied. The muscle hook prevents damage to the canaliculi and puncta while tying the tubes together. A drip pad is placed beneath the nose if necessary. Generally, nasal packing is not required but can be used if warranted.

Intravenous steroids, usually 8 mg of dexamethasone, are given intraoperatively to suppress inflammation. In cases of dacryocystitis, an intravenous antibiotic such as 1 g of cephalexin is also administered.

Postoperatively, efforts are made to suppress edema, infection, and fibrosis to prevent stenosis of the ostium. The patient is placed on oral antibiotics for 10 days, topical antibiotic/steroid drops for 2 weeks, and a tapering steroid dose of dexamethasone (Medrol Dosepak®; Pharmacia & Upjohn Co., Kalamazoo, MI) for 6 days if not medically contraindicated. Saline nasal spray is used four times daily for 1 month, and intranasal steroids are used once daily for a month. The patient is asked to refrain from nose-blowing for a few weeks.

The STENTubes are left in place for up to 3 months and irrigation is performed postoperatively at approximately 1 month. If an endoscope is available in the office, intranasal cleaning of the ostium can be performed monthly until the tubes are removed. The patients are placed on antibiotic–steroid drops for 1–2 weeks after removal of the stent tubes. Occasionally, oral steroids and antibiotics are given if there are signs of infection or inflammation.

The success rate of the procedure in experienced hands is comparable to that of external DCR. Failures can be reoperated on using the 5-mm balloon via a canalicular approach with or without reintubation with stent tubes.

20

Radiofrequency Dacryocystorhinostomy

Reynaldo M. Javate, Susan Irene E. Lapid-Lim, and Ferdinand G. Pamintuan

Surgical specialists worldwide are rapidly acquiring expertise in radiosurgery or radiofrequency surgery. Many praise its superior results over conventional scalpel surgery. It is particularly gaining ground in the field of ophthalmic oculoplastic and orbital surgery. The authors, for instance, have used radiosurgery in repair of upper lid retraction in thyroid eye disease, transconjunctival blepharoplasty, ptosis repair, endoscopic forehead lift, biopsy excisions, and orbital surgeries including procedures involving optic nerve gliomas, among others.[1] In this chapter, emphasis is given to the authors' evolving approaches to radiofrequency-assisted dacryocystorhinostomy (DCR) surgery.

History

Ancient Egyptians evidently used heated metal instruments for surgical tissue destruction and hemostasis. Over recent centuries, electrosurgery emerged as a method to cut and coagulate tissues. The electrically heated, traditional platinum electrode wire produced residual tissue destruction, third-degree burns, prolonged healing, and poor cosmetic results. Low-frequency alternating current also caused muscle contractions in humans (the Faraday effect). In the late 1800s, Jacques d'Arsonval used high-frequency (>10,000 Hz) currents and a solenoid coil to heat tissues while avoiding the muscle spasms. In the 1920s, surgeon George Wyeth first used incisional electrosurgery, whereas William Bovie, a Harvard physicist, designed a machine for simultaneous cutting and coagulation of tissues. Today, the Bovie cautery or diathermy machine exists in practically every operating theater. Modern electrosurgical or diathermy machines have "step up" transformers to generate voltages higher than household, commercial current, and electric oscillating circuits to increase electric circuit oscillations.

In standard diathermy, a high-frequency electric current is passed through the patient. A "passive" electrode (large plate) is moistened and strapped to the patient's leg or back, and an "active" electrode is used to touch tissues. The electrical "density" of tissues determines the heating effect: current spread over a large surface area generates minimum heat, but current concentrated at a small point produces enough heat to cut, coagulate, or destroy tissue. Dr. Irving Ellman, in 1975, patented a lightweight, solid-state radiosurgery instrument to filter fully rectified waves. Its handpiece transmitted a pure frequency signal of 3,800,000 cycles per second. Maness et al. confirmed that a filtered wave produces less tissue alterations and that the optimum frequency for cutting soft tissues was 3.8 million cycles per second (MHz) and this frequency is still used in modern radio-units.

Definition of Radiosurgery

High-frequency (500 KHz and 4 MHz) radio waves are transmitted through soft tissue from a handpiece (thin wire tungsten "active" electrode) and focused through soft tissues by a passive electrode (insulated ground plate/antenna plate that does not need contact with the patient).[2] Water molecules in tissues exert a natural resistance to the passing radio signals, generating heat to volatize the cells. Sebben[3] described this sudden expansion of microbubbles of steam within the tissues; in effect, the passing electrode tip leaves a trail of cellular dehydration and destruction with virtually no hemostasis. This cutting effect (electrosection) exerts no manual pressure or crushing because soft tissues split apart with razor-sharp precision. Alternatively, a coagulating current produces molecular oscillations to induce heat buildup that coagulates and dehydrates tissue without volatilization. This electrocoagulation is important for surgical hemostasis.

Comparison with Electrocautery, CO_2 Laser Surgery, and Incisional Surgery

Incisional surgery with the scalpel still remains the gold standard. It produces no thermal damage but does not provide hemostasis. Radiosurgery has been shown to be superior over electrocautery because it results in less lateral thermal damage to tissues. It also produces significantly less tissue damage than KTP, YAG, or pulse CO_2 laser surgeries. An added advantage is that the electrodes are also self-sterilizing. Sebben differentiated the two high-frequency modalities. In electrocautery, the filament resists an electric current passing through it and becomes red-hot. This heat (not the electric current) transfers from filament to the tissues. In electrosurgery (radiosurgery), electromagnetic radiation is passed to the patient and converted to heat because of the resistance offered by the tissue cells. Whereas electrocautery operates optimally within the frequency range of 0.5–1.5 MHz, radiosurgery obtains best results within 3.8–4.0 MHz. There is less trauma to cells, less fibrous scarring, and less postoperative discomfort because a radiofrequency of 4MHz is very gentle on the tissues with the active electrode remaining cold.[2]

Radiosurgery Waveforms

A transformer in all radiosurgery units changes the main voltage input to a high-voltage, high-frequency current. Further filtering and rectification produces any of the following waveforms. A microsmooth pure cut (fully filtered, fully rectified, 90% cut/10% coagulation) waveform is ideal for initial skin incisions, grafting, and biopsies where excess bleeding is not expected. This waveform gives the least tissue damage from lateral heat. A blended current (fully rectified 50% cut/ 50% coagulation) cut/coagulation waveform balances the minimal tissue injury of a pure cut with the hemostasis induced by coagulation as needed for subcutaneous dissections and lesion excisions (e.g., of verrucae, nevi, skin tags, papillomas, keloids, and keratoses) where slight bleeding is expected.

The authors, likewise, reserve this waveform for transconjunctival blepharoplasty. Direct/indirect, spot coagulation with minimal lateral heat spread requires a partially rectified (10% cut/90% coagulation) waveform to adequately control bleeding vessels up to 2mm in diameter. The authors use this waveform in resection of orbicularis muscle and orbital fat in procedures such as blepharoplasty, ptosis repair, correction of lid retractions, and lesion excisions (e.g., telangiectasias and spider veins). This is also used in external, mini-incision, and endonasal DCR. Fulguration uses a spark gap current which generates significant lateral heat (similar to unipolar diathermy [Hyfrecator]) mainly used for electro-desiccation as in superficial hemostasis and destruction of small basal cell carcinomas or cysts. The bipolar waveform (1.7MHz), which avoids tissue adherence to the forceps tip, is ideal for wet-field cautery, very precise hemostasis, and for control of individual bleeding vessels in microsurgery.

Electrodes

There are different types of electrodes available for use with the radiosurgery units. The choice of electrode is dependent on type of surgery to be performed, anticipated bleeding, and desired cosmetic results. There are extra-fine empire electrodes (for thin skin incisions with very minimal scarring), fine-wire electrodes (for extremely fine excisions and incisions), round-loop electrodes (for excision of small lid neoplasms/biopsy specimens from bigger neoplasms), triangular- or oval-loop electrodes (for excision of pedunculated and raised skin lesions), and ball electrodes (for coagulation).

The authors use the endoscopic forehead lift electrode for endoscopic radiofrequency-assisted forehead (ERAF) lift. The Ellman-Javate DCR electrodes (Figure 20.1), however, are preferred for endonasal DCR, mini-incision DCR, and standard-external DCR.[4]

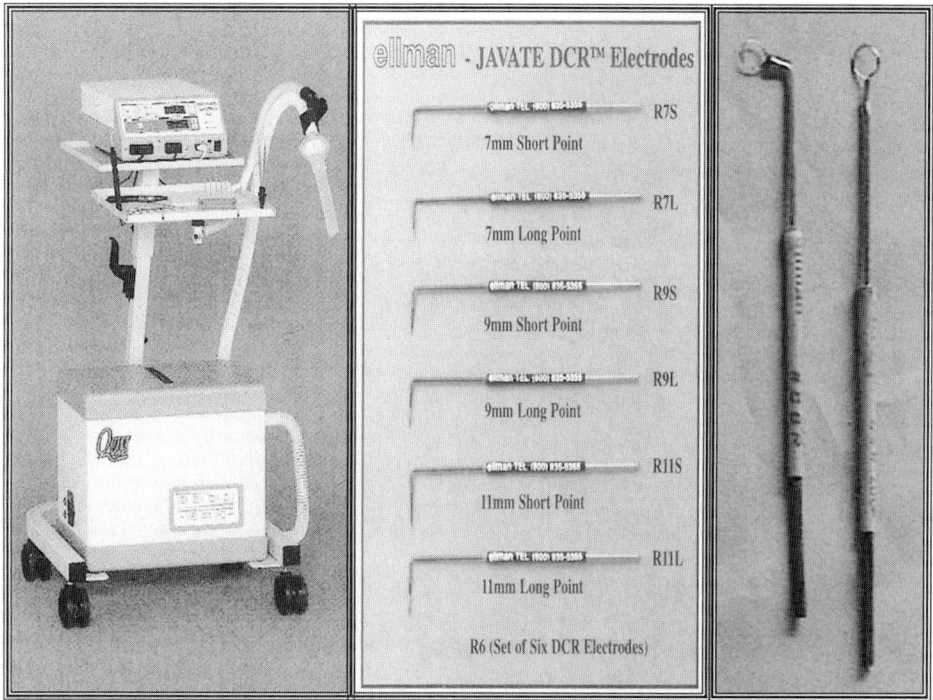

FIGURE 20.1. Ellman Dual Radiofrequency Surgitron Unit and Ellman-Javate DCR Electrodes.

Radiosurgery in Dacryocystorhinostomy

The authors use an Ellman Surgitron Dual Frequency Unit (Ellman International, Hewlett, Long Island, NY) and all settings and waveforms refer to this machine. For more than 10 years, the initial techniques have undergone several modifications that have helped achieve surgical success.[5]

External Dacryocystorhinostomy and Mini-Incision Dacryocystorhinostomy with the Radiofrequency Unit

In external DCR, the authors reserve radiosurgery for skin incisions, creation of lacrimal sacs and nasal mucosal flaps, and hemostasis. They recently introduced the mini-incision DCR[6] for better cosmetic results. The Ellman-Javate DCR electrode (attached to the Ellman Surgitron unit set in the cut mode) is used to make an 8- to 10-mm incision set about 7–8 mm below the lower lid margin (Figure 20.2A). It starts at a point slightly inferior to the medial canthal tendon, extending just into the anterior lacrimal crest, and continuing laterally in a horizontal direction following the periorbital relaxed skin tension lines. This offers less bowstringing and postoperative scarring in contrast to incisions positioned 3–4 mm beneath the lower lid margin which can cause ectropion from wound contracture or orbital fat prolapse when incisions are placed just above the orbital septum.[7] Radiofrequency also provides excellent hemostasis because individual bleeding points are

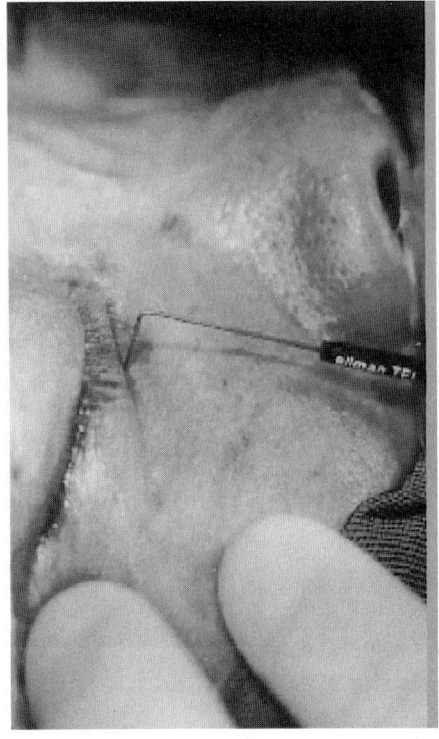

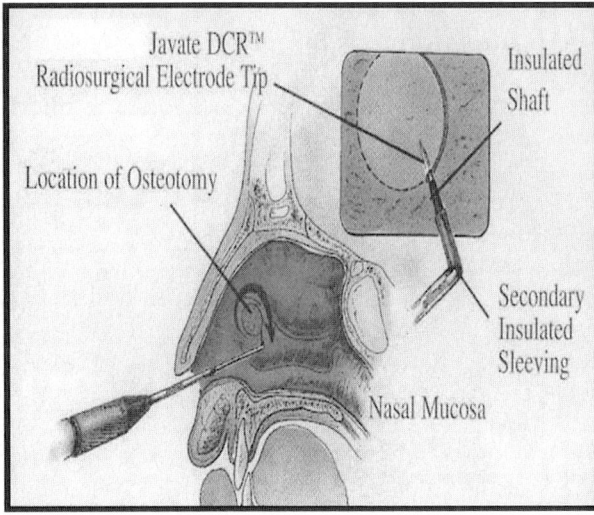

FIGURE 20.2. (A) Mini-incision DCR: (left) an 8- to 10-mm-long skin incision is place approximately 7–8 mm beneath the lower eyelid margin, using the Javate DCR electrodes attached to a radiosurgery unit. **(B)** ERA-DCR: (right) diagrammatic representation showing incision of the nasal mucosa with the Javate DCR electrodes.

controlled by the electrodes. Tissue anatomy is not obscured by hemorrhage, thereby providing better visualization and shortened operative time. Patients wearing spectacles also report greater comfort immediately after mini-incision DCR surgery. This is not only attributable to less postoperative pain and inflammation but also the spectacle nose pads usually do not rest on the resulting incision site. The rapid postoperative recovery allows an earlier return to normal daily activities and work.

Blunt scissors are then used to dissect down to the anterior lacrimal crest. Bleeders are coagulated to markedly decrease postoperative periorbital ecchymosis. The DCR electrode is then used to incise through the periosteum overlying the anterior lacrimal crest. After the osteotomy is created, the nasal mucosal flaps are made using the electrode set in coagulation mode. The remainder of the procedure is generally similar to the gold standard external techniques.

Endoscopic Radiofrequency-Assisted Dacryocystorhinostomy

A patient undergoing endoscopic radiofrequency-assisted (ERA)-DCR is placed in a supine position with the head slightly elevated to decrease venous pressure at the operative site. Although local anesthesia is an option, general endotracheal anesthesia is preferred because of the copious volume of irrigation used to completely irrigate the mitomycin from the nasal passage. Nasal preparation includes packing with cotton soaked in 0.05% oxymetazoline hydrochloride along the lateral nasal wall to initiate mucosal decongestion. A 4-mm 0-degree rigid Karl Storz Hopkins endoscope (Karl Storz GmbH and Co., Tuttlingen, Germany) is used for visualization as submucosal injection of 2% lidocaine hydrochloride with epinephrine (1:100,000) is placed in the middle turbinate and the lateral nasal wall just anterior to the attachment of the turbinate. In some patients, the middle turbinate limits access to the lacrimal sac fossa. In such patients, the middle turbinate is infractured medially instead of removing its anterior portion. The entire procedure is performed with a videocamera attached to the endoscope. The assisting surgeon is able to observe the surgery on a video monitor.

A 20-G retinal light pipe lubricated with antibiotic ointment is inserted through the dilated superior canaliculus. To ensure that its tip reaches the most inferodependent portion of the lacrimal sac, a 0- or 30-degree rigid Karl Storz Hopkins endoscope is introduced into the nose to visualize the area anterior to the middle turbinate. The light from the endoscope is then kept at minimum setting to enhance the illumination visualized from the retinal light pipe. A diffuse glow indicates inadequate apposition of the light pipe to the lacrimal bone. A discrete area of light marks the intended area of rhinostomy along the lateral nasal wall. When the glow from the tip is adequately positioned at the posteroinferior wall of the sac (where the overlying bone is thinnest), the light pipe is held in place using sterile tape. The overlying mucosa is injected with the lidocaine-bupivacaine-epinephrine solution under endoscopic guidance. A 20-mm area of this nasal mucosa is incised using an assortment of electrode points of varying lengths (Ellman-Javate DCR electrodes) with the Ellman Surgitron Dual Frequency Unit set in coagulation mode at a power setting of 50–60 (Figure 20.2B). In the past, the authors used the straight electrode for this step. However, they have recently adapted the loop electrode for scraping the nasal mucosa with greater facility. The incised mucosa is then lifted off with a Freer periosteal elevator.

The initial puncture into the intended rhinostomy site is made with a curette and the ostium is further enlarged to a 10- to 15-mm diameter size using a Kerrison punch. This rhinostomy includes part of the frontal process of the maxilla (anterior lacrimal crest).

A retinal light pipe inserted into the lacrimal sac facilitates the demarcation of the posterior-inferior and anterior-inferior walls of the sac through visible indentations. These indentations ensure that incisions in these areas made with the Ellman-Javate DCR electrodes will create the ideal 5- to 10-mm openings. A lacrimal sac that is difficult to visualize (e.g., because of cicatrization) is dilated with Aquagel Lubricating Gel (Parker Laboratories, Inc., Fairfield, NJ) introduced through the canaliculus to help prevent injury to the common canaliculus during incision. Shorter DCR electrodes are used for normal-sized or enlarged lacrimal sacs, whereas the longer electrodes are necessary to reach cicatrized lacrimal sacs. Additional marginal sac tissue is removed with a Blakesley nasal forceps. The Ellman-Javate DCR electrodes and the Blakesley nasal forceps, when used under endoscopic visualization, permit the direct biopsy of the lacrimal sac, not possible in cases performed with laser DCR.

Once the nasal mucosa, rhinostomy, and lacrimal sac openings are judged adequate in size, cotton balls soaked in a 0.5 mg/mL solution of mitomycin C are applied for 3 minutes over the surrounding mucosa with the purpose of inhibiting fibroblastic proliferation. Residual mitomycin is then copiously irrigated from the operative site and nasal cavity with sterile normal saline.[4,8] Bicanalicular intubation of the nasolacrimal fistula is completed using a BD Visitec (Franklin Lakes, NJ) modified 5013 lacrimal intubation set with a retriever device to bring the tubes out through the external nares. A Griffiths nasal catheter (Griffiths Nasal Catheter 5206), with the probes of the canalicular tubes passed through it, is pushed superiorly through the nostril to straddle the bony opening using alligator forceps.[9] This is a nasolacrimal catheter designed for temporary retention in the lacrimal fossa to ensure the patency of the intranasal ostium (Figure 20.3). The canalicular tubes are tied into two square knots, further secured by a 5–0 silk suture, and cut to an appropriate length within the nose. Patency of the fistula is then confirmed endoscopically through visualization of lacrimal irrigation around the silicone stents in the nose. Oxidized, regenerated cellulose is placed at the tip of the middle turbinate with a bayonet forceps to control operative and postoperative hemorrhage. The material absorbs spontaneously. Table 20.1 details the different instruments that the authors use for a usual case of ERA-DCR.

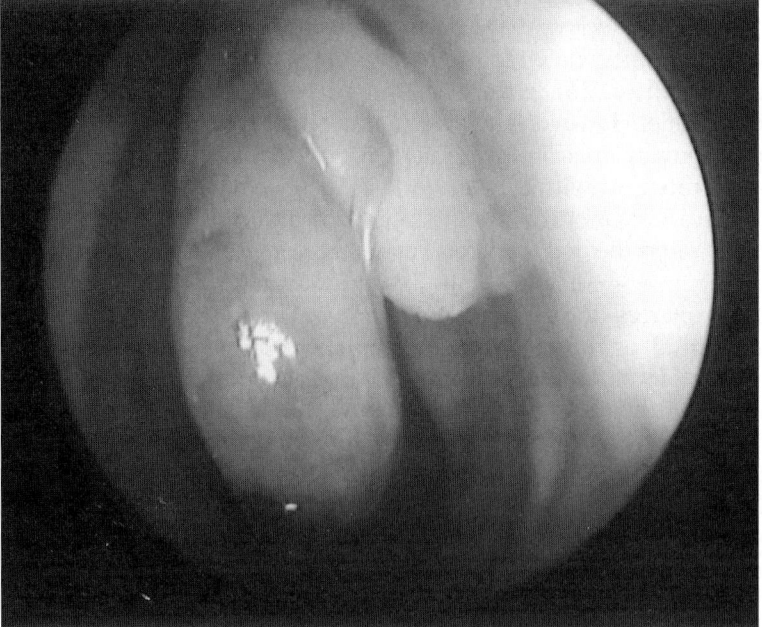

FIGURE 20.3. Endoscopic photograph showing bicanalicular silicone tubes emerging from the central lumen of the Griffiths nasal catheter.

TABLE 20.1. Instruments used in ERA-DCR.

1. Headlight	11. Retinal light pipe
2. Bayonet forceps	12. Ellman-Javate DCR electrodes (Ellman International, Hewlett, Long Island, NY)
3. Nasal speculum	
4. Cotton balls	13. Suction machine (Vapor-Vac Ellman International, Inc) with tip
5. Oxymetazoline hydrochloride 0.05% solution	14. Bone curette
6. Spinal anesthesia needle	15. Kerrison punch
7. Lidocaine 2% with epinephrine (1:100,000) solution; lidocaine 4% solution; bupivacaine 0.75% solution	16. Becton-Dickinson Visitec Lacrimal intubation set with retrieval device
	17. Mitomycin C solution (2 mg/mL)
8. Karl Storz Hopkins 0- and 30-degree Rigid Endoscopes (Karl Storz GmbH and Co., Tuttlingen, Germany)	18. Corneal eyeshields
	19. Becton-Dickinson Griffiths nasal catheter no. 5206
9. Karl Storz Blakesley nasal forceps	20. Collagen absorbable hemostat
10. Aquagel (lubricating gel; Parker Laboratories, Inc., Fairfield, NJ)	21. Suction tip

Postoperative Care

Postoperative regimen after external DCR, mini-incision DCR, and ERA-DCR includes a broad-spectrum oral antibiotic, antibiotic ophthalmic solution (Ofloxacin; Santen Pharmaceutical Co. Ltd., Osaka, Japan) applied topically four times daily, and nasal saline irrigation three times daily.

The postoperative care of patients after external DCR procedures is simpler, consisting of three to four follow-up visits where skin sutures and silicone tubes are removed at appropriate times. In contrast, endonasal DCR needs more frequent postoperative visits at intervals of 1–2 weeks. Lacrimal saline irrigation and meticulous endoscopic-guided removal of nasal debris and mucus at the rhinostomy site are performed when indicated. Steroid nasal spray (Fluticasone propionate Nasal Spray; Glaxo Smith Kline, Philippines) is used during the first postoperative week. The Griffiths nasal catheter is removed 2–3 months after surgery, whereas the silicone tubes are removed 3–6 months after surgery (Figure 20.4). Postoperative ostium patency is assessed by lacrimal irrigation and by endoscopic documentation of fluorescein dye flowing from the tear meniscus into the nose through the surgical ostium (Figure 20.5). Surgical success is further based on the relief of preoperative signs and symptoms of nasolacrimal obstruction.

The primary advantages of endoscopic lacrimal surgery (ERA-DCR) are elimination of external scarring and limited injury to the nasolacrimal fistula. Other advantages include less surgical trauma and bleeding, minimal operative and postoperative morbidity, rapid recovery, and patients' earlier return to work or school. ERA-DCR, likewise, allows the identification and correction of any intranasal pathology that may cause DCR failure, lacrimal sac biopsy under direct visualization, and success rates approaching 98%[10] for long-term patency of the intranasal ostium.

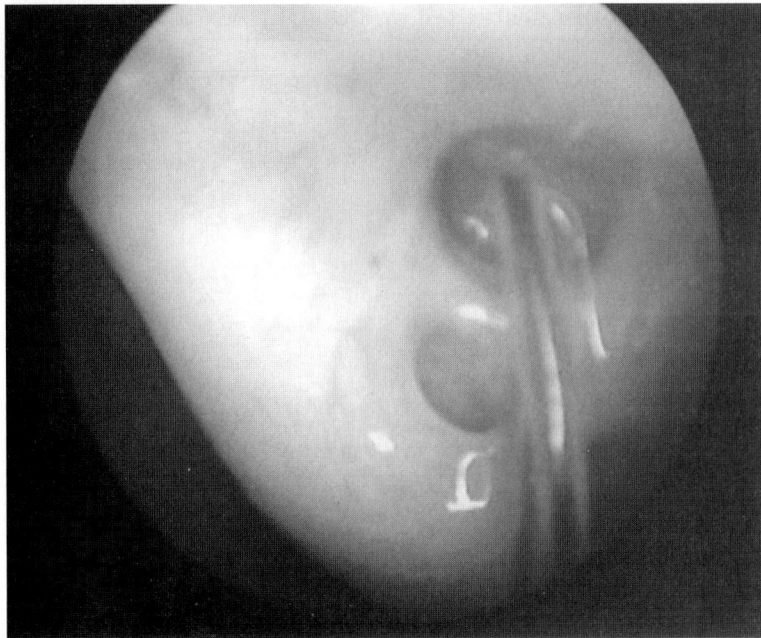

FIGURE 20.4. Endoscopic photograph showing large, healed, intranasal ostium 2 months after removal of the Griffiths nasal catheter and with bicanalicular silicone tubes still in place.

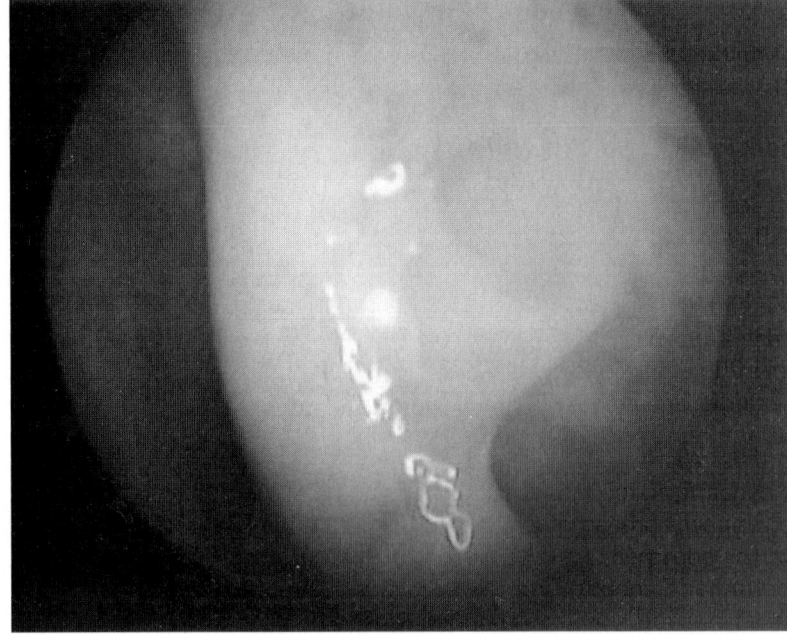

FIGURE 20.5. Endoscopic photograph taken 1 year postoperatively showing fluorescein dye flowing through the surgical ostium after lacrimal irrigation.

Postoperative Complications

Any DCR procedure may present with possible complications. Epistaxis or infections in the nose or orbit are possible with the latter and may require antibiotics. Adhesions between the intranasal ostium, the middle turbinate, and the nasal septum may be avoided by meticulous surgery and regular cleaning of the intranasal cavity at the site of the ostium created during endonasal DCR. Placement of the Griffiths nasal catheter, likewise, may lessen the incidence of these adhesions. Although ERA-DCR with the Griffiths nasal catheter may be complicated by granulation tissue formation between the nasal mucosa and the edge of the distal flange of the button, this is not necessarily associated with ostium occlusion. Cheese-wiring of the canaliculi may occur if the stenting is too tight, necessitating stent loosening or removal. If the stent is too loose, however, prolapse of the stent onto the eye may occur; this may be avoided by tightening the stent. Sump syndrome may occur if the rhinostomy is too small in size and high up in the lacrimal sac, causing tears and mucus to accumulate in the sac and to discharge onto the eye. Pyogenic granulomas may form at the puncta or the rhinostomy site if the tubing is left in place too long. This necessitates tube removal. Persistent watering or epiphora may indicate scarring of the rhinostomy and reoperation may be necessary.

Precautions in the Use of Radiofrequency Units

The radiosurgical instrument should never be used in the presence of flammable or explosive liquids or gases. It is contraindicated in patients with pacemakers, unless prior clearance is given by their primary physicians or cardiologists and steps are taken to ensure that the pacemaker is shielded from the high-frequency interference. Whenever the electrode is changed, always remember to deactivate the handpiece by releasing pressure on the foot pedal to avoid injury to the surgeon, the patient, and other personnel.

References

1. Bosniak SL, Javate RM, Aquino MS, et al. Radiosurgery: a new approach to eyelid, orbital, and lacrimal surgery. Int J Aesthetic Restorative Surg 1995;3:9–15.
2. Aimino G, Davi G. Principles of radiofrequency in oculoplastics. Oculoplast Surg Radiofrequency 1999;1:13–22.
3. Sebben JE. Electrosurgery: high-frequency modalities. J Dermatol Surg Oncol 1988;14(4):367–371.
4. Javate RM, Campomanes BS, Co ND, et al. The endoscope and the radiofrequency unit in DCR surgery. Ophthal Plast Reconstr Surg 1995;11:54–58.
5. Javate RM, Lapid-Lim SIE, Pamintuan FG. New waves in dacryocystorhinostomy. Oculoplast Surg Radiofrequency 1999;18:99–104.

6. Javate RM, Chua H, Pelayo J. Mini-incision DCR using the radiosurgery unit, oculoplastic and reconstructive surgery. Ocular Surgery News Europe/Asia-Pacific Edition, January 2001;19:20,137–138.
7. Harris GJ, Sakol PJ. Relaxed skin tension line incision for dacryocystorhinostomy. Am J Ophthalmol 1989;108:742–743.
8. Kao SCS, Liao CL, Tseng JHS, et al. Dacryocystorhinostomy with intraoperative mitomycin-C. Ophthalmology 1997;104:86–89.
9. Griffiths JD. Nasal catheter use in dacryocystorhinostomy. Ophthal Plast Reconstr Surg 1991;7:177–186.
10. Javate RM, Pamintuan FG. Endoscopic radiofrequency assisted DCR (ERA-DCR) with double stent: a personal experience. Orbit 2005;24(1): 15–22.

21

Powered Endoscopic Dacryocystorhinostomy

Peter John Wormald and Angelo Tsirbas

Endoscopic dacryocystorhinostomy (DCR) was first described by McDonogh and Meiring[1] in 1989. In that article, they describe the identification of the frontal process–lacrimal bone junction as the key landmark for identification of the lacrimal bone. The technique involved the removal of as much of the bone of the frontal process as possible before opening the lacrimal sac. There was no attempt to achieve full lacrimal sac exposure or nasal and lacrimal sac mucosal apposition. The sac was then carefully sutured to the mucosa of the lining of the nose, achieving apposition of the lacrimal and nasal mucosa.

Other authors subsequently have described the use of punches and chisels for bone removal.[2,3] The success rate for these techniques was approximately 80%.[1–4] If the literature is reviewed, it is apparent that external DCR by dedicated oculoplastic surgeons could achieve success rates of between 90% and 95%.[3,5] It is also apparent with review of the literature that one of the keys to success for external DCR surgery is the creation of the largest possible bony ostium with full exposure of the lacrimal sac.[6,7]

To enable these principles to be achieved via an endoscopic route, the intranasal relationships of the lacrimal sac and nasal anatomy needed to be better understood.[8] This was achieved by a study in our department using computed axial tomography dacryocystography (CT DCG) to define the limits of the lacrimal sac and to establish the relationship of the lacrimal sac with the middle turbinate.[8] Descriptions in the past have shown that the lacrimal sac sits anterior to the middle turbinate and the fundus of the sac ends just above the insertion of the middle turbinate onto the lateral nasal wall.[1–4] This insertion is termed the axilla of the middle turbinate.[8] The CT study showed that the lacrimal sac extended between 8 and 10 mm above the axilla of the middle turbinate.[8] In addition, the axial scans revealed that the bone of the frontal process of the maxilla progressively thickened toward the fundus of the sac and reached up to 15 mm in some patients. Initial cadaver dissections indicated it was not possible in the majority of patients to remove the bone above the axilla with a punch. Chisels were not reliable and could damage the underlying skin.

Fortunately, the understanding of the anatomy of the lacrimal sac and the need for precise bone removal coincided with the development of the powered instruments for standard sinus surgery. Powered instruments were first used for sinus surgery in the late 1980s. As the technology improved and the torque of the motor driving the instruments improved, drills were implemented. Initially, cutting burrs were used, and although they quickly and aggressively removed the bone overlying the lacrimal sac, any contact between the burr and the mucosa of medial lacrimal sac wall tended to damage the wall. Often, this resulted in a significant defect of the medial wall of the sac.

The goal of the new surgical technique is to preserve all sac mucosa so that the sac can be marsupialized into the lateral nasal wall. To avoid such damage, a rough diamond DCR burr was developed for powered endoscopic DCR surgery.[9] The technique, described below, has been specifically designed to duplicate the external DCR technique with complete exposure of the lacrimal sac so that the sac stands above the lateral nasal wall.[9,10] The sac is opened by an H-incision which preserves all the lacrimal sac mucosa and allows approximation of the lacrimal mucosa with the preserved mucosa of the nasal cavity. This achieves first intention healing rather than secondary intention healing, which is similar to that achieved with an external DCR with suturing of the lacrimal flaps.[9,10]

Surgical Technique[9,10]

A decongestant solution is prepared with 2 mL of 10% cocaine solution, 1 mL of 1:1000 epinephrine, and 4 mL of 0.9% saline. Half of this solution is used to soak six neurosurgical cottonoids (2 × 1 cm) and the other half placed on four cottonoids for use during the surgery if bleeding is problematic. After the patient has been anesthetized but before the patient has been draped, one of the six cottonoids is placed between the middle turbinate and septum, one under the middle turbinate, one above the middle turbinate, and the remaining three anterior to the middle turbinate. If the procedure is to be done under local anesthetic, these packs are placed for 10 minutes before infiltration of the anesthetic is performed.

Local anesthetic infiltration is done using a dental syringe with 2% lidocaine and 1:800,000 epinephrine. If the patient is under general anesthetic, 2 mL is used to infiltrate the lateral nasal wall above and anterior to the middle turbinate and the anterior end of the middle turbinate. If the procedure is to be performed under local anesthetic, the lacrimal sac, nasal septum, and upper lip are also infiltrated.

After nasal decongestion but before surgery, the surgeon needs to assess the access to the region anterior and above the insertion of the middle turbinate. The less experienced the surgeon, the larger amount of space required. If the septum is deviated toward this region and compromises access, a limited septoplasty should be performed before the DCR. The septum is accessed via a Killian's incision placed about a centimeter behind the anterior mucocutaneous junction. A muco-perichondrial flap is raised, and the cartilaginous bony junction of the septum identified. The suction Freer is used to separate the cartilage from the bone and a mucoperiosteal flap is formed on both sides of the bone. The deviated bony septum is resected until sufficient access to the middle turbinate insertion on the lateral nasal wall is achieved. After the DCR has been completed, a 3-0 Vicryl Rapide® (Ethicon, Somerville, NJ) plication suture is placed through the septum. This obliterates the potential space created by raising the flaps and prevents a postoperative septal hematoma from forming.

The first and one of the most important steps in powered endoscopic DCR is the mucosal incision. The incision is performed with a number 15 blade on a number 7 handle and starts 8–10 mm above and behind the insertion of the middle turbinate into the lateral nasal wall (the so-called "axilla of the middle turbinate"). The incision is brought horizontally forward 8–10 mm anterior to the axilla of the middle turbinate. The blade is turned vertically and the incision is carried down the prominent frontal process of the maxilla until the insertion of the inferior turbinate into the lateral nasal wall. This is about two-thirds of the way down the anterior edge of the middle turbinate (Figure 21.1A).

The blade is turned horizontally and the insertion continued posteriorly until the insertion of the uncinate process is reached (Figure 21.1B). If this incision is properly placed, it provides accurate margins for the correctly sized bony ostium and for complete exposure of the lacrimal sac. A 30° endoscope is turned so that the view captures the lateral nasal wall. The endoscope is pushed high into the nasal vestibule and all instruments are passed under the endoscope. At no time should the endoscope and instruments cross.

A suction Freer is used to elevate the mucosal flap, making sure that the tip of the Freer is on bone at all times during this process. The frontal process is rounded and its posterior aspect falls away, and if care is not taken to maintain contact between the bone and the elevator, the surgical plane will be lost. The 30° endoscope allows the tip of the Freer to be visualized as the dissection proceeds around the frontal process of the maxilla toward the insertion of the uncinate. The flap is elevated up to the insertion of the uncinate but no further. The thin lacrimal bone is sought between the insertion of the uncinate and the posterior aspect of the frontal process of the maxilla. A round blade is used to palpate the hard bone of the frontal process of the maxilla until the soft lacrimal bone is clearly identified. This palpation is best done in the region directly above the insertion of the inferior turbinate into the lateral nasal wall in the inferior aspect of the raised flap. The round blade is used to elevate the thin lacrimal bone over the posterior inferior aspect of the lacrimal sac. This allows the forward

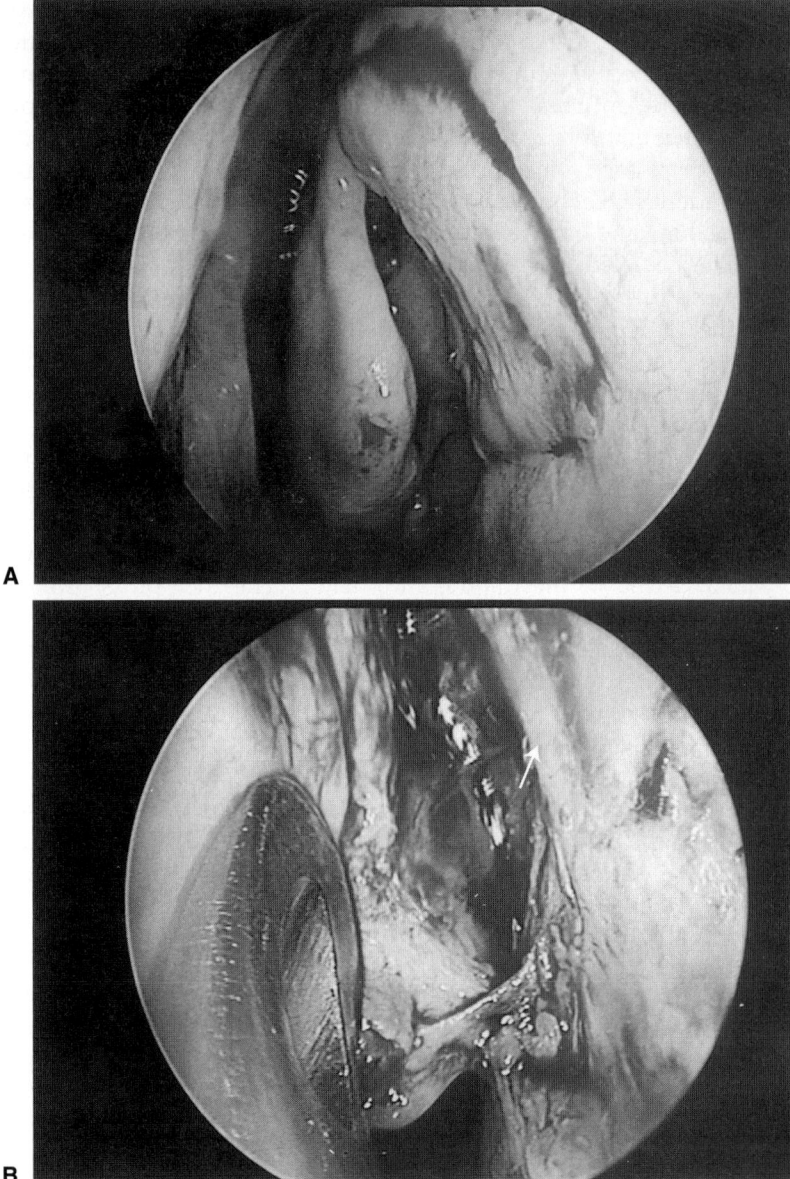

FIGURE 21.1. **(A)** The mucosal incisions on the left lateral nasal wall are shown for endoscopic DCR. **(B)** The nasal mucosal flap is elevated by a suction dissector with exposure of the lacrimal bone (white arrow).

biting Hajek-Kofler punch (Karl Storz, Tuttlingen, Germany) to be inserted. The tip of this instrument is placed on the exposed sac where the lacrimal bone had been removed, and as the instrument is engaged, the tip pushes the lacrimal sac away. This allows the bone over the anterior inferior aspect of the lacrimal sac to be removed (Figure 21.2).

Removal of bone is continued superiorly until the punch can no longer be seated. At this point (about halfway up toward the superior incision), the bone becomes too thick for the punch to be able to grip. A powered 15° endoscopic DCR burr is attached to a microdebrider handpiece (Medtronic Xomed, Jacksonville, FL) and used to remove the residual bone covering the lacrimal sac (Figure 21.3).

First, the residual bone exposed by elevation of the flap is thinned. Once the bone is thin, then the burr is moved to the bone–lacrimal sac

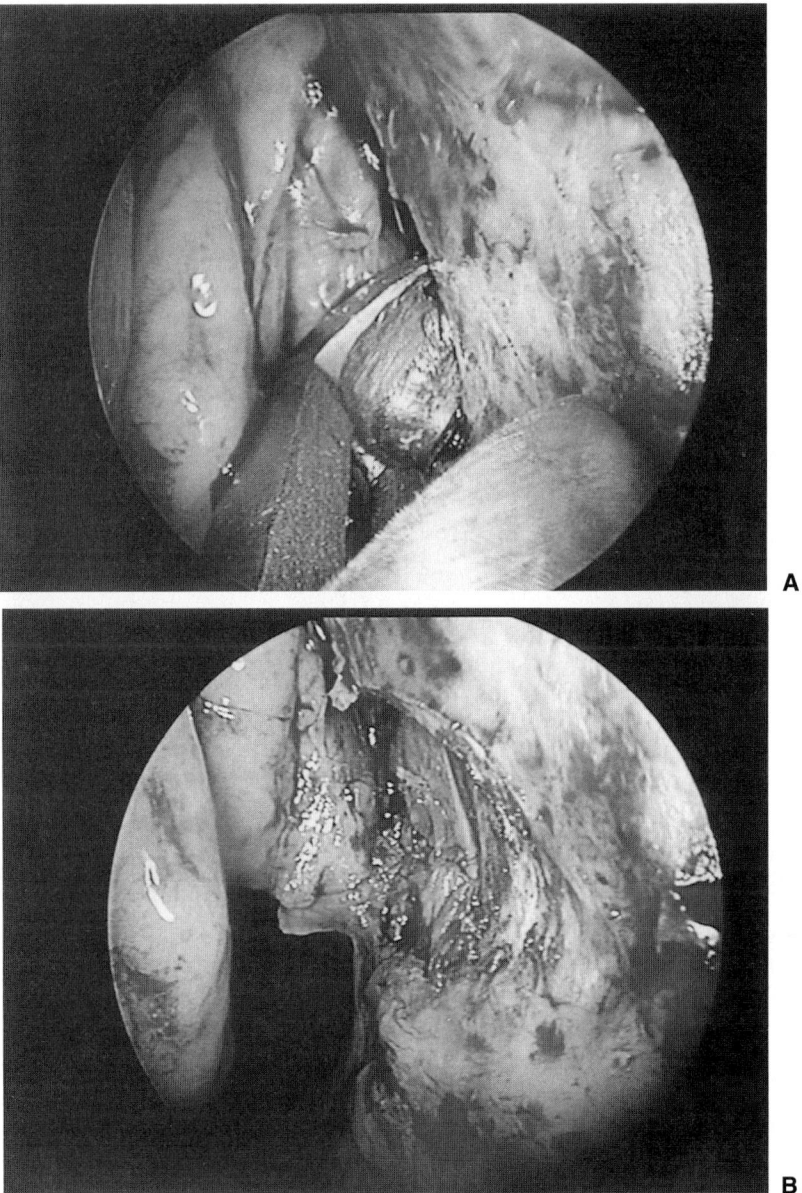

FIGURE 21.2. **(A)** The Hajek Koefler punch is used to remove the bone over the anterior inferior aspect of the lacrimal sac. **(B)** After the first bite, the anteroinferior lacrimal sac is seen.

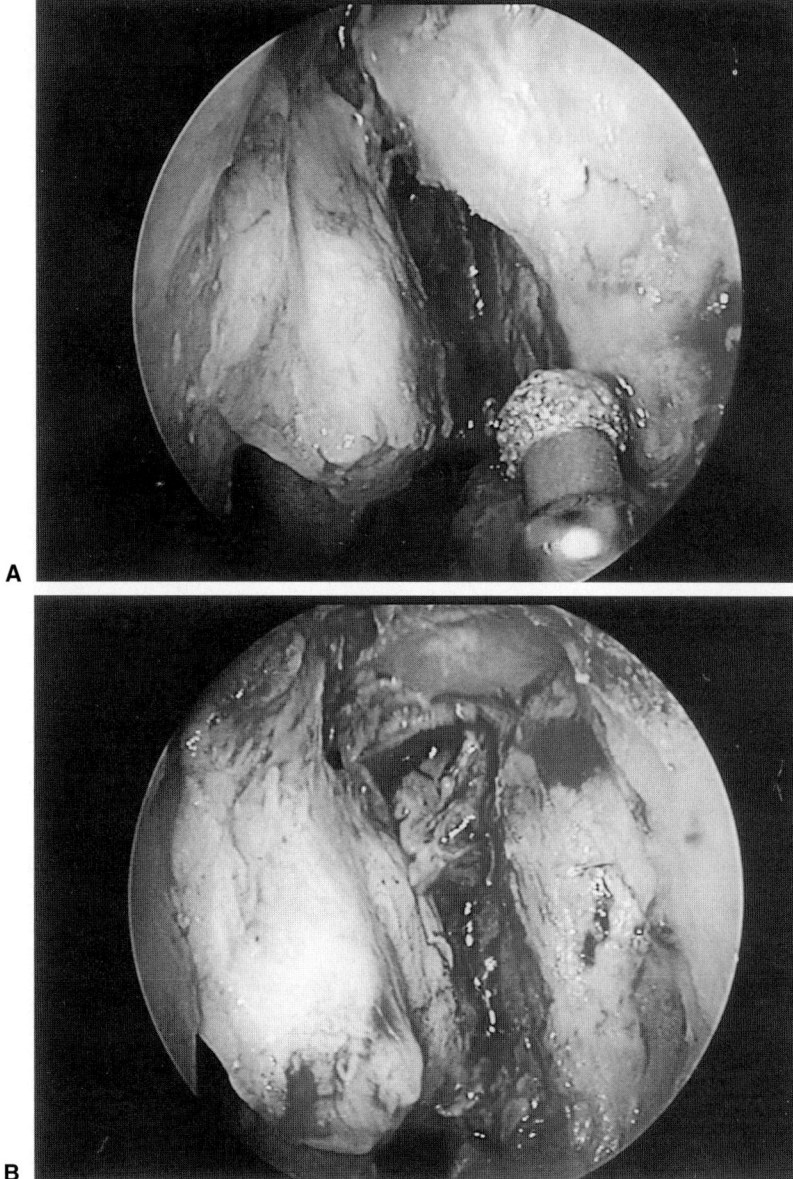

FIGURE 21.3. **(A)** A rough diamond DCR burr is used to remove all bone over the remaining lacrimal sac up to the superior incision. **(B)** Bowman lacrimal probe is used to tent the medial wall of the lacrimal sac.

junction and the remaining lacrimal sac is exposed. Care should be taken not to push the burr too far under the edge of the bone because this creates significant pressure on the lacrimal sac and the burr will create a hole in the sac. However, the sac wall is able to withstand light pressure as long as the entire burr can be visualized during the dissection. As the bone is removed in the region of the posterior superior region, the underlying mucosa of the agger nasi cell is exposed. This is routinely done as the superior portion of the lacrimal sac is constantly related to the agger nasi cell. In addition, a small amount of skin is routinely exposed just anterior to the lacrimal sac indicating complete bony removal and defining the anterior aspect of the lacrimal sac. Once the bony removal is complete, the lacrimal sac should stand above the lateral nasal wall. This allows the sac to be completely marsupialized into the lateral nasal wall. A Bowman's lacrimal probe is placed into the lacrimal sac and the medial wall of the sac is tented (Figure 21.4).

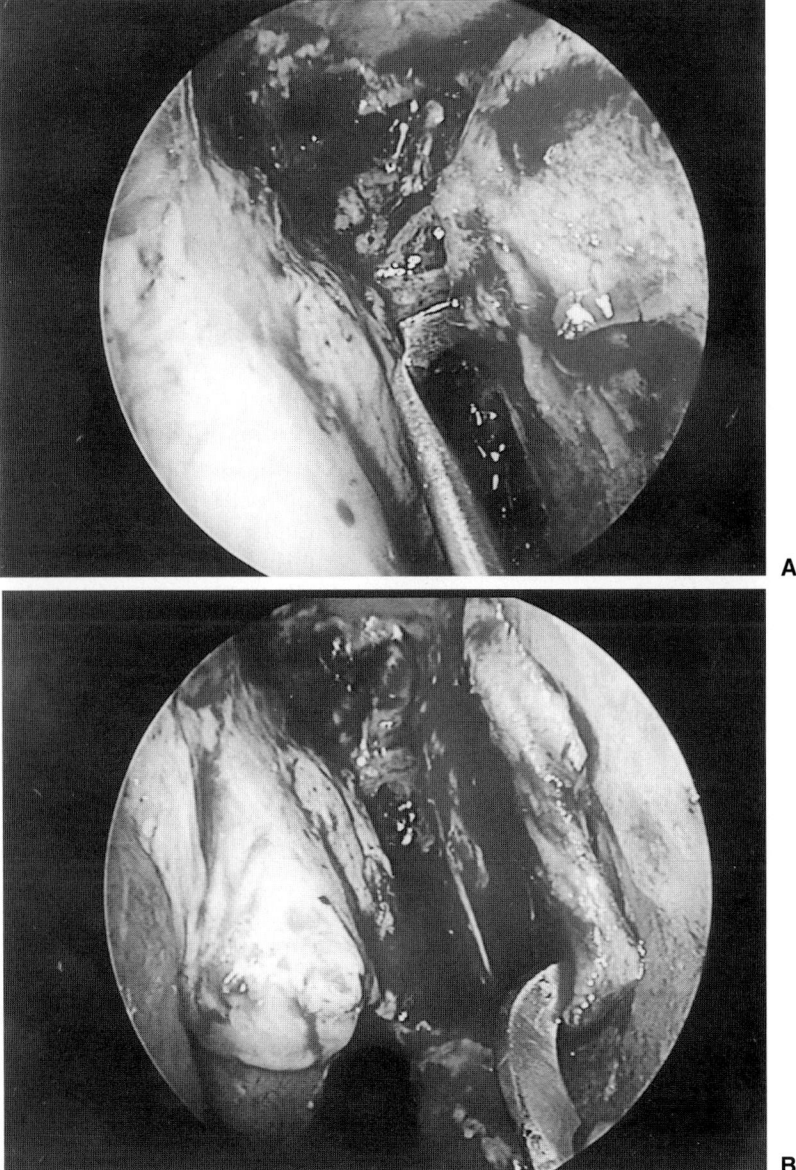

A

B

FIGURE 21.4. **(A)** The DCR spear knife is used to make the initial incision into the lacrimal sac. Note the Bowman's probe tenting the sac wall. **(B)** The mini-sickle knife is used to make anterior superior and inferior releasing incisions to enable the anterior lacrimal mucosal flap to be rolled out.

The tip of the probe should be clearly visualized before incision of the sac is attempted. If the tip of the probe is at the common canaliculus entry to the sac, it may appear as if the probe is in the sac, as the sac will still move when the probe is moved. Incision in this scenario can potentially injure the common canaliculus' opening into the sac. The sac is opened using a DCR spear knife (Medtronic Xomed). The knife is introduced into the sac lumen directly under the tip of the probe and the sac opened by rotating the spear knife. The whole blade should not be inserted into the sac lumen, rather only the cutting edge should be inserted. The sac is opened from top to bottom. The DCR mini-sickle knife (Medtronic Xomed) is used to create a releasing incision at the superior and inferior extent of the vertical incision, allowing the anterior lacrimal mucosal flap to be rolled anteriorly toward the anterior nasal mucosal incision. Microscissors are used to make posterior releasing incisions at the top and bottom of the vertical incision. This allows the posterior lacrimal flap to be rolled posteriorly with complete marsupialization of the lacrimal sac. A standard sickle knife is used to make a vertical incision into the mucosa of the agger nasi cell and to roll this mucosa anteriorly until it meets the mucosa of the posterior lacrimal flap with mucosa to mucosa apposition. The original nasal mucosal flap is trimmed with pediatric through-biting forceps, creating a superior limb of mucosa the same size as the space between the superior incision and the lacrimal mucosa (Figure 21.5).

In addition, the nasal mucosa is trimmed until it approximates the posterior lacrimal flap. An inferior limb can also be created if there is a space between the lower portion of the opened lacrimal sac and the inferior incision. This should allow approximation of nasal mucosa and lacrimal mucosa superiorly, posteriorly, and inferiorly. The only area where lacrimal and nasal mucosa will usually not be approximated is anteriorly, where the anterior lacrimal mucosa will often fall a few millimeters short of the anterior incision. Silastic O'Donaghue lacrimal intubation tubes are placed through the upper and lower canaliculus into the nose. A 4-mm silastic tube cut to 1.5 cm is slid over the O'Donaghue tubes to act as a spacer (Figure 21.6A). A loop of silastic tubing is pulled in the medial canthal region to ensure that there is no tension on the tubing. If the tubes are tight, they can cheese-wire through the superior and inferior puncta. Once the silastic tubing is tension-free, Ligar clips are placed endoscopically behind the 4-mm silastic spacer. A rectangular piece of Gelfoam® (Pharmacia & Upjohn, Kalamazoo, MI) is slid up the tubes onto the lacrimal mucosa. The silastic tubes are cut. Gelfoam® is lifted and the position of the flaps verified before the Gelfoam® is replaced (Figure 21.6B). The operation is complete.

Postoperative Care

All patients receive systemic antibiotics (amoxicillin/clavulanic acid or cefuroxime) for 5 days as well as antibiotic eye drops (Chloromycetin), one drop four times per day for 3 weeks. Nasal saline spray and douche

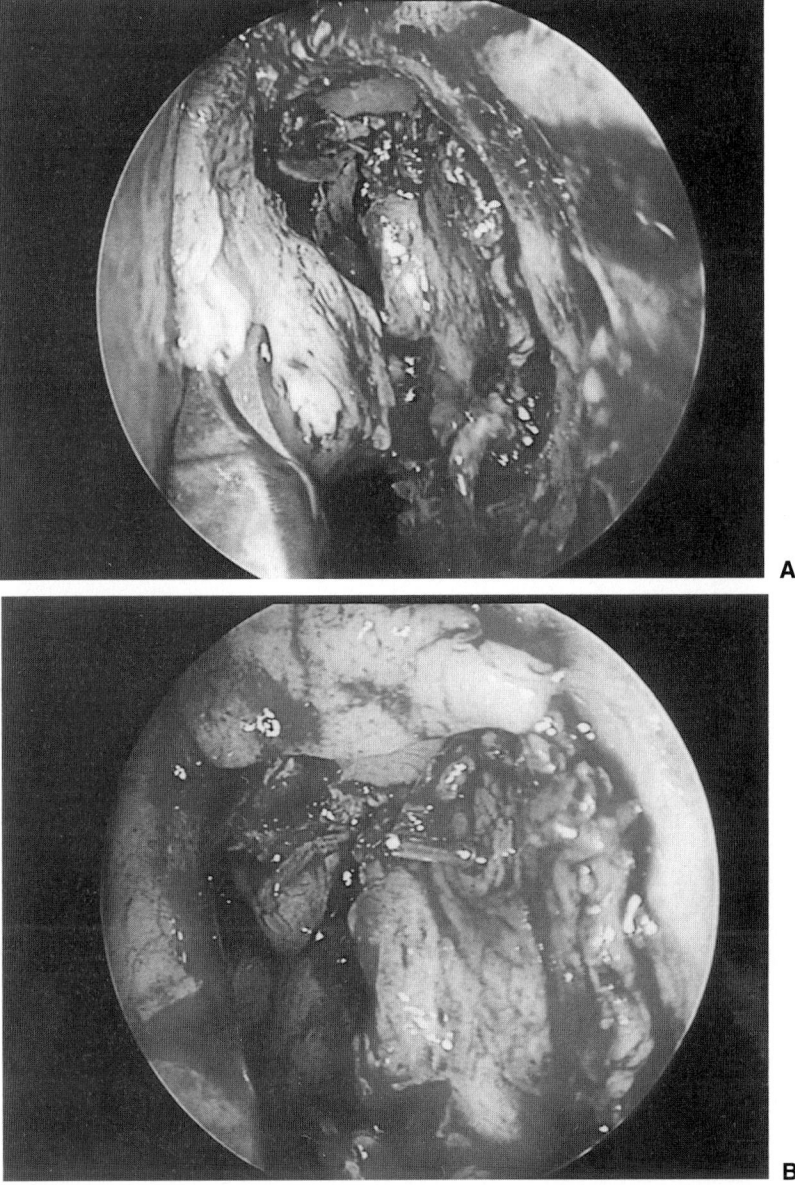

FIGURE 21.5. (A) The pediatric through-biting Blakesley is used to trim the nasal mucosal flap to allow apposition with the lacrimal sac mucosa. **(B)** Mucosal apposition is achieved superiorly between the nasal mucosa and lacrimal mucosa, posterosuperiorly between the agger nasi cell mucosa and lacrimal mucosa, posteroinferiorly and inferiorly between the nasal and lacrimal mucosa. A small gap will often remain anteriorly.

are started within 24 hours of surgery. This helps to remove blood clots from the nose and creates a clear nasal passage. It also prevents mucous from accumulating around the O'Donaghue tubes, which can create a medium for secondary infection. The patient is reviewed at 4 weeks

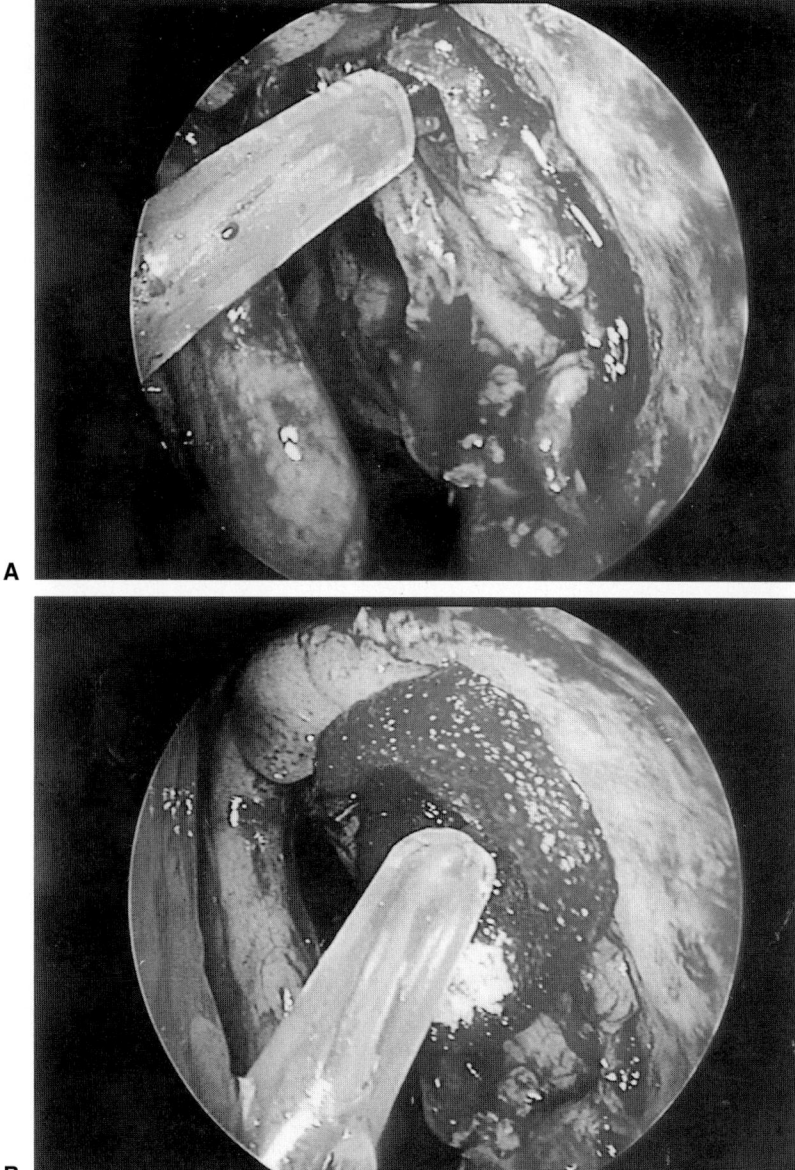

FIGURE 21.6. **(A)** Silastic tubes are in place and the spacer (silastic tubing) has been secured. **(B)** Gelfoam® is slid over the silastic tubes, and the position of the flaps is checked before the Gelfoam® is replaced.

and the O'Donaghue tubes are removed. A nasal endoscopy is performed and the lacrimal ostium observed. In most cases, it is well healed. However, if there are any granulations present, these are removed. Fluorescein is placed in the conjunctiva and nasal penetration is confirmed.

Results

The results of lacrimal surgery should be reported with reference to patient symptoms as well as to the anatomic surgical success of creating a functioning pathway between the conjunctiva and the nose. For a patient to be deemed to have a successful powered endoscopic DCR in our department, the patient needs to be asymptomatic with a functioning patent lacrimal ostium. This is confirmed endoscopically by the immediate draining of fluorescein from the conjunctiva into the healed lacrimal ostium. These criteria classify any patient with residual symptoms as a failure irrespective of an improvement in symptoms or the state of the lacrimal ostium. In addition, if the patient was completely asymptomatic and did not have an endoscopically visible ostium and if there was no fluorescein visible in the nose, the procedure was considered a failure. Using these strict outcome criteria, the results of powered endoscopic DCR have been reported in several publications.

Primary Dacryocystorhinostomy[9-11]

In the most recent analysis of 128 consecutive DCRs, the overall success rate was 95%. Of the failures, there were three DCRs that had no visible lacrimal ostium and no fluorescein in the nose. Four of the failures had a patent lacrimal sac with a free flow of fluorescein from the conjunctiva to the nose but were still symptomatic. All these patients said that their symptoms had improved after surgery. If the patients are divided into patients who had an anatomic nasolacrimal obstruction as defined by an obstructed DCG and scintigraphy (n = 87), the success rate was 98%.[11] Only two patients in this group failed with obstruction of the lacrimal ostium. Those patients with a functional patent had stenosis of the lacrimal ostium and four had a patent ostium with free flow of fluorescein nasolacrimal obstruction, defined by a patent system on DCG and impeded or absent nasal penetration on scintigraphy (n = 41), had a success rate of 88%.[11] Five of these patients failed. Of the four patients who had a patent lacrimal ostium, all believed that their symptoms had significantly improved. One patient with an anatomic failure was asymptomatic but was classified as a failure. The other anatomic failures all had significant symptoms and went on to have revision surgery.

Revision Dacryocystorhinostomies

If the results of patients undergoing powered endoscopic revision DCR are reviewed (n = 17), we note that the success rate decreases to 76.5%. We also found that the failures in this group were largely those patients who had undergone two or more previous DCRs. This is thought to result from the scarring and cicatrization of the lacrimal sac and the increased difficulty of achieving a marsupialized lacrimal sac with good nasal and lacrimal mucosa apposition.

Pediatric Dacryocystorhinostomies

Pediatric DCR was defined as a patient younger than 13 years of age undergoing an endoscopic powered DCR. The average age of the patients was 6.5 years (range, 2–13 years, standard deviation, 3.3). All patients had been diagnosed as having congenital nasolacrimal duct obstruction. The success rate was 14 of 16 (89%). The two failures occurred in a patient who had bilateral congenital nasolacrimal duct obstruction and had undergone three previous external DCRs on each side.

Conclusion

Powered endoscopic DCR allows the lacrimal sac to be fully exposed so that it stands proud of the lateral nasal wall after dissection. By fully preserving all the lacrimal mucosa during opening of the sac, the sac can be marsupialized into the lateral nasal wall, becoming part of the lateral nasal wall. This marsupialization is different from creating an ostium into the sac. Complete marsupialization decreases the likelihood of closure of the sac. In addition, preservation of the nasal mucosa allows this mucosal flap to be trimmed so that the nasal and lacrimal mucosa can be opposed to ensure primary intention healing rather than secondary intention healing and potentially lessens the risk of fibrosis and subsequent closure of the lacrimal ostium. Results of this procedure have proved to be reliable in primary, revision, and in pediatric DCRs.

References

1. McDonogh M, Meiring J. Endoscopic transnasal dacryocystorhinostomy. J Laryngol Otol 1989;103:585–587.
2. Metson R. Endoscopic surgery for lacrimal obstruction. Otolaryngol Head Neck Surg 1991;104:473–479.
3. Hartikainen J, Jukka A, Matti V, et al. Prospective randomized comparison of endonasal endoscopic dacryocystorhinostomy and external dacryocystorhinostomy. Laryngoscope 1998;108:1861–1866.
4. Wormald PJ, Nilssen E. Endoscopic DCR: the team approach. Hong Kong J Ophthalmol 1998;1:71–74.
5. Javate RM, Campornanes BS, Nelson D, et al. The endoscope and the radiofrequency unit in DCR surgery. Ophthal Plast Reconstr Surg 1995;11(1):54–58.
6. Linberg J, Anderson R, Busted R, Barreras R. Study of intranasal ostium external dacryocystorhinostomy. Arch Ophthalmol 1982;100:1758–1762.
7. Welham R, Wulc A. Management of unsuccessful lacrimal surgery. Br J Ophthalmol 1987;71:152–157.
8. Wormald PJ, Kew J, Van Hasselt CA. The intranasal anatomy of the nasolacrimal sac in endoscopic dacryocystorhinostomy. Otolaryngol Head Neck Surg 2000;123:307–310.
9. Wormald PJ. Powered endonasal dacryocystorhinostomy. Laryngoscope 2002;112:69–71.

10. Tsirbas A, Wormald PJ. Endonasal dacryocystorhinostomy with mucosal flaps. Am J Opthalmol 2003;135(1):76–83.

11. Wormald PJ, Tsirbas A. Investigation and treatment for functional and anatomical obstruction of the naso-lacrimal duct system. Clin Otolaryngol 2004;29:352–356.

22

Laser Dacryocystorhinostomy: Part 1. Laser-Assisted Endonasal Endoscopic Dacryocystorhinostomy

Michael Mercandetti

Laser-assisted dacryocystorhinostomy (DCR) has been performed with argon, potassium titanyl phosphate (KTP), holmium:YAG, CO_2, Nd:YAG, erbium, and diode lasers. These lasers create the ostium from an intranasal, transcanalicular, or combined approach. In these approaches, microscopes, loupes, or endoscopes have been utilized.

Laser-assisted DCR was first reported in the literature by Massaro and colleagues[1] in 1990. This report involved one patient on whom the argon laser was used and the success rate was 100%. An operating microscope was used for intranasal visualization. Gonnering and colleagues[2] in 1992 described the use of the CO_2 laser in conjunction with the endoscope. Fifteen patients were treated and the success rate was again 100%. Woog and colleagues[3] had an 83% success rate in 40 patients with the use of the holmium:YAG laser. Of the 34 cases presented by Metson and colleagues,[4] seven patients had revision DCRs. Table 22.1 shows the success rates of various reported studies performing intranasal laser-assisted DCRs.

Some of the laser-assisted studies reported used adjunctive equipment or medication. In the study by Kong and colleagues,[5] the drill and the radiofrequency unit were used in addition to the laser. In the study reported by Camara and Santiago,[6] no mitomycin C was used. In the 2000 report by Camara and associates,[7] mitomycin C was used.

Doyle and colleagues[8] reported on a pediatric population of six patients and a 0% success rate.

As with all reports of success after DCR, the definition of success must be clearly delineated. Tripathi and colleagues[9] reported a 91.3% success rate in their series, but only 65.2% of the patients declared themselves cured.

Postoperative care is more involved with any endonasal and laser-assisted procedure than a conventional external DCR. The ostium must be examined and debrided as necessary. The low-intensity helium-

TABLE 22.1. Intranasal laser-assisted DCR success rates.

Author	Year	Laser	Cases	Rate of Success
Massaro et al.	1990	Argon	1	100
Gonnering et al.	1992	CO2:KTP	15	100
Woog et al.	1993	Holmium:YAG	40	83
Reifler	1993	KTP	19	68
Metson et al.	1994	Holmium:YAG	34	82
Seppa et al.	1994	CO2/Nd:YAG	12	83
Kong et al.	1994	Holmium:YAG/Nd:YAG	92	77
Tutton and O'Donnell	1995	Nd:YAG	6	100
Sadiq et al.	1996	Holmiun:YAG	86	59
Mickelson et al.	1997	KTP	12	100
Szubin et al.	1999	Argon or Holium:YAG	28	96
Camara and Santiago	1999	Holmium:YAG	48	90
Camara et al.	2000	Holmium:YAG	123	99
Doyle et al.	2000	KTP	6	0
Caversaccio et al.	2001	Erbium:YAG	12	75
Piaton et al.	2002	Diode	363	92
Tripathi et al.	2002	Holmium:YAG	40	91
Moore et al.	2002	Holmium:YAG	33	71
Mirza et al.	2002	KTP	76	64
Liu et al.	2002	Semiconductor	7	86
Morgan et al.	2004	Holmium:YAG	9	67

neon laser[10] has been reported to diminish healing time because of its antiinflammatory properties. The treatment was also noted to retard the propagation of granulation tissue.

The success rate of laser-assisted DCRs ranges from 0% to 100%. Limitations of the procedure include damage to tissue surrounding the ostium from the heat generated by the laser. Additionally, the size of the ostium is limited because of the power of the laser. The expense of the equipment, training of personnel, and safety issues are also factors that must be considered in the use of the lasers. However, the ability to perform the surgery quickly, under local anesthesia, and with potentially less bleeding is appealing.

Acknowledgment. The author appreciates the work of Vickie Hase, who assisted in preparation of this chapter.

References

1. Massaro BM, Gonnering RS, Harris GJ. Endonasal laser dacryocystorhinostomy: a new approach to nasolacrimal duct obstruction. Arch Ophthalmol 1990;108(8):1172–1176.
2. Gonnering RS, Lyon DB, Fisher JC. Endoscopic laser-assisted lacrimal surgery. Am J Ophthalmol 1991;111(2):152–157.
3. Woog JJ, Metson R, Puliafito CA. Holmium:YAG endonasal laser dacryocystorhinostomy. Am J Ophthalmol 1993;116(1):1–10.
4. Metson R, Woog JJ, Pulafito CA. Endoscopic laser dacryocystorhinostomy. Laryngoscope 1994;104(3 pt 1):269–274.

5. Kong YT, Kim TI, Kong BW. A report of 131 cases of endoscopic laser lacrimal surgery. Ophthalmology 1994;101(11):1793–1800.

6. Camara JG, Santiago MD. Success rate of endoscopic laser-assisted dacryocystorhinostomy. Ophthalmology 1999;106(3):441–442.

7. Camara JG, Bengzon AU, Henson RD. The safety and efficacy of mitomycin C in endonasal endoscopic laser-assisted dacryocystorhinostomy. Ophthal Plast Reconstr Surg 2000;16(2):114–118.

8. Doyle A, Russell J, O'Keefe M. Paediatric laser DCR. Acta Ophthalmol Scand 2000;78(2):204–205.

9. Tripathi A, Lesser TH, O'Donnell NP, White S. Local anaesthetic endonasal endoscopic laser dacryocystorhinostomy: analysis of patients' acceptability and various factors affecting the success of this procedure. Eye 2002; 16(2):146–149.

10. Beloglazov VG, At'kova EL, Nurieva SM, Khvedelidze EP. Low-intensity helium-neon laser in the treatment of patients after endonasal dacryocystorhinostomy. Vestn Oftalmol 2004;120(5):7–12.

23

Laser Dacryocystorhinostomy: Part 2. Laser-Assisted Endonasal Endoscopic Dacryocystorhinostomy with the Holmium:YAG Laser

Ajay Tripathi and Niall P. O'Donnell

The endonasal approach to dacryocystorhinostomy (DCR) offers various advantages over the external approach, such as minimal tissue injury, lack of cutaneous scar, excellent hemostasis, minimal operative and postoperative morbidity, shorter surgery time, ease of surgery under local anesthesia, and no interference with lacrimal pump function. The improvement in fiberoptic endoscopes ensures excellent visualization during nasal surgery and has resulted in a revival of interest in endonasal DCR. The use of a laser to perform the surgery rather than using surgical instruments has become popular in view of the ease of the procedure and has proved a viable alternative in cases of nasolacrimal duct obstruction. It is important for the surgeon to be familiar with the normal nasal anatomy and its variants. The authors always undertake laser-assisted endonasal DCR in conjunction with otorhinolaryngologists because of their expertise in endonasal surgery and the ability to manage unexpected nasal problems which may otherwise result in abandoning the procedure once started.

Patient Preparation

Laser-assisted endoscopic DCR is only indicated in obstructions to tear drainage distal to the lacrimal sac. It is mandatory to inquire about previous nasal trauma and surgery. A history of recurrent nasal infections indicates nasal pathology which must be addressed before undertaking DCR.

Prior to the patient arriving in the operating room, the appropriate side of the nasal cavity is sprayed with a combination of lidocaine hydrochloride 5% and phenylephrine hydrochloride 0.5%. The procedure is performed under local anesthesia with an injection of 2.5 mL of 2% lidocaine combined with 1:200,000 epinephrine via a postcaruncular approach to the medial orbital wall region. A Merocel (Medtronic Xomed, Jacksonville, FL) nasal packing is inserted into the appropriate nasal cavity and the lidocaine/phenylephrine (Aurum Pharmaceuticals, Essex, UK) combination instilled into the nasal cavity to ensure good contact with the nasal mucosa at the expected operative site. The authors do not undertake skin preparation preoperatively. The surgical area is draped using a fenestrated ENT drape. Once in the operating room, the nasal packing is removed and three Codman surgical pads, which have been soaked in 10% cocaine, are inserted into the proposed surgical site to further decongest and anesthetize the nose.

Technique

A fiberoptic light source is passed, after punctal dilatation, through the lower lacrimal punctum, into the inferior canaliculus, and advanced along the canaliculus into the lacrimal sac. The light source is then inclined inferonasally to locate the most inferior aspect of the sac. It is then secured in position over the drape with the help of a small artery clip. Nasal endoscopy using a 0- or 30-degree scope is performed and the lacrimal sac is identified by observing the illumination within the sac.

A holmium:YAG laser (PowerSuite, wavelength 2100 nm; Lumenis Corp., London, UK) is applied via a handheld fiberoptic wire under direct endoscopic visualization. The nasal mucosa is opened and a bony ostium is formed at the site of the illuminated lacrimal sac. The usual settings of the laser are 0.6–0.8 Joules/Hz (equivalent of 6–8 watts) for mucosal application and 1.0 Joules/Hz (equivalent of 10 watts) for application to bone. Once the connection between the lacrimal sac and the nasal cavity is established, the nasolacrimal system is intubated in the usual manner with a bicanalicular stent, which is secured in the nose by passing the stent through a Watzke sleeve [retinal implant silicone sleeve (0.76 mm); Labtichna Ophthalmics Corp., Canada]. The stent is left in place for 12 weeks. After stent removal, a sac washout is performed to assess patency of the new channel.

Complications

Complications after endonasal laser DCR are relatively infrequent. These can be:

1. Stent prolapse occurs infrequently because the mucosal and bony ostium diameters are narrower than the diameter of the Watzke sleeve encapsulating the stent. A prolapsed stent should ideally be repositioned and only in rare cases will it need to be removed prematurely.

2. Granulomas may develop at the operative site.

3. Local hematoma formation in the lids or cheek area can result from local anesthetic injection.

4. "Cheese-wiring" of the lacrimal puncta caused by excessive tension on the bicanalicular stent.

5. False passage formation as the light source is advanced along the lacrimal canaliculus.

6. Incorrect localization of the sac illumination and subsequent incorrect location.

7. Failure of the procedure is usually attributed to a complete healing of the nasal mucosa, which looks previously untouched when these patients are endoscopically reviewed. Alternatively, an adhesion between the site of the nasal mucosal opening and the middle turbinate may lead to a surgical failure.

8. Systemic reaction to topical cocaine used to aid nasal anesthesia/decongestion.

The anatomic success rate after the procedure varies between 90% and 95%. Most series suggest up to 60% of patients have complete resolution of symptoms with another 20% noticing an improvement in symptoms to a tolerable level. Lower eyelid malposition and lacrimal pump failure may result in less than satisfactory outcomes in some patients. The authors have observed that success rates are higher in younger patients, in those with a shorter duration of symptoms, and in those without any previous surgical intervention.

The keys to success are proper positioning and size of the ostium and prevention of late closure of the nasal mucosal opening. Variation in nasal anatomy or previously undetected nasal pathology may make surgery technically difficult and one would be best advised to undertake such surgery with an otorhinolaryngologist.

The ease of the surgical procedure from the surgeon's point of view and the ability to perform rapid and, when required, bilateral surgeries make laser-assisted endonasal DCR an acceptable alternative to external DCR in suitable patients.

Acknowledgment. The authors appreciate the work of Vickie Hase, who assisted in preparation of this chapter.

24

Laser Dacryocystorhinostomy: Part 3. Laser-Assisted Endonasal Endoscopic Dacryocystorhinostomy with the Potassium Titanyl Phosphate Laser

Showkat Mirza, Andrew K. Robson, Marco Carvessacio

Preoperative Assessment

Patients are seen by both a consultant ophthalmologist and otolaryngologist in a joint epiphora clinic and undergo a full assessment including palpation of the lacrimal sac, probing and irrigation of the canaliculi and lacrimal sac, dye disappearance test, and nasal endoscopy. In cases where the site of obstruction is not obvious, a macrodacryocystogram is performed to confirm nasolacrimal duct obstruction. If there is a suspicion of lacrimal sac neoplasm or evidence of a severe posttraumatic bony deformity of the lacrimal sac, then an external surgical approach is selected.

Endonasal Potassium Titanyl Phosphate Laser Dacryocystorhinostomy Technique

The endonasal laser dacryocystorhinostomies are performed by both a consultant ophthalmologist and otorhinolaryngologist. Patients are placed under either a general anesthetic or under local anesthetic with intravenous sedation. In all cases, cophenylcaine nasal spray is applied to the nasal mucosa as a decongestant and local anesthetic. For cases under local anesthesia, topical anesthetic drops are instilled into the eye, and lidocaine 2% with epinephrine is infiltrated subcutaneously in the medial canthus. The canaliculi are dilated with a probe and then a vitreoretinal light probe is passed through the upper or lower canaliculus into the lacrimal sac, thereby transilluminating the lateral nasal wall. The position of the light is viewed endonasally and the illuminated area of the middle meatus is infiltrated using lidocaine 2% with epinephrine (1:100,000) submucosally, followed by packing of the area with pads soaked in epinephrine (1 : 100,000). An Orion™ Laser System KTP/532 (Laserscope Ltd., Cwmbran, South Wales, UK) with 0.4-mm fiber is used.

Under the guidance of a 4-mm, 0° rigid nasal endoscope, the laser probe is directed at the area of transillumination along the lateral nasal wall. The nasal mucosa, bone, and lacrimal sac mucosa are ablated with a laser power setting of 5–10 W on super pulse mode. "Cold steel" techniques rather than laser ablation, particularly around the lacrimal sac, may avoid excessive scarring and improve rhinostomy patency rates. A rhinostomy of 0.5–1.0 cm in diameter is formed. Stenting is performed by inserting the ends of a silicone tube through the superior and inferior canaliculi. The ends are then retrieved from the nose with fine nasal forceps and tied.

Postoperatively, patients are instructed to use saline nasal spray. The stent is removed after 3 months. Patients are assessed at this time and then after a further 6 months with irrigation of the canaliculi and/or the fluorescein test.

Minor complications include epistaxis requiring packing, conjunctivitis, stent infection, surgical emphysema, and sinusitis.

Acknowledgment. The authors appreciate the work of Vickie Hase, who assisted in preparation of this chapter.

25

Revision Dacryocystorhinostomy

Adam J. Cohen, F. Campbell Waldrop, and David A. Weinberg

Patients with residual tearing after dacryocystorhinostomy (DCR) can be quite challenging with regard to diagnosing the cause of surgical failure and determining appropriate management. Both the surgeon and patient are understandably quite frustrated with a "wet" eye after DCR.

For primary external and endoscopic DCR, the failure rate has been reported to be 5%–10% or less[1,2] and 20%–40%,[1,2] respectively. Several authors have reported much lower failure rates for primary endoscopic DCR,[3] but most studies thus far have shown that endonasal DCR, using a variety of techniques, carries a higher failure rate when compared with external DCR. The most common cause of DCR failure is occlusion of the rhinostomy site by soft tissue, common canalicular obstruction,[4] cicatricial ostium closure, formation of synechiae between the ostium and the middle turbinate or the septum, and granuloma formation at the ostium.[5] Most endonasal DCR techniques described do not use mucosal flaps, and it is unclear whether or not this predisposes to rhinostomy closure, because flaps have not been proven to increase surgical success rates in external DCR.[6]

There are two broad categories of patients who have undergone DCR and complain of tearing and/or lacrimal discharge postoperatively. The first category includes those who were misdiagnosed with NLDO (nasolacrimal duct obstruction) preoperatively, but instead have a different etiology of tearing, such as reflex tearing or canaliculitis. The second category comprises patients with failure of the surgical procedure despite a correct diagnosis of NLDO.

NLDO is only one of many possible causes of tearing or lacrimal discharge, and a complete history and careful eye examination should direct the surgeon to the correct diagnosis. A thorough evaluation includes detailed questioning with regard to the character of the tearing or discharge. For example, is the tearing seasonal? Is there itching? These inquiries may suggest an allergic component. Is the tearing worse with reading or watching television, or at the end of the day, or associated with eye discomfort, e.g., foreign body sensation? An answer may indicate dry eye syndrome with reflex tearing.

Other etiologies of tearing include eyelid and punctal malposition, eyelash misdirection, punctal occlusion, conjunctivochalasis, canalicular obstruction or infection (canaliculitis), medications (glaucoma and antiviral ophthalmic drops, 5-fluorouracil,[7] or docetaxel[8]) causing dry eye syndrome or punctal and/or canalicular stenosis, blepharitis and dry eye syndrome, ocular surface disease, uveitis, or an embedded corneal or eyelid foreign body, to name a few. One of the non-ocular causes of tearing is aberrant regeneration of the facial nerve secondary to nerve injury from prior facial trauma or surgery leading to gustatory epiphora ("crocodile tears"). Sinorhinitis, endoscopic sinus surgery with insult to the nasolacrimal sac or duct, and radiotherapy for head and neck malignancies resulting in dry eye and keratopathy with reflex tearing or scarring of the nasolacrimal system are other non-ocular causes of excess tearing.

Certain medical conditions may increase the likelihood of failure after DCR. Lymphoma, sarcoidosis, and vasculitides, such as Wegener's granulomatosis, are disorders that may produce an NLDO. Sarcoidosis and Wegener's granulomatosis may require prolonged and intense immunosuppression to achieve optimal results.[9,10] Many surgeons believe that the optimal timing for surgery coincides with disease quiescence in cases of Wegener's granulomatosis.[10,11] Whereas wound necrosis and nasocutaneous fistulas have been reported,[12] others have reported DCR to be effective in treating these patients.[10,11,13,14] DCR failure may result also from an inadequate or misplaced osteotomy, misdirected tear drainage (fistula) into the ethmoid sinus, fibrosis across the fistula, obstruction of the fistula site by the middle turbinate or adhesions to the nasal septum, pyogenic granuloma, incomplete opening of the lacrimal sac at the time of surgery ("sump syndrome"), or canalicular obstruction, especially at the common canaliculus.[2,3]

Along with a detailed history, careful examination to establish the etiology of DCR failure is critical. Close inspection of the tear lakes may reveal a disparity between the eyes. If a patient has a unilateral increased tear lake on the side ipsilateral to the previous DCR, this is suggestive of decreased tear outflow but may also herald a contralateral dry eye with ipsilateral reflex tearing that overwhelms a partially stenotic ostium. A basal tear secretion test and the 5-minute dye disappearance test, as described in Chapters 6 and 7, may help in discriminating between reflex tearing and impaired lacrimal drainage. In unclear cases, a trial of ocular lubricants in the dry eye may render the patient asymptomatic, thereby avoiding surgery.

If the ipsilateral eye is found to have an increased retention of dye (delayed dye disappearance), it is likely the fistula is significantly stenosed or occluded and indicates the need for reoperation of some sort. There could be a component of lacrimal pump failure attributable to significant lower eyelid laxity, which will also cause dye retention. For that reason, the surgeon may wish to horizontally tighten a significantly lax lower lid at the same time as the DCR. Lacrimal irrigation should also help to differentiate the two, along with nasal endoscopy to evaluate the size and location of the DCR fistula and the presence and amount of dye in the nose.

In a patient with normal tear production, increased tear lake, and dye retention, three scenarios may exist. The first is a compromised fistula, i.e., an anatomic obstruction necessitating revisional surgery. The blockage may be at the level of the canaliculi or the rhinostomy, and irrigation will assist in this determination. The second is a functional or physiologic obstruction, in which the fistula is patent on probing and irrigation (discussed in Chapters 7 and 8). The fistula is anatomically patent, indicating the likely etiology is lacrimal pump dysfunction, which is often associated with orbicularis weakness and/ or lower eyelid laxity. This is usually responsive to horizontal eyelid tightening, although lacrimal pump dysfunction secondary to a seventh nerve palsy may not improve that easily. The third possibility is a combination of the first two scenarios, requiring concomitant eyelid surgery and revision of the fistula. If there is punctal stenosis or eversion, then that needs to be addressed during eyelid tightening because this represents a true obstructive lesion and not a functional component of NLDO.

Nasal endoscopy is an important diagnostic modality that can be performed in the office. It permits the clinician to directly visualize the rhinostomy and passage of fluorescein into the nasal vault. This examination is greatly facilitated by videoendoscopy. The nose may be anesthetized with cetacaine spray (Cetyline Industries, Pennsauken, NJ) or cophenylcaine, which provides not only anesthesia but also mucosal vasoconstriction and decongestion. The surgeon may perform a modification of the Jones dye tests, which were originally described with regard to the evaluation of the unoperated lacrimal drainage system. After instilling fluorescein into the inferior fornix and waiting several minutes, the surgeon can inspect the rhinostomy site and nasal vault for the presence of fluorescein dye.

If present, this confirms patency of the fistula. A minimal amount of dye reaching the inside of the nose suggests stenosis of the canaliculi or rhinostomy. If no dye is seen with a regular light source, it may be appreciated with a cobalt blue light source, the Jones 1E test.[15] If no dye is detected, irrigation with a fluorescein solution under gentle pressure may result in the presence of dye in the nose. A quantitative assessment of the dye present in the nasal vault should be made to better qualify the patency, i.e., size of the fistula. If sparse fluorescein is found in the nose, this is likely the result of a highly stenotic fistula, which can be easily overwhelmed by normal tear production or reflex tear production, resulting in symptomatic tearing. If dye is easily visualized after irrigation, then it is more likely that a dysfunctional lacrimal pump is the cause of recidivistic tearing.

Several ancillary diagnostic tests may assist in the evaluation of a failed DCR. It should be noted that although these diagnostic tools exist, many oculofacial surgeons do not routinely use them because most of the information necessary to effectively treat most patients can be obtained on examination in the office. Nonetheless, these special tests may be particularly helpful in selected cases.

Dacryocystography may discern a canalicular stricture or the "sump syndrome," where a collection of dye can be seen to pool in the residual nasolacrimal sac that was not opened at the time of the DCR.[16] Dacryoscintillography is a technetium scan that provides information on physiologic tear drainage because the radioactive tracer is drawn into the lacrimal drainage system via the lacrimal pump rather than being injected into the canaliculi via syringe, as in dacryocystography. It is particularly useful in cases of functional obstruction, i.e., lacrimal pump failure, or partial obstruction, either of which can present as intermittent epiphora with normal syringing or minimal reflux of the irrigant. Computed tomography has been used by some to delineate the relationship between the surgical ostium and the surrounding soft tissues, allowing for detection of fistula obstruction by soft tissue, scarring, neoplasia, bone, or turbinate.[17] Nevertheless, nasal endoscopy in the office can also provide much of the same information without the expense, radiation exposure, and risk of an IV dye reaction, e.g., in diabetics with nephropathy, associated with computed tomographic scanning.[18]

Management

After the patient has been evaluated, and it has been determined that the DCR has failed, several tests can be performed in the office to determine how the problem can be corrected. Nasal videoendoscopy, in conjunction with probing and irrigation, may help determine if the DCR fistula is stenotic or obliterated, and where the osteotomy and fistula are located. If there is significant reflux through the opposite punctum on lacrimal irrigation, then the DCR fistula is inadequate or occluded. If it refluxes through the same punctum, then there is a canalicular obstruction. It is important to know if there are any intranasal anatomic factors that might contribute to failure of a repeat DCR, e.g., a markedly deviated septum, severe intranasal scarring, a nasal polyp, or another mass. If so, then those issues should be addressed before or concurrent with any further attempts to reestablish lacrimal drainage, such as DCR or conjunctivodacryocystorhinostomy (CDCR).

A therapeutic trial of frequently used artificial tears should be used before proceeding with repeat surgery if a component of reflex tearing is suspected. Punctal malposition and lid laxity may also need to be addressed, and that can be done at the same time as repeat tear duct surgery. The status of the canaliculi is critical in determining the next step. If at least one canaliculus is completely patent, then balloon dilatation or repeat DCR may be pursued. If both canaliculi are occluded, then one may consider canaliculodacryocystorhinostomy if at least 5–7 mm of one or both canaliculi are patent. If there is less than 5 mm of patent canaliculus, then the next appropriate step may be a CDCR and placement of a Jones or Gladstone-Putterman tube.

Surgical Intervention for Failed Dacryocystorhinostomy

Once it has been established that DCR was unsuccessful and the patient is symptomatic, some form of surgical intervention will likely be necessary. It is possible that the patient may only be intermittently symptomatic because of reflex tearing that overwhelms the lacrimal drainage system at certain times, typically outdoors in windy or cold weather. In that case, one could consider botulinum toxin injection to the lacrimal gland.[19] There may be a component of lacrimal pump failure because of eyelid laxity that requires horizontal lower eyelid tightening. Canalicular narrowing or stenosis may contribute to DCR failure. That problem may need to be addressed by any one of the following: protracted canalicular intubation with or without canalicular trephination, canaliculodacryocystorhinostomy, or complete bypass of the occluded canaliculi via CDCR with a Jones or Gladstone-Putterman tube.

Any significant nasal septal deviation causing marked narrowing of the nasal passage or encroachment of the middle turbinate on the DCR fistula should be corrected in order to improve the likelihood of success of the revision surgery, and the same is true for any significant intranasal scarring involving the turbinate and nasal septum.

Balloon Dilatation[20]

The stenotic or occluded DCR fistula can often be managed successfully with balloon dilatation. A balloon catheter is inserted through the upper or lower canaliculus (the superior canaliculus may be preferable, to avoid damage to the functionally more important inferior canaliculus). Under endoscopic guidance, the balloon is positioned within the DCR fistula. If the DCR fistula is completely occluded, then a new opening must be created from the lacrimal sac into the nose. This may be accomplished with a trephine or large Bowman's probe. Protocols may vary for the balloon dilatation, but the authors have routinely inflated the balloon to 8 atmospheres for 90 seconds, followed by reinflation for 60 seconds. After dilating the fistula, the authors suggest silicone intubation with large-diameter larger tubing such as the LacriCath® STENTube (Quest Medical, Inc. Allen, TX) which may serve to more effectively stent the stenotic or occluded DCR fistula. The stent may be left in place as briefly as 4–6 weeks, but longer duration stenting, perhaps a few months, may possibly confer more protection of the fistula. Techniques for silicone intubation and fixation of the silicone tube have already been discussed earlier in this text. The authors have found balloon dilatation with silicone intubation to be highly successful in patients with stenosis of the DCR fistula.

Repeat Dacryocystorhinostomy

Should DCR fail, the procedure may need to be repeated, either from an external or internal (transnasal) approach, particularly if the DCR fistula is completely occluded. This will also permit obtaining a histopathologic specimen if that is deemed appropriate. The external approach may be undertaken via a skin (Lynch) incision, transcaruncular route, or transcanalicular avenue using a small-diameter laser probe. Repeat DCR may be performed via the transnasal route, either laser-assisted or not. Probing of the occluded DCR fistula concurrent with nasal videoendoscopy may demonstrate the site of the osteotomy and fistula intranasally by visualizing the tenting lateral nasal mucosa over the probe.

External Approach via Skin Incision

The nose is packed with cottonoids lightly soaked with cocaine or phenylephrine/lidocaine solution. The medial canthal region is infiltrated with local anesthetic containing epinephrine. An inferior Lynch skin incision is made with a scalpel, and this may be placed directly over the scar from the previous surgery, if a skin incision was used.

The initial portion of the DCR reoperation is the same as a primary DCR, including blunt dissection down to the inferomedial orbital rim, incising periosteum, and developing a subperiosteal plane anterior and medial to the lacrimal sac. However, scar tissue from previous surgical dissection will be encountered medial to the lacrimal sac, particularly at the site of the stenosed or occluded DCR fistula. The cicatrix will make reoperation more challenging because the surgeon will often encounter more bleeding, less effective local anesthesia, and obliteration of natural tissue planes. It may be helpful to place a Bowman's probe into the lacrimal sac to help demonstrate where the osteotomy and previous fistula are located. The surgeon can make a vertical incision onto the Bowman's probe through the wall of the fistula, while staying close to the medial orbital wall to prevent inadvertent injury to the canaliculi.

If the osteotomy location is known in advance, an incision can be made through periosteum and soft tissue several millimeters anterior to the osteotomy, and subperiosteal dissection can be performed posteriorly toward the osteotomy. The osteotomy should be examined for adequacy. If it is too small or poorly positioned, the osteotomy can be enlarged, in the appropriate directions, with a Kerrison rongeur, after using a periosteal elevator to lift soft tissue away from the bony margins. The superior margin of the osteotomy should be at least a few millimeters above the level of the common internal punctum, if possible. As always, particularly with the superior edge of the osteotomy, one should avoid twisting the rongeur, which could extend a crack into the cribriform plate and produce a cerebrospinal fluid leak.

If there is obstruction at the common internal punctum, where the common canaliculus enters the lacrimal sac, then any soft tissue obstructing the opening into the nose should be resected, while saving anterior mucosal flaps on the nasal and lacrimal sac sides to anastomose once a satisfactory channel into the nose has been created. If the middle turbinate encroaches on the osteotomy, then the portion of the turbinate obstructing the osteotomy is resected after infiltrating it with local anesthetic solution for analgesia and hemostasis. Light cautery may be applied to any visible bleeding vessels within the turbinate stump, and Surgicel (Johnson & Johnson, Inc., Piscataway, NJ) can be placed if there is only mild diffuse oozing of blood without any focal source.

Bleeding is always a potential challenge during DCR, and other maneuvers to control bleeding include placing a cottonoid, gauze, or Gelfoam® (Pharmacia & Upjohn, Kalamazoo, MI) soaked in local anesthetic with epinephrine or thrombin, or the application of Avitene® (C.R. Bard, Inc., Murray Hill, NJ). If there is vigorous bleeding, an active attempt should be made to find the source. It may be necessary to place a Merocel® sponge (Medtronic Xomed, Jacksonville, FL) soaked in antibiotic solution in the nose at the end of the case to tamponade persistent venous bleeding, but this will likely be insufficient to address active arterial bleeding.

The surgeon should avoid unnecessary trauma to the nasal mucosa, including overexuberant cautery, in order to limit postoperative scarring that may impact the success of the surgery. Care should be taken to protect the nasal and lacrimal sac mucosal flaps while working within the DCR fistula and nose.

Silicone tubing is frequently used to stent the reopened fistula, although some surgeons have recommended placement of a larger stent in the fistula. The two ends of the tubing may be sutured together with a slowly dissolving suture, such as Monocryl®, Dexon®, or Vicryl® (Ethicon, Inc., Somerville, NJ), placed just medial to the common internal punctum. This tube fixation technique facilitates tube removal and helps prevent lateral tube prolapse postoperatively, which can necessitate premature removal of the tubing. The authors advocate suturing the two anterior flaps together because there is less tissue contraction associated with primary intention healing, as opposed to secondary intention healing (without a mucosal anastomosis). There should be little laxity in the anastomosed flaps to avoid their being drawn into the fistula and contributing to obstruction of the osteotomy.

If the sutured flaps seem somewhat loose and floppy, this can be addressed by suturing the flaps down to overlying periosteum anterior to the fistula. The cutaneous incision is closed in a layered manner. A "moustache" dressing may be placed below the nose at the end of the case, particularly if there is visible oozing of blood in the nose intraoperatively. In addition to intraoperative antibiotics, intraoperative and/or postoperative systemic corticosteroids may help temper the cicatricial response to surgery, especially for reoperation, where the fibroblasts may be "geared up" for a more emphatic response.

Endoscopic-Assisted Endonasal and Transcanalicular Approaches

Endoscopic-assisted approaches to failed DCR have allowed the surgeon to directly visualize intranasal anatomy as it relates to the previously formed surgical ostium without incising the skin. Two modalities are used today: the more common endonasal approach and the transcanalicular approach.

The endoscopic endonasal approach to primary lacrimal bypass surgery has been described previously. The authors have found the endonasal approach coupled with balloon dilatation to be highly effective in treating failed DCR.

Direct visualization of a lacrimal probe passed anterograde through the previously created ostium allows for enhanced understanding of why the prior DCR failed. Initially, the surgeon should evaluate the ostium for stenosis or complete obstruction. If this is the case, the lacrimal probe may be passed through the stenotic or obstructed ostium at several points. These defects may be coalesced to form a larger defect with a Dandy nerve hook, or Blakesley forceps can be used to strip away the tissue. If the nasolacrimal sac was incompletely opened, an angled beaver blade can be used to fillet the sac open or Blakesley forceps can be used to remove any part of the medial sac which is not completely open.

The middle turbinate is easily identified with nasal endoscopy and may contribute to DCR failure. If the middle turbinate appears to be abutting the ostium, a Freer elevator can be used to gently infracture this bone. The surgeon should remain cognizant that overzealous manipulation of the middle turbinate may result in cerebrospinal fluid rhinorrhea. If the lacrimal sac lies behind (lateral to) the middle turbinate, it may be necessary to resect the anterior portion of the turbinate to increase the chances of surgical success.

The septum is easily inspected with nasal endoscopy. Deviation and scarring of the septum may result in adhesions to the middle meatus and possible failure of DCR. If a deviated septum is identified, septoplasty and lysis of any adhesions should be undertaken. Straightening of the septum will allow for easier endoscopic intranasal manipulations and debriding of the ostium.

After intranasal revision, balloon dacryoplasty may be performed, as described earlier.

The transcanalicular laser-assisted approach to DCR has been described in an exemplary manner (Chapter 13). Advantages include avoidance of skin incisions, short operating times, and lower risk of hemorrhage. When dealing with a common canalicular obstruction, this modality is ideal for revisional surgery because direct visualization is possible with the endoscope. In addition, dealing with a stenosis or completely obstructed ostium is possible, given the approach and endoscopic visualization.

Mitomycin C

Topical application of mitomycin C to the DCR fistula at the time of reoperation has been advocated by some surgeons, who have noted enhanced success compared with DCR performed without mitomycin C.[21-27] Nevertheless, not all investigators have found an improved surgical success rate with the use of mitomycin C.[28]

Mitomycin C is an antineoplastic antibiotic, isolated from *Streptomyces caespitosus*, that inhibits DNA and RNA replication, cell division, protein synthesis, and fibroblast proliferation. This agent has a long history of ophthalmic usage in glaucoma filtering surgery. Its usage results in looser, hypocellular subepithelial connective tissue. Various protocols have been used in DCR, including concentrations of mitomycin C ranging from 0.2 to 1 mg/mL and exposure times of 2.5–30 minutes (usually 5 minutes or less). No major complications have been reported relative to the usage of mitomycin C in DCR surgery, and it does not substantially increase the cost of surgery. One should be very careful to avoid the mitomycin C coming into contact with the skin edges of the wound, or this may result in impaired wound healing and possible postoperative wound dehiscence, as noted by Liao et al.[24]

Silicone Intubation

Although many surgeons incorporate silicone intubation into primary and secondary (revision) DCR procedures, this remains somewhat controversial. Not only is it unclear whether silicone intubation improves the success rate of surgery, but silicone intubation has been associated with certain surgical complications, including peripunctal granulation tissue, chronic infection, canalicular laceration (slitting of the punctum), stent prolapse, discomfort, and corneal abrasions.[29] In fact, Allen and Berlin[30] reported an increased failure rate in DCR patients in whom a silicone tube was placed at the time of surgery. Some authors have recommended silicone intubation in selected patients, such as those with common canalicular scarring; patients with a small, contracted, scarred lacrimal sac; or when the lacrimal sac-nasal mucosal flap anastomosis is suboptimal.[25] As to whether silicone intubation is more important for a DCR reoperation remains unclear. A variety of DCR fistula stents have been used and it is uncertain if a larger-diameter silicone tube (or other stent) makes any difference.

Conclusion

With a careful, systematic approach to the patient with tearing after DCR, the appropriate management usually eliminates the epiphora. It is extremely important to identify all etiologic factors contributing to the DCR failure so that they can be properly addressed. Nasal endoscopy is essential because it may reveal a deviated septum, synechiae, or a middle turbinate blocking the DCR fistula. If the DCR fistula is stenotic or occluded, then the fistula can be reopened via an external, transcanalicular, or transnasal approach, either with or without the assistance of a laser. Often, simple balloon dilatation, with or without silicone intubation, is successful. Occasionally, repeat DCR is necessary, and mitomycin C may be used to enhance the likelihood of surgical success. If the canaliculi and DCR fistula appear patent to fluorescein dye and lacrimal irrigation (syringing), then one may be dealing with reflex tearing caused by a dry ocular surface or lacrimal pump failure secondary to lower eyelid laxity. The former is treated with artificial tears, whereas the latter typically responds to horizontal tightening of the eyelid. Success can usually be assured once the etiology of the DCR failure is determined and appropriately treated.

References

1. Hartikainen J, Antila J, Varpula M, Puuka P, Seppa H, Grenman R. Prospective randomized comparison of endonasal endoscopic dacryocystorhinostomy and external dacryocystorhinostomy. Laryngoscope 1998;108: 1861–1866.

2. Hartikainen J, Grenman R, Puukka P, Seppa H. Prospective randomized comparison of endonasal endoscopic dacryocystorhinostomy and external dacryocystorhinostomy. Ophthalmology 1998;105:1106–1113.

3. Camara JG, Bengzon AU, Henson RD. The safety and efficacy of mitomycin C in endonasal endoscopic laser-assisted dacryocystorhinostomy. Ophthal Plast Reconstr Surg 2000;16:114–118.

4. Allen KM, Berlin AJ, Levine HL. Intranasal endoscopic analysis of dacryocystorhinostomy failure. Ophthal Plast Reconstr Surg 1988;4:143.

5. Woog JJ, Kennedy RH, Custer PL, Kaltreider SA, Meyer DR, Camara JG. Endonasal dacryocystorhinostomy. A report by the American Academy of Ophthalmology. Ophthalmology 2001;108:2369–2377.

6. Schepler TR, Davenport OR, Neuhaus RW, Shore JW. Dacryocystorhinostomy: flap versus no flap. Presented at the ASOPRS Fall meeting, New Orleans, October 2004.

7. Eiseman AS, Flanagan JC, Brooks AB, Mitchell EP, Pemberton CH. Ocular surface, ocular adnexal, and lacrimal complications associated with the use of systemic 5-fluorouracil. Ophthal Plast Reconstr Surg 2003;19(3): 216–224.

8. Esmaeli B, Valero V, Ahmadi MA, Booser D. Canalicular stenosis secondary to docetaxel (taxotere): a newly recognized side effect. Ophthalmology 2001;108(5):994–995.

9. Chapman KL, Bartley GB, Garrity JA, Gonnering RS. Lacrimal bypass surgery in patients with sarcoidosis. Am J Ophthalmol 1999;127(4): 443–446.

10. Hardwig PW, Bartley GB, Garrity JA. Surgical management of nasolacrimal duct obstruction in patients with Wegener's granulomatosis. Ophthalmology 1992;99(1):133–139.

11. Kwan AS, Rose GE. Lacrimal drainage surgery in Wegener's granulomatosis. Br J Ophthalmol 2000;84(3):329–331.

12. Jordan DR, Miller D, Anderson RL. Wound necrosis following dacryocystorhinostomy in patients with Wegener's granulomatosis. Ophthalmic Surg 1987;18:800–803.

13. Glatt JH, Putterman AM. Dacryocystorhinostomy in Wegener's granulomatosis. Ophthal Plast Reconstr Surg 1990;6:207–210.

14. Wong RJ, Gliklich RE, Rubin PA, Goodman M. Bilateral nasolacrimal duct obstruction managed with endoscopic techniques. Arch Otolaryngol Head Neck Surg 1998;124(6):703–706.

15. Enzer YR, Shorr N. The Jones IE test: cobalt blue endoscopic primary dye test of lacrimal excretory function. Ophthal Plast Reconstr Surg 1997; 13:204–209.

16. Welham RAN, Wulc AE. Management of unsuccessful lacrimal surgery. Br J Ophthalmol 1987;71(2):152–157.

17. Mauriello JA, Vadehra V, Fleckner M, Shah C. Correlation of orbital computed tomographic findings with office probing and irrigation in 17 patients after successful and failed dacryocystorhinostomy. Ophthal Plast Reconstr Surg 1999;15(2):116–120.

18. Allen KM, Berlin J, Levine HL. Intranasal endoscopic analysis of dacryocystorhinostomy failure. Ophthal Plast Reconstr Surg 1988:4(3):143–145.

19. Whittaker KW, Matthews BN, Fitt AW, Sandramouli S. The use of botulinum toxin A in the treatment of functional epiphora. Orbit 2003; 22(3):193–198.
20. Becker BB, Berry FD. Balloon catheter dilatation in lacrimal surgery. Ophthalmic Surg 1989;20:193–198.
21. Selig YK, Biesman BS, Rebeiz EE. Topical application of mitomycin C in endoscopic dacryocystorhinostomy. Am J Rhinol 2000;14:205–207.
22. Yeatts RP, Neves RB. Use of mitomycin C in repeat dacryocystorhinostomy. Ophthal Plast Reconstr Surg 1999;15:19–22.
23. Camara JG, Bengzon AU, Henson RD. The safety and efficacy of mitomycin C in endonasal endoscopic laser-assisted dacryocystorhinostomy. Ophthal Plast Reconstr Surg 2000;16:114–118.
24. Liao SL, Kao SCS, Tseng JHS, Chen MS, Hou PK. Results of intraoperative mitomycin C application in dacryocystorhinostomy. Br J Ophthalmol 2000; 84:903–906.
25. You Y, Fang C. Intraoperative mitomycin C in dacryocystorhinostomy. Ophthal Plast Reconstr Surg 2001;17:115–119.
26. Ugurbas SH, Zilelioglu G, Sargon MF, Anadolu Y, Akiner M, Akturk T. Histopathologic effects of mitomycin C on endoscopic transnasal dacryocystorhinostomy. Ophthalmic Surg Lasers 1997;28:300–304.
27. Yalaz M, Firinciogullari E, Zeren H. Use of mitomycin C and 5-fluorouracil in external dacryocystorhinostomy. Orbit 1999;18:239–245.
28. Zilelioglu G, Ugurbas SH, Anadolu Y, Akiner M, Akturk T. Adjunctive use of mitomycin C on endoscopic lacrimal surgery. Br J Ophthalmol 1998; 82:63–66.
29. Walland MJ, Rose GE. The effect of silicone intubation on failure and infection rates after dacryocystorhinostomy. Ophthalmic Surg 1994;25:597–600.
30. Allen K, Berlin AJ. Dacryocystorhinostomy failure: association with nasolacrimal silicone intubation. Ophthalmic Surg 1989;20:486–489.

26

The Adjunctive Use of Mitomycin C in Dacryocystorhinostomy

Jorge G. Camara, Mary Ann Yasay-Luis, and Irene D. Enriquez

Since the development of ophthalmologic surgery, the process of healing has occasionally befuddled ophthalmologists in surgical procedures in which a new opening is created. Examples of this include closure of the sclerotomy site in glaucoma filtration surgery, and of the aperture created in optic nerve sheath fenestration surgery; and scarring of the osteotomy site in dacryocystorhinostomy (DCR). To address this setback, ophthalmic surgeons have used mitomycin C (MMC) (Mutamycin; Bristol-Myers Squibb, Princeton, NJ) to improve the success rate of these procedures, especially where there is a high likelihood of failure. This chapter illustrates the adjunctive use of MMC to keep the osteotomy site patent in DCR.

MMC is an alkylating chemotherapeutic agent derived biosynthetically from 3-amino-5-hydroxybenzoic acid (AHBA), d-glucosamine, and carbamoyl phosphate. It was first isolated from the broth of *Streptomyces caespitosus* by Hata et al. in 1955. It exhibits its cytotoxic effects by the cross-linking of DNA during mitosis. It inhibits RNA replication, cell division, protein synthesis, and fibroblast proliferation.

DCR is the procedure of choice for the surgical correction of lacrimal drainage system obstruction distal to the common canaliculus in adults. It involves fistulization of the lacrimal sac through an osteotomy into the nasal cavity. The most common cause of DCR failure is closure of the osteotomy site. This is attributed to fibrous tissue growth, scarring, and granulation tissue formation over the osteotomy site.[1]

In 1997, Kao et al.[2] showed the effectiveness of using intraoperative MMC during external DCR in maintaining a larger osteotomy site and found that the patency rate of the lacrimal drainage system with MMC after 6 months was 100% compared with the 87.5% success rate in DCR without MMC.

In external DCR, a skin incision is made, then blunt dissection of the periosteum overlying the lacrimal crest is performed. The periosteum is incised and elevated off the lacrimal sac fossa. The osteotomy is created over the lacrimal fossa with an electric drill or a chisel and mallet. The lacrimal sac is opened in a longitudinal manner to form anterior and posterior flaps. The nasal mucosa is cut in a similar manner

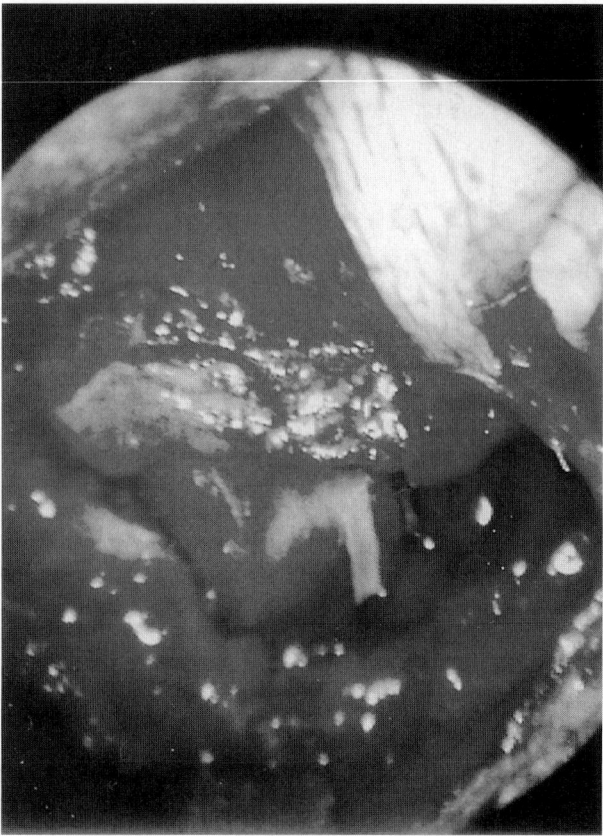

FIGURE 26.1. A neurosurgical cottonoid saturated with 0.2 mg/mL MMC is placed over the anastomosed posterior flaps and osteotomy site, with the anterior flaps visible. (Photo courtesy of Shine C.S. Kao, MD and Shu L. Liao, MD.)

to the lacrimal sac incisions. The posterior nasal and lacrimal sac flaps are joined together with 5-0 Vicryl suture (Ethicon, Somerville, NJ). A silicone tube is used to intubate the lacrimal system and the ends are tied together intranasally with a 4-0 silk suture.

A piece of neurosurgical cottonoid, attached to a long thread and saturated with 0.2 mg/mL MMC, is placed over the anastomosed posterior flaps and osteotomy site with the long thread passing out through the nostril (Figures 26.1 and 26.2).

The anterior nasal and lacrimal sac flaps are closed with additional 5-0 Vicryl sutures, as are the periosteum and orbicularis muscle. The skin incision is sutured with a running 6-0 nylon suture. The MMC saturated cottonoid is removed transnasally after a 30-minute soak by pulling the long thread out from the nostril. The silicone tube is removed at 6 months after surgery.[2]

The recommended use of MMC in endonasal endoscopic DCR, whether performed with or without the laser, is as follows. First, the superior punctum is dilated and a transilluminator is introduced via the superior canaliculus into the lacrimal sac (Figure 26.3). The nasal mucosa anterior to the lacrimal sac and to the nasolacrimal duct is revealed with the transilluminator and is incised with a sickle knife. The incision is carried just superior to the level of the lacrimal sac. Then the nasal mucosa is elevated off the underlying bone with a Freer elevator. The mucosa is then removed with a Blakesley endoscopic forceps. The bone overlying the lacrimal sac and nasolacrimal duct is now transilluminated using the endoilluminator in the superior canaliculus. The bone is removed with a high-speed drill. The intensity of the light source increases as the bone overlying the lacrimal sac is thinned. The bone is removed until the lacrimal sac mucosa is visualized.

The lacrimal sac mucosa is then incised with a sickle knife, allowing visualization of the transilluminator through the opening that has been created. The ostium is made to be approximately 8 mm or more in diameter. Silicone tubing is then placed into each canaliculus through

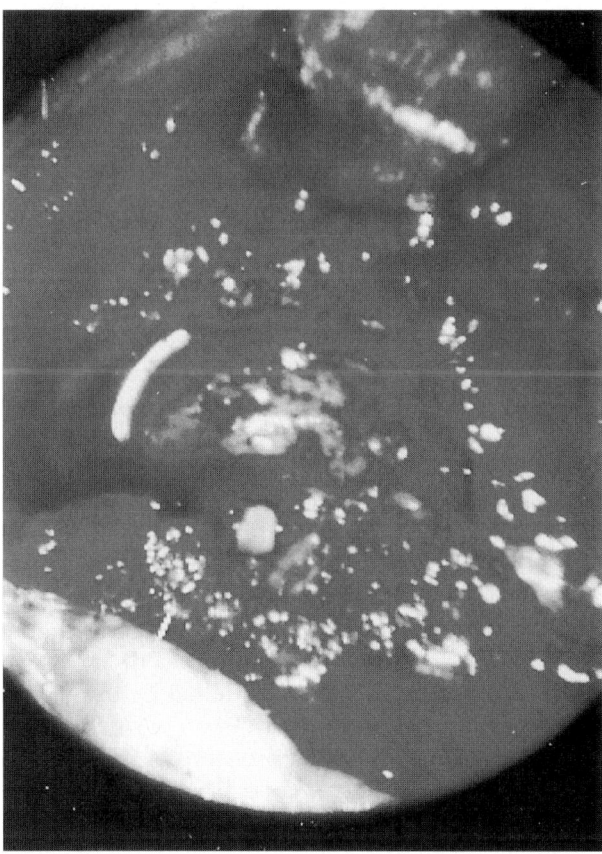

FIGURE 26.2. The anterior flaps are sutured over the neurosurgical cottonoid. (Photo courtesy of Shine C.S. Kao, MD and Shu L. Liao, MD.)

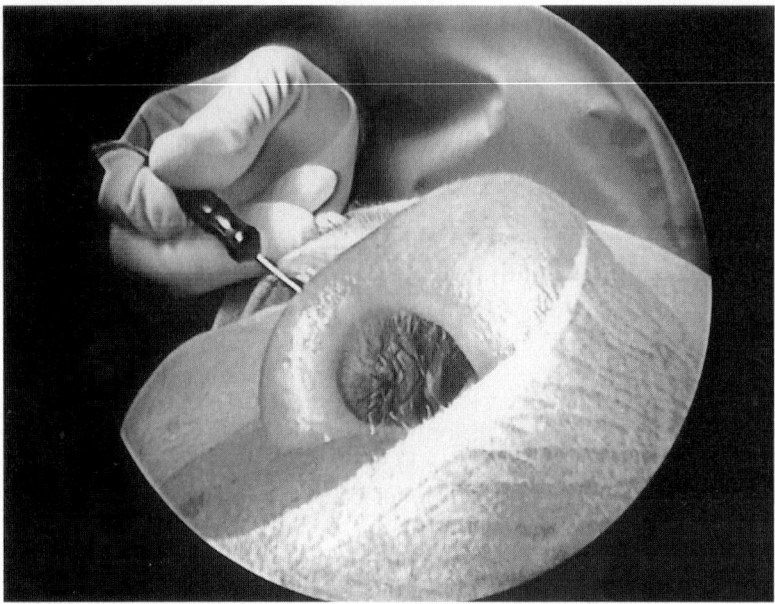

FIGURE 26.3. The transilluminator is introduced into the canaliculus and is seen illuminating the nasal mucosa overlying the lacrimal sac.

the newly created ostium into the middle meatus. The probes are retrieved from the intranasal ostium under endoscopic visualization.[3] The patency of the ostium is confirmed by irrigation of each canaliculus with fluorescein-containing saline solution.[3] A cotton ball permeated with 0.1 mL of a 0.5 mg/mL solution of MMC held with a mosquito clamp is then introduced into the nostril and placed on the osteotomy site for 5 minutes. The MMC is not washed away. The silicone tubing is then tied in the nasal vestibule. The silicone tube is removed between 6 weeks and 6 months, depending on the preference of the individual surgeon.

In endoscopic laser-assisted DCR, the inferior punctum is dilated and a 20-gauge fiberoptic lacrimal light pipe (Trek Medical Products, Mukwonago, WI) is introduced into the canaliculus and threaded into the lacrimal sac. A 0-degree-diameter nasal endoscope (Karl Storz, Tuttlingen, Germany) with an attached endoscopic camera (Smith & Nephew Dyonics, Andover, MA) is placed into the nostril. Using the video monitor, the source of transilluminated light marks the site of the intended rhinostomy.

The power setting used for the procedure is 0.5 Joules per pulse, delivered at a rate of 5 pulses per second. The laser energy is delivered through a 365-μm-diameter bare fiber passed through a laser-delivery handpiece with an opening for the laser fiber at its tip, and a suction port (Figure 26.4).

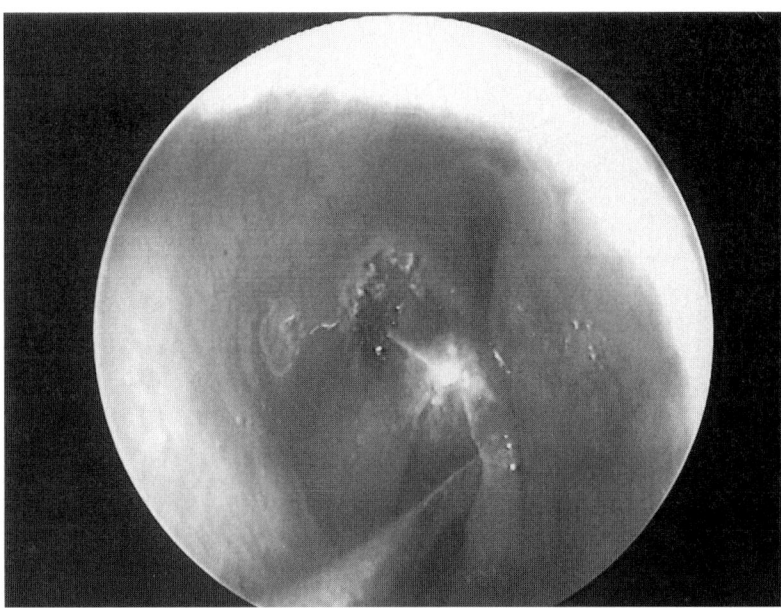

FIGURE 26.4. The light pipe can be seen exiting through the newly created osteotomy site as a Freer elevator infractures the middle turbinate.

Vaporization of the nasal mucosa, followed by ablation of lacrimal bone, is performed. A sinus curette is used to remove charred bone to visualize clearly the medial wall of the lacrimal sac (Figure 26.5). After exposure of the lacrimal sac, its medial wall is removed using either the laser or the angled endoscopy forceps, if a biopsy is considered necessary.

With the development of the osteotomy, the light pipe can be visualized entering the lateral nasal cavity. A bony opening of approximately 6–8 mm in diameter is created. Silicone tubing is guided through the superior and inferior canaliculi and retrieved with forceps under endoscopic visualization. A cotton ball permeated with a 0.5 mg/mL solution of MMC held with a mosquito clamp is then placed on the osteotomy site for 5 minutes[4] (Figure 26.6). The MMC is not washed away.

The silicon stents are tied in a square knot and encircled using a 6-0 nylon suture. Tobramycin-dexamethasone ophthalmic solution (Tobra-Dex; Alcon Laboratories, Inc., Fort Worth, TX) is irrigated through the inferior canaliculus and out into the nasal cavity through the osteotomy. The silicone tubing is removed after 3 months.[4]

The use of MMC intraoperatively in external DCR or in endonasal endoscopic DCR has been shown in several scientific articles to increase the success rate of the procedure by preventing excessive scar tissue formation at the osteotomy site. There have been no reported complications relative to its use in DCR.

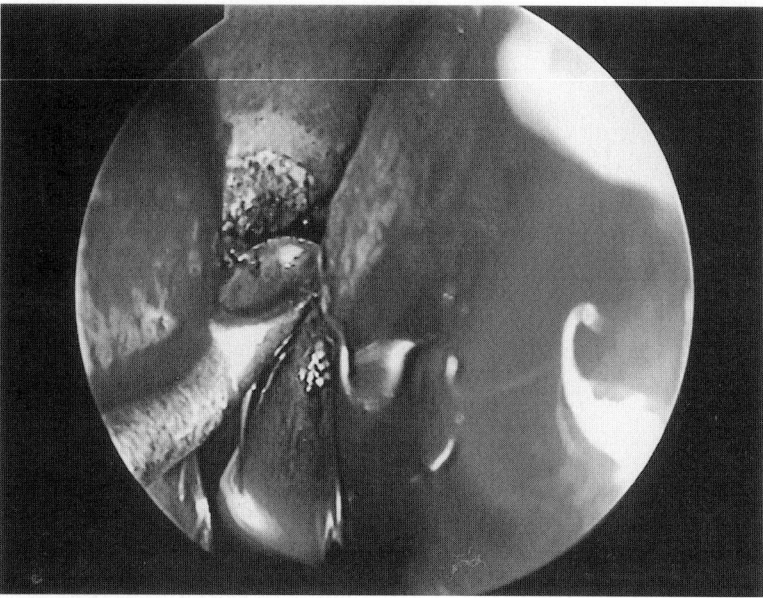

FIGURE 26.5. A nasal curette is used to enlarge the osteotomy and remove fragments of charred bone.

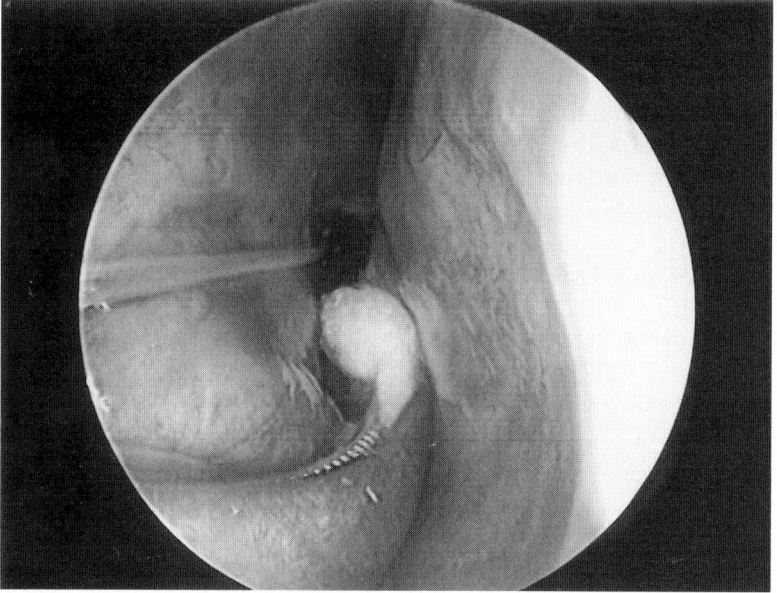

FIGURE 26.6. A cotton tip soaked with a 0.5 mg/mL solution of MMC and held by mosquito forceps is placed over the osteotomy site for 5 minutes.

References

1. Allen K, Berlin AJ. Dacryocystorhinostomy failure: association with nasolac-rimal silicone intubation. Ophthalmic Surg 1989;20:486–489.
2. Kao S, Liao CL, Tseng JH, Chen MS, Hou PK. Dacryocystorhinostomy with intraoperative mitomycin C. Ophthalmology 1997;104:86–91.
3. Woog JJ. Endoscopic dacryocystorhinostomy and conjunctivodacryocysto-rhinostomy. In: Manual of Endoscopic Lacrimal and Orbital Surgery. Philadelphia: Elsevier; 2004:105–120.
4. Camara JG, Bengson AU, Henson RD. The safety and efficacy of mitomycin C in endonasal-endoscopic laser assisted dacryocystorhinostomy. Ophthal Plast Reconstr Surg 2000;16(2):114–118.

27

The Griffiths Nasolacrimal Catheter

John D. Griffiths

Since the initial description of dacryocystorhinostomy (DCR) in 1904,[1] the modern day DCR has been modified many times. A common cause of failure of the DCR is closure of the nasal ostium as a result of cicatricial soft tissue obstruction. Attempts at keeping this nasal ostium patent have resulted in many modifications and they have included the use of various forms of packing, suturing of flaps, nonsuturing of flaps, and a variety of alloplastic stents and other devices. The device that will be described here has evolved after multiple previous attempts at improving the patency of the DCR fistulous tract. None of the previous modifications have been as successful as the use of this nasolacrimal catheter.

Methods

The Griffiths Nasolacrimal Catheter is an alloplastic material that is shaped like a collar button (Figure 27.1). This is a self-retaining device made from a soft silicone-like material and can be used in either the external approach[2] or the endonasal approach[3] DCR. Once standard canalicular intubation tubes have been placed, the nasolacrimal catheter can be inserted. By passing the canalicular probes through the lumen of the nasolacrimal catheter, the catheter can then be advanced along the path of the tubing and passed into the nostril with a small bayonet forceps (Figure 27.2). The proximal collar of the catheter is then pulled through the nasal ostium with a toothed forceps, if an external approach is used. This system is diagrammed in Figure 27.3. The proximal collar of the catheter is then placed into the lacrimal sac fossa under the orbicularis muscle (Figure 27.4). The nostril is then inspected with a nasal speculum or endoscope to see that the distal collar is overlying the nasal mucosa (Figure 27.5). This combination of canalicular tubes and nasolacrimal catheter is then left in place for 6 months.

Removal of these tubes and catheter is accomplished in the office. The canalicular tube is divided with scissors in the medial canthus.

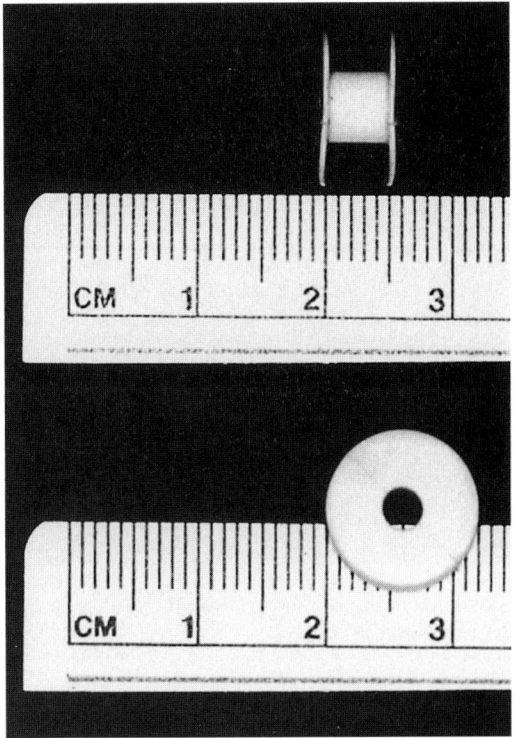

FIGURE 27.1. Collar button design of the Griffiths Nasolacrimal Catheter.

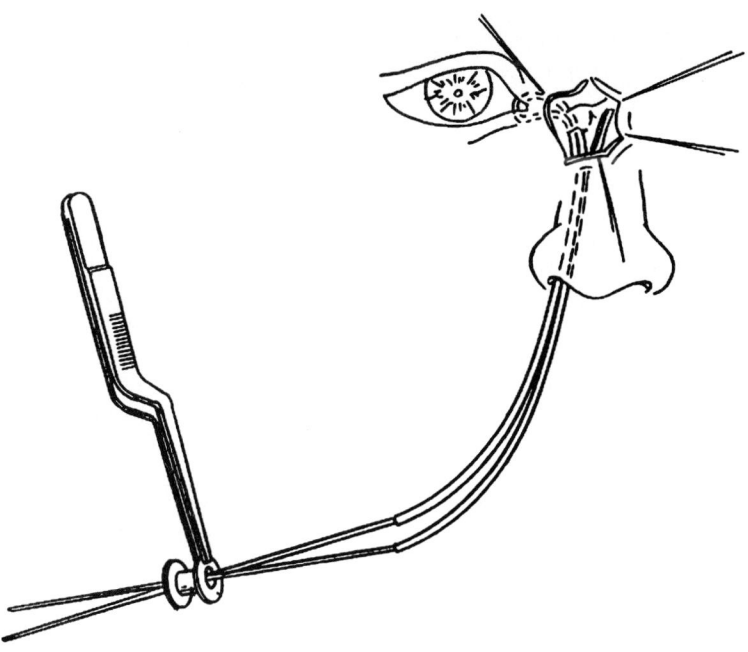

FIGURE 27.2. Diagram depicting placing the nasolacrimal catheter over the canalicular probe and tubes.

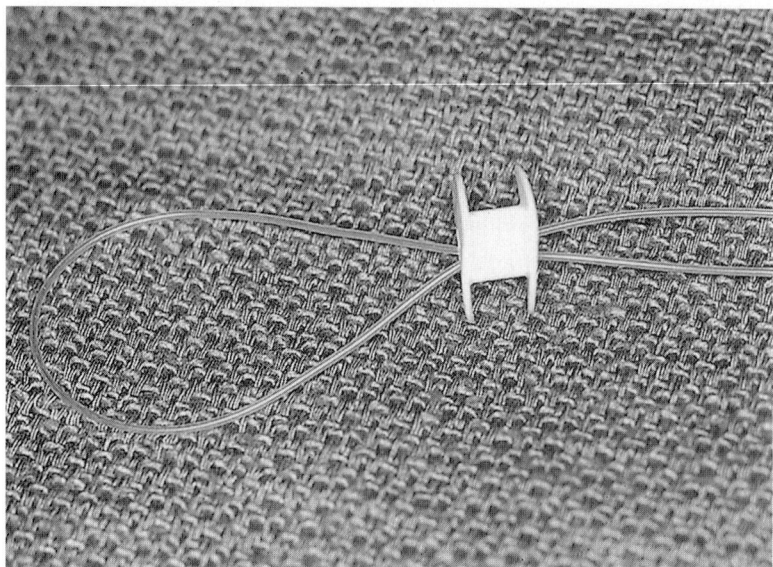

FIGURE 27.3. Demonstration of the position of the nasolacrimal catheter and the canalicular intubation system.

The distal collar of the catheter is then grasped in the nostril with a forceps or hemostat and both are pulled out through the nostril (Figure 27.6). Because the catheter material is soft and pliable, this causes little or no discomfort to the patient. Removal is performed

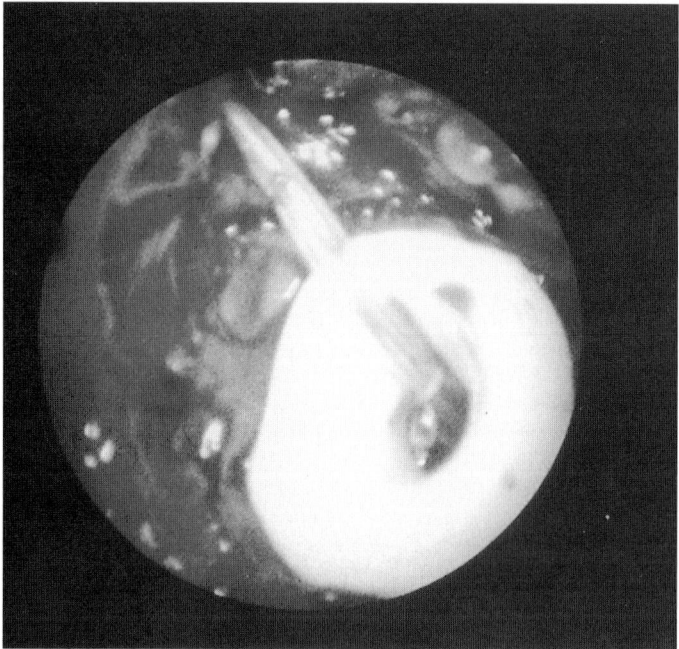

FIGURE 27.4. Surgical photograph demonstrating the proximal collar of the nasolacrimal catheter in the lacrimal sac fossa showing the canalicular tubes passing through the central lumen.

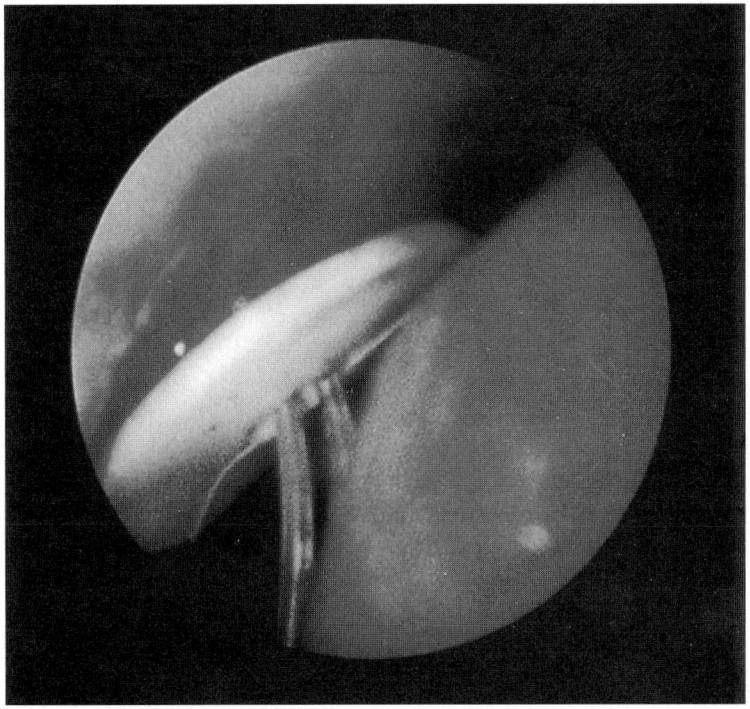

FIGURE 27.5. Endoscopic photo demonstrating the proper position of the proximal collar in the right nostril with the collar overlying the lateral nasal wall mucosa, the middle turbinate to the right of this collar, and the canalicular tubing being present in the lumen of the catheter.

FIGURE 27.6. Diagrammatic representation of removal of the canalicular tubes by dividing them with scissors at the interpalpebral commissure and grasping the catheter and tubing with hemostat of foreign body forceps in the right nostril.

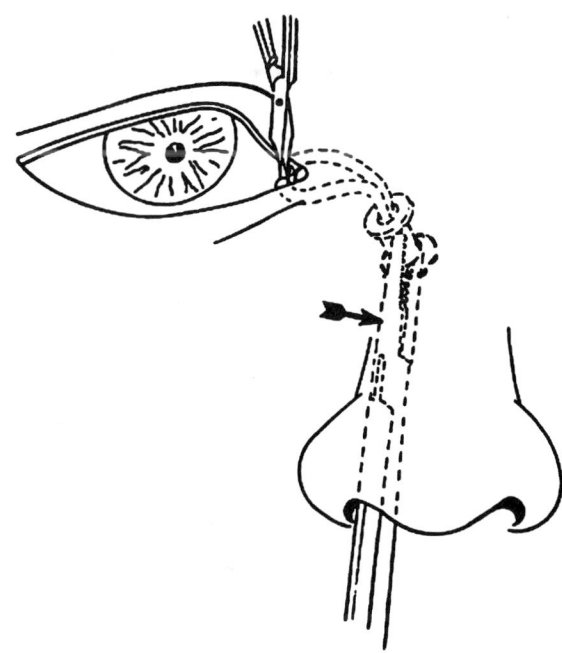

with topical anesthesia in adults. In the pediatric age group, sedation or a brief mask anesthesia may be required in the outpatient surgery setting.

Discussion

The material used in this nasolacrimal catheter is known as C-Flex (Consolidated Polymer Technologies, Inc., Clearwater, FL). It is a thermoplastic elastomer similar to silicone, but it has a higher degree of tensile strength, a greater degree of elasticity, and a coefficient of friction less than half that of silicone.[4] For this reason, it is highly biocompatible and well tolerated by the patient. No cases of pyogenic granuloma have been encountered with this material, as is sometimes seen with the standard silicone material. A few patients that have been lost to follow-up and then returned some 2–3 years later have shown no signs of inflammatory reaction from this C-Flex material.

Originally, this catheter was used only for previously failed DCRs in which there was no flap material to suture. Because this technique was so successful in these cases, this surgeon has used this device in virtually all DCR patients – in primary or in previously failed DCRs. The flap material then lines up along the shaft of the catheter and heals quite nicely without suturing. Once the technique of placing the nasolacrimal catheter is learned, it is easier, faster, and has a higher success rate than sewing flaps in this surgeon's hands.

The Griffiths Nasolacrimal Catheter is available in two sizes. The regular or standard size has a collar diameter of 12 mm and is the preferred size in the adult external approach. The small size has a collar diameter of 8 mm and is preferred in the infant pediatric patient and in the endonasal approach. This smaller size collar is easier to position through the smaller nasal ostium typical of those patients. The inside diameter of the lumen and the outside diameter of the catheter itself are the same in both collar sizes.

Conclusion

This nasolacrimal catheter has been extremely successful and is now the standard technique in the author's hands. It is simpler, faster, and more successful than other methods of maintaining nasal ostium patency in DCR surgery. It is well tolerated by the patient and is easily removed in the office setting.

The Griffiths Nasolacrimal Catheter is available from BD Visitec (Franklin Lakes, NJ) in the Standard size (12-mm collar) and the Pediatric/Endonasal size (8-mm collar). The author has no financial interest in this device.

References

1. Toti A. Nuovo metodo conservatore di cura radicale delle supporazioni chronicle dell sacco lacrimale. Clin Mod Firenze 1904;10:385–389.
2. Woog J, Metson R, Puliafito C. Holmium YAG endonasal laser dacryocysto-rhinostomy. Am J Ophthalmol 1993;116:1–10.
3. Griffiths JD. Nasal catheter use in dacryocystorhinostomy. Ophthal Plast Reconstr Surg 1991;7:177–186.
4. Mardis HK. Evaluation of polymeric materials for endourologic diseases. Semin Int Radiol 1987;4:36–45.

28

The Sisler Lacrimal Canalicular Trephine

Hampson A. Sisler

The use of the canalicular minitrephine known as the Sisler trephine was reported in 1990.[1,2] The minitrephine was developed to allow for opening a canaliculus that was occluded distally. Lacrimal trephines had been used earlier but were for different purposes, such as opening an occluded punctum or proximal canalicular obstruction and were larger in diameter.[3]

Anatomy

The lacrimal drainage system begins at the puncta in the medial aspect of the upper and lower eyelids, where they meet in the blink cycle. The proximal, vertical canaliculi merge into a sacculation at the point of right angle bend into the horizontal portion and, at said sacculation point, achieve their largest diameter of 1.5 mm. The upper and lower canaliculi continue horizontally, gradually narrowing to 0.15 mm in diameter, and then either join together at the point of entry into the lacrimal sac or enter it separately. It is in this distal canaliculus that obstruction occurs most frequently and is, because of its miniscule size, the most difficult to repair.

Instrumentation

The minitrephine is 16 mm long and 0.81 mm in diameter (sold by BD Visitec, Franklin Lakes, NJ) (Figure 28.1A and B). It has a plastic hub affixed to the shaft proximally by which it can be grasped and rotated. An intraluminal stylet, provided with it, is removable (Figure 28.2). The hub is fashioned for a Luer lock, whereby it can be attached to a syringe, which can also be provided with a spring device for retracting the plunger when the rotating trephine to which it is attached gains entry into the patent lacrimal sac (Figure 28.3).

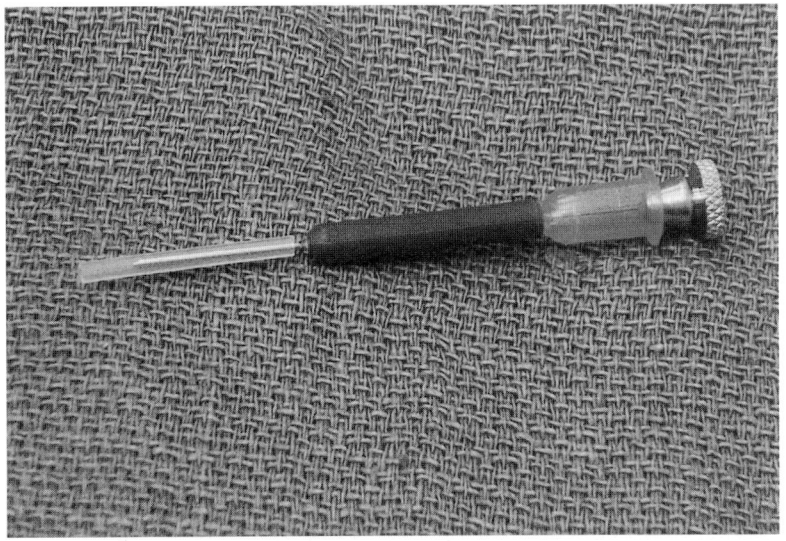

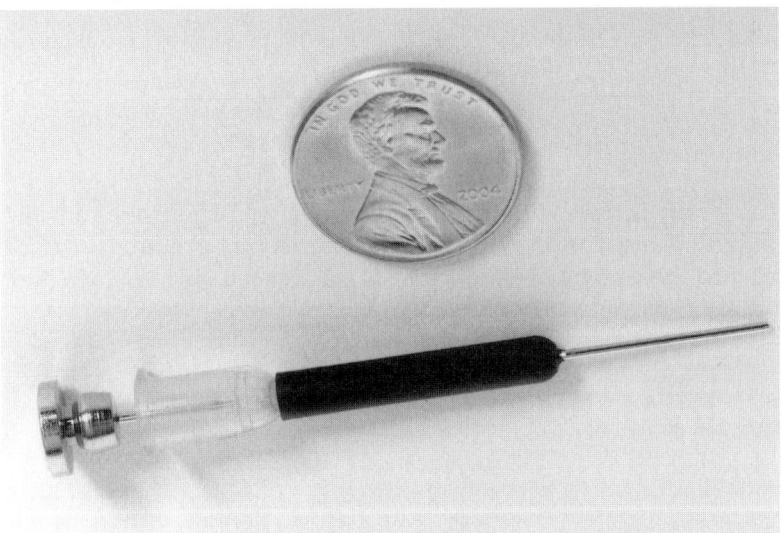

FIGURE 28.1. (A and **B)** The Sisler minitrephine.

Technique

Topical anesthesia is first placed on the eye. A nasociliary nerve block is achieved by injection of 1 mL of anesthetic through a 30-gauge needle directly along the nasal wall of the orbit, starting just above the medial canthal tendon and extending back 2 cm. The trephine is lubricated and made to enter the previously dilated proximal canaliculus and passed to the obstruction site (Figure 28.4). The trephine is rotated in a boring manner until the tip emerges into the lacrimal sac, at which time the spring-weighted plunger pops back and a cylinder of scar tissue passes into the lumen of the trephine or back into the barrel of the syringe.

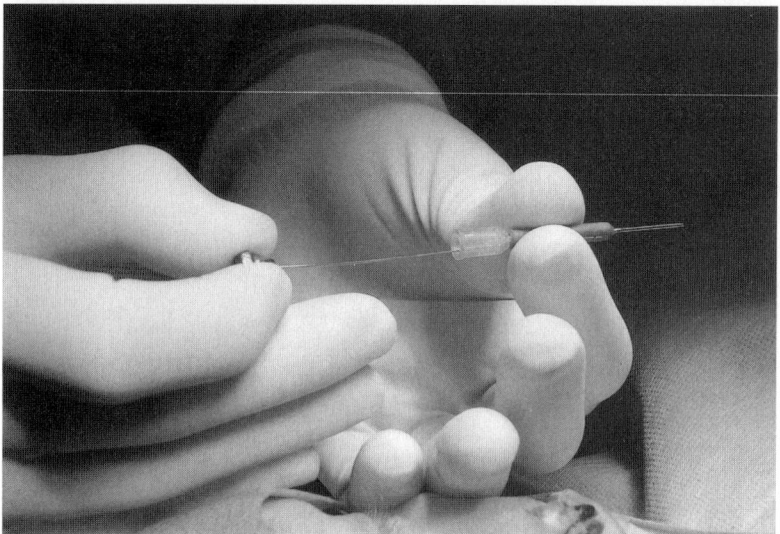

FIGURE 28.2. The Sisler minitrephine with partially removed intraluminal stylet. (Photo courtesy Adam J. Cohen, MD.)

The assembly is then withdrawn. This is followed by stenting by any preferred means. Postoperatively, antibiotic/steroid eye drops may be applied to the conjunctival cul-de-sac four times a day, or as desired. Stents are typically left in place for about 6 weeks.

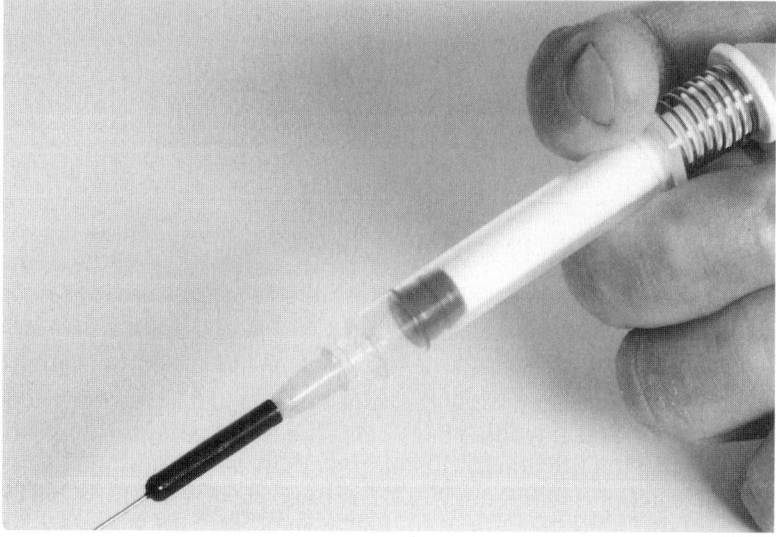

FIGURE 28.3. The Sisler minitrephine with syringe and spring device. (Photo courtesy of Hampson A. Sisler, MD.)

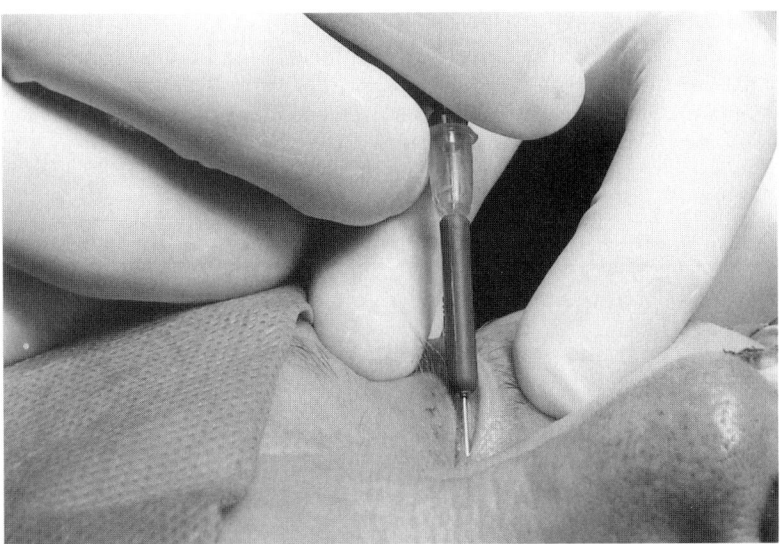

FIGURE 28.4. The Sisler minitrephine passed into the left lower eyelid canaliculus. (Photo courtesy of Adam J. Cohen, MD.)

Complications

Possible complications include damage to the proximal, nondiseased
canaliculi by the invading trephine. Herein, prophylactic trephine
lubrication is important. Before this, dilation of the proximal, normal
canaliculus needs to be done carefully, following the normal anatomy
to avoid trauma to it. The creation of a false passage with either instrument is to be avoided, and finalization in the lacrimal sac needs to be
proven by irrigation of the passages on through the nasolacrimal duct
before the emplacement of the stent or by the popping back of the
plunger at the moment of entry. Moreover, the trephine should not be
forcibly advanced, in order to minimize surgical trauma to these delicate structures.

Conclusion

The Sisler trephine makes recanalization of a distally blocked lacrimal
canaliculus an office procedure as opposed to major surgical microdis-
section in an operating room setting. The uniform, cylindrically shaped
bolus of scar tissue removal makes for a sculptured passageway
through the previous obstruction which, with its smooth and clean
edges, is less likely to reocclude with time.

References

1. Sisler HA, Allarakhia L. A new ophthalmic microtrephine. Ophthalmic Surg
   1990;21:656–657.

2. Sisler HA, Allarakhia L. New microtrephines make lacrimal canalicular rehabilitation an office procedure. Ophthal Plast Reconstr Surg 1990;6: 203–206.
3. Veirs ER. Stenosis of the common canaliculus. Correction with a canalicular rod. Arch Ophthalmol 1969;81:569–570.

Index